Contemporary Health Studies

To
Alex, Maia, Milana and Meadow
Ronald and Yvonne Dunn

Contemporary Health Studies

An Introduction

Louise Warwick-Booth, Ruth Cross and Diane Lowcock

polity

First published in 2012 by Polity Press
Reprinted 2014, 2015 (Twice), 2017 (Twice)

Polity Press
65 Bridge Street
Cambridge CB2 1UR, UK

Polity Press
350 Main Street
Malden, MA 02148, USA

ISBN-13: 978-0-7456-5021-0 (hardback)
ISBN-13: 978-0-7456-5022-7 (paperback)

A catalogue record for this book is available from the British Library.

Typeset in 10.5 on 13 pt Quadraat Regular
by Servis Filmsetting Ltd, Manchester
Printed and bound in Italy by Rotolito Lombarda S.p.A.
The publisher has used its best endeavours to ensure that the URLs for external websites referred to in this book are correct and active at the time of going to press. However, the publisher has no responsibility for the websites and can make no guarantee that a site will remain live or that the content is or will remain appropriate.

Every effort has been made to trace all copyright holders, but if any have been inadvertently overlooked the publisher will be pleased to include any necessary credits in any subsequent reprint or edition.

For further information on Polity, visit our website: www.politybooks.com

Contents

Detailed contents		vii
Foreword		xiv
Acknowledgements		xvi
List of figures		xvii
List of tables		xviii
List of case studies		xix
List of learning tasks		xx
How to use this book		xxii
	Introduction	I
Part I	**Understanding and Promoting Health**	5
1.	What is Health?	7
2.	Contemporary Threats to Health	29
3.	Investigating Health	52
Part II	**Disciplinary Context**	85
4.	Sociology and Health	87
5.	Social Anthropology and Health	109
6.	Health Psychology	130
7.	Health Promotion	150
Part III	**Influences upon Health**	173
8.	Individual Characteristics and their Influence upon Health	176
9.	Social and Community Characteristics and their Influence upon Health	194
10.	The Physical Environment and its Influence on Health	212
11.	Policy Influences upon Health	229

12.   The Global Context of Health   251
13.   Synthesizing Perspectives: Case Studies for
      Action   272

      Glossary   294
      References   316
      Index   351

Detailed contents

Introduction   1

Part I   Understanding and Promoting Health   5

1.   What is Health?   7

     Key learning outcomes   7
     Overview   7
     Definitions of health   7
     Theoretical perspectives   12
         The medical model   13
         The social model   14
         The holistic model   16
         The biopsychosocial model   16
         Different perspectives   17
         Social construction   17
         A moral phenomenon   17
     Lay perspectives   18
         Understandings according to culture   20
         Understandings across the lifespan   22
     Why is this important for understanding health?   25
     Summary   27
     Questions   28
     Further reading   28

2.   Contemporary Threats to Health   29

     Key learning outcomes   29
     Overview   29
     Conceptualizing the identifying of threats   30
         Nature and determinants of health   30
         Magnitude and severity   33
         Media construction and moral panics   33
         Communicable and non-communicable diseases   35
         Contemporary threats   40
     Why and how is all this important?   48
     Summary   50
     Questions   50
     Further reading   50

3.   Investigating Health   52

     Key learning outcomes   52
     Overview   52
     What is research?   53
     Philosophical frameworks   54
     Research question/s   55
     Quantitative research   58
          Nature of quantitative research   58
          Quantitative methods   58
          Quantitative sampling   59
          Steps in quantitative sampling   59
          Quantitative analysis   64
     Qualitative research   67
          Nature of qualitative research   67
          Qualitative methods   69
          Qualitative sampling   69
          Qualitative analysis   74
     Differences between quantitative and qualitative
          research   75
     Ethics of research   77
     Evidence-based practice   78
          Finding evidence   79
          Appraising evidence   79
          Applying evidence to practice   80
     Why is understanding research important?   83
     Summary   83
     Questions   83
     Further reading   84

Part II   Disciplinary Context   85

4.   Sociology and Health   87

     Key learning outcomes   87
     Overview   87
     What is sociology?   87
     Sociology of health and illness   89
          Functionalist theory   90
          Symbolic interactionism   91
          Marxist theory   94
          Feminist theory   96
          Social constructionism   96
          Post structuralism   98
          Society as a determinant of health   99
     Sociological critique of health promotion   104
     Why is this important for understanding health?   105

Summary   107
Questions   107
Further reading   107

5.   Social Anthropology and Health   109

     Key learning outcomes   109
     Overview   109
     What is social anthropology?   109
     Culture and health   110
     Experiencing illness   115
     Culture and treatment   117
     Cultural representations   120
     Culture and mental illness   122
     Cultural influences upon health   124
     Why is this important to health studies?   126
     Summary   128
     Questions   128
     Further reading   128

6.   Health Psychology   130

     Key learning outcomes   130
     Overview   130
     What is health psychology?   131
         Health behaviour   132
         Different kinds of behaviour   134
         Determinants of behaviour   135
         Self efficacy   136
         Beliefs about control   136
         The Health Belief Model   137
         Research and the Health Belief Model   139
         The Theory of Planned Behaviour   139
         Research and the Theory of Planned
             Behaviour   140
         Protection Motivation Theory (PMT)   140
         The Stages of Change Model   142
         Critiques of theory   143
         Health Action Model   144
     How is health psychology important?   146
     Critical perspectives   148
     Summary   148
     Questions   148
     Further reading   148

7.   Health Promotion   150

Key learning outcomes   150
Overview   150
What is health promotion?   151
Origins of health promotion   152
Tools for understanding health promotion   154
     Tannahill's (1985) model   154
     Beattie's (1991) model   155
     Naidoo and Wills' (2000) typology   158
     Tones and Tilford's (1994) empowerment model   160
     Caplan and Holland's (1990) four perspectives   162
Principles and values   164
     Focus on upstream approaches   165
     Non- victim blaming approaches   165
     Evidence base   166
     Participation and empowerment   166
     Equity   167
     Ethical practice   167
     Focus on salutogenic models   168
Critiques of health promotion   168
Contribution of health promotion   169
Summary   171
Questions   171
Further reading   172

Part III   Influences upon Health   173

8.   Individual Characteristics and their Influence upon
     Health   176

Key learning outcomes   176
Overview   176
What is this all about?   177
How do individual characteristics influence health?   177
     Foetal development   177
     Foetal programming   178
     Age   181
     Biology and biological sex   181
     Gender   183
     Hereditary and genetic factors   183
     Personality   184
     Self-esteem   187
     Nature/nurture debate and individual characteristics   188
What does this mean?   189
A life span perspective   189
How is this relevant?   192

Summary   192
Questions   193
Further reading   193

9. Social and Community Characteristics and their Influence
    upon Health   194

    Key learning outcomes   194
    Overview   194
    Social and community networks   195
    Social support   196
    Relationship between social support and health   196
    Social capital   198
    Measuring social capital   198
        Trust and reciprocity   200
        Civic engagement   200
        Social networks   200
    Relationship between social capital and health   201
    Settings for social and community networks   204
        The family   204
        Faith-based organizations   205
    Implications for policy and practice   206
    Social and community networks   209
    Summary   209
    Questions   211
    Further reading   211

10. The Physical Environment and its Influence on Health   212

    Key learning outcomes   212
    Overview   212
    What is this all about?   213
    Physical environment (living and working
        conditions)   214
        Agriculture and food production   214
        Water and sanitation   217
        Housing   218
        The working environment   220
        Unemployment   221
        Education   223
        Health care services   224
    What does this mean?   225
    How is this relevant?   225
    Summary   227
    Questions   227
    Further reading   227

11.   Policy Influences upon Health   229

       Key learning outcomes   229
       Overview   229
       What is social policy?   230
       Social policy as a determinant of health   233
       Current policy issues   235
       The British Welfare State   236
       Ideological and political values   239
       Health services as a determinant of health   242
       Healthy public policy   243
       The broader policy environment   244
       The importance of fiscal policy   246
       Social policy and health studies   247
       Summary   249
       Questions   249
       Further reading   249

12.   The Global Context of Health   251

       Key learning outcomes   251
       Overview   251
       Why is global health important?   251
       How does the global context influence health?   252
            Globalization   252
            Migration   254
            Trade   255
            The environment   258
            Inequalities   259
            Financing and health care   262
            Health governance and policy   264
       Why is all of this important?   268
       Summary   270
       Questions   270
       Further reading   270

13.   Synthesizing Perspectives: Case Studies for Action   272

       Key learning outcomes   272
       Overview   272
       Malaria case study   273
            Strategies to tackle malaria   273
       Cervical cancer case study   277
            Strategies to tackle cervical cancer   277
       Health and neighbourhoods case study   282
            Strategies to improve neighbourhood health   284
       The determinants of health 'rainbow'   287

Key strengths of the rainbow model   288
How the rainbow model might be improved   289
Summary   293

Foreword

Some years ago Ruth Cross and I travelled on the overnight flight to Zambia to teach a module on the Leeds Met MSc Public Health course delivered at Chainama College of Health Sciences. For reasons which we never managed to fathom, we were upgraded. We fully enjoyed the additional perks of being on the right side of the 'curtain' for once and had a much easier and more relaxing journey than we would otherwise have done. Nonetheless this experience served as a metaphor for the more fundamental lottery of life which determines who is fortunate enough to be born into, or live in, conditions likely to sustain their health and support healthy behaviour and, importantly, who is not. Health is acknowledged to be a basic human right. It follows therefore that inequalities in health which are avoidable and result from the unfair distribution of life chances are unjust.

The nature of health continues to be the subject of considerable discussion. It is generally accepted that it is more than the absence of disease and includes positive well-being. One of the particular strengths of *Contemporary Health Studies* is that it brings a broad, multi-disciplinary approach to understanding the nature of health and its determinants. The authors of this book draw on their extensive experience of teaching undergraduate courses in health studies and other related subjects and postgraduate courses in health promotion to consider the nature of health and the factors which influence it. They make explicit the four major disciplines which inform their discussion: notably sociology, anthropology, health psychology and health promotion. While the authors are supportive of a social model of health they also consider alternative conceptualizations and encourage readers to take a critical approach to defining health and identifying the factors which impact upon it.

The use of Dahlgren and Whitehead's model as a framework for considering the key influences on health is interesting for two principal reasons. Firstly, it stems from their early work clarifying the concept of health equity as a basis for considering strategies to address the problem and particularly the role of policy. Considering the factors which cause inequality in health is a theme which permeates the whole of this text. Secondly, rather than viewing the various determinants of health as separate and discrete variables, clustering the determinants within each other from micro-level, through meso-level to macro-level, clearly demonstrates the interconnectedness of the various levels of influence. Health, therefore, is seen to be the product of complex causal pathways rather than simple linear ones. It is all too easy to blame individuals for their health behaviour such as smoking, poor diet and too little exercise rather than considering the web of inter-related factors which result in that behaviour. This text considers factors ranging from the personal through to the global.

The use of case studies illustrates the application of the key principles and theories discussed in the text and their relevance to tackling contemporary challenges to health. Throughout, the authors encourage the active involvement of the reader by posing questions for reflection and through various learning tasks. This book should become a core text for health studies students and will also be of value to students on nursing courses, professions allied to medicine, environmental health and all those involved in multi-disciplinary public health. By developing a broad understanding of health and its determinants among readers it should increase their understanding, motivation and capacity to work towards improving health and tackling inequity.

Jackie Green
Emeritus Professor of Health Promotion, Leeds Metropolitan University

Acknowledgements

The authors would like to thank the following people:

The reviewers for providing helpful and constructive comments on the development of the book proposal, draft chapters and the final manuscript.

The members of the Health Promotion Group in the Faculty of Health and Social Sciences at Leeds Metropolitan University for their support and encouragement.

Sally Foster and Professor Jackie Green for reviewing selected draft chapters.

Dr James Woodall for writing the case study on prisoner family health.

The many students we have taught who have helped us to develop and refine our ideas – we have learned as much from you as we hope you have from us.

Our editor, Emma Hutchinson, for all her timely advice, answering all our questions and generally keeping us on track.

Figures

0.1 Dahlgren and Whitehead determinants of health rainbow   3

2.1 Population pyramids and projected growth   42

3.1 Schema outlining the philosophical
underpinnings of research   56

3.2 Representative sampling   62

6.1 The Health Belief Model   138

6.2 The Theory of Planned Behaviour   140

6.3 The Health Action Model   146

7.1 Tannahill's Model of Health Promotion   155

7.2 Beattie's Model of Health Promotion   157

7.3 Tones and Tilford's Model of Health Promotion   162

7.4 Caplan and Holland's Model of Health Promotion   163

8.1 The health career   190

9.1 Proposed mechanisms of action for social support   197

9.2 How social networks impact upon health   203

13.1 Factors influencing malaria using Dahlgren
and Whitehead's model as a framework for
understanding determinants   274

13.2 Factors influencing cervical cancer using
Dahlgren and Whitehead's model as a framework
for understanding determinants   279

13.3 Factors influencing neighbourhood health using
Dahlgren and Whitehead's model as a framework
for understanding   284

13.4 Barton and Grant's (2006) 'health map' – an
extension of Dahlgren and Whitehead's model   292

Tables

1.1	Classifications and sub-classifications of 'health' (adapted from Johnson, 2007: 46–60)	12
1.2	The medical model of health compared with the social model of health	15
2.1	Changing patterns of disease, health and illness	38
2.2	Effects of climate change upon health	40
2.3	The impact of safety and security upon health	44
3.1	Generating research questions	56
3.2	Example research questions and methodological approaches	57
3.3	An overview of quantitative data collection techniques	60
3.4	Levels of measurement	65
3.5	An overview of qualitative data collection techniques	70
3.6	Overview of qualitative sampling approaches	73
3.7	Differences between quantitative and qualitative research	76
3.8	Types of research question and associated methodological design	81
4.1	Summary and critique of explanations of health inequalities	102
6.1	Different types of behaviour (adapted from Hubley & Copeman, 2008).	135
6.2	General critiques of behaviour change models in health psychology	145
7.1	Different types of models	154
11.1	Ideological positions and their implications for health	240
12.1	Comparison of life expectancy and healthy life expectancy	260
12.2	Disparities in the global incidence of HIV/AIDS	261
12.3	The key actors in global policy-making	265
12.4	Overview of the Millennium Development Goals	267
13.1	The determinants of malaria	274
13.2	The determinants of cervical cancer	278
13.3	The determinants of unhealthy neighbourhoods	283

Case studies

Chapter	Case study	
1	Conflicting perspectives on the phenomenon of 'binge-drinking'	27
2	Bovine Spongiform Encephalopathy (BSE) and variant Creutzfelt-Jakob Disease (vCJD) 'Mad cow disease panic of the 1990s'	49
3	Understanding philosophical frameworks of research: application to the study of pain	82
4	The gendering of mental health	106
5	Anti-social behaviour, ADHD and the role of culture	127
6	The practice of sunbathing and using sunbeds	147
7	Using Caplan and Holland's model to consider different approaches to addressing domestic violence in women	170
8	Individual characteristics and the experience of HIV/AIDS	191
9	Zambian Open Community Schools, Lusaka	210
10	The physical environment, health and health experience in a South African context	226
11	Challenges to health in times of recession	248
12	Women's powerlessness and health outcomes	269
13	Malaria	273
14	Cervical cancer	277
15	Neighbourhoods	282

Learning tasks

1.1 Question 8
1.2 Activity 11
1.3 Activity 14
1.4 Activity 24
2.1 The significance of health threats 30
2.2 Diabetes and health 32
2.3 Contraceptive use and media reports 36
2.4 Analysing trends in life expectancy 39
3.1 Where do I begin in thinking about my research project? 53
3.2 Choosing an appropriate method for your project 72
3.3 Sampling for your project 74
3.4 Appraising evidence for your project 80
4.1 Developing your sociological thinking about health 88
4.2 Stigma and health: biographical disruption 94
4.3 The social construction of disability 99
4.4 Thinking about social influences upon health 100
5.1 Positive cultural influences 111
5.2 Lay beliefs 117
5.3 Healthworld as culture 119
5.4 Cultural representations of mental illness 123
6.1 Reflective exercise 131
6.2 Lifestyle factors 133
6.3 Determinants of health behaviour 135
6.4 Limitations of models of behaviour change 144
7.1 What do you think health promotion is? 151
7.2 Applying Beattie's model of health promotion 158
7.3 Behaviour change campaigns 160
7.4 Ethics in health promotion 168
8.1 Individual characteristics and health 178
8.2 The Avon Longitudinal Study of Parents and Children 180
8.3 Personality and motivation 187
8.4 The nature/nurture debate and individual differences 189
9.1 Your social network map 195
9.2 Measuring social capital 199
9.3 Example of a connected community? 203
9.4 The Big Society debate – will it improve social capital? 208
10.1 The physical environment and health 213

10.2	Food scares and health	216
10.3	Community-led total sanitation (CLTS)	217
10.4	The influence of the working environment on health	220
11.1	The UK media and MMR	231
11.2	Making health policy work	234
11.3	Ideological beliefs	242
11.4	Policy sectors and health implications	246
12.1	Globalization debate	254
12.2	Transnational corporations, health and ethics	258
12.3	Climate change and health	259
12.4	Financing health care	263
13.1	Using Dahlgren and Whitehead as an analytical tool	281
13.2	Strategies for tackling health problems	286
13.3	Evaluating Dahlgren and Whitehead's model of determinants of health	287
13.4	Building on the rainbow model of health.	291

How to use this book

This section is designed to help you to decide how to get the most out of this book. The book aims to provide an in-depth multi-disciplinary overview of the field of 'health studies'. *Contemporary Health Studies* focuses on what health studies is about as a discipline, examining how health is conceptualized in various ways and how it might be understood from a variety of different disciplinary perspectives. Health is known to be strongly influenced by social factors as well as individual ones and this book aims to explore this idea in some depth.

The book does not promote a particular theoretical viewpoint because health studies as a discipline draws upon a range of theoretical stances to allow for different perspectives to be applied to health-related issues. Indeed, the discipline encourages students to engage critically in the numerous discourses surrounding health. The book therefore examines, throughout the text, human experience of health as it is mediated by individual, societal and global contexts, putting particular emphasis on the social, political and environmental dimensions of health. An understanding of these issues is absolutely essential for contemporary health practitioners. Thus, the book contains a strong, up-to-date, social-scientific focus all the way through. The book is primarily geared towards undergraduate students undertaking a health studies course. However, it will also be very useful for undergraduate students studying a wide range of generic health-related courses including clinical programmes such as dietetics, environmental health and nursing. Students studying health promotion will also find this book invaluable. Students at all levels of undergraduate study will be able to engage with the content and it should prove to be a useful companion to undergraduate programmes other than health studies. Whatever the specific 'health' focus of their course this book should enable students to engage actively with their learning, and with contemporary debates about health, by providing meaningful opportunities for them to learn and reflect.

The book is designed to be used in several different ways. It can be read as a whole – from start to finish – since the chapters are organized in a logical sequence. Alternatively, readers might wish to select certain chapters for attention, depending on their interest or concerns and what might be relevant to them. Sections of each chapter that relate to other parts of the book have been highlighted in the text through cross-referencing, so that the reader can follow ideas and topic areas without having to read the whole book from cover to cover. The book is an introductory level text and so offers a comprehensive and contemporary framework of key topic areas within the discipline of health studies. It contains useful references to further reading, resources and additional material available on the companion website, allowing scope for those who wish to explore in more depth.

The book is also divided into three coherent parts and each part can be read independently of the whole. The *first* part sets the context for the book, exploring what health is, contemporary threats to health and how we investigate it; the *second* part focuses on disciplinary perspectives such as sociology, anthropology, health psychology and health promotion; the *third* part looks at influences on health, ending with a set of contemporary case studies that brings everything together.

Part I

Chapter 1 – What is Health?

Chapter 1 will be useful to students on *any* health-related and health professional courses as it explores the fundamental question 'What is health?' providing an overview of how health is conceptualized and understood. Understanding different perspectives and theories on health is foundational to learning about health and training, in any profession, to promote health. This chapter is also a necessary read in order to contextualize the debate within subsequent chapters.

Chapter 2 – Contemporary Threats to Health

This chapter identifies and explores contemporary threats to health. It is a useful and interesting read for all of those working in the public health field because it helps to identify public health objectives within the UK and globally. The chapter also provides insight into the nature of those threats and the factors that influence specific issues being identified as such threats. Hence, it encourages thought about the processes associated with defining contemporary threats to health and also identifies threats that are less obvious, such as terrorism. Ultimately, this chapter is a unique summary of the contemporary threats to health.

Chapter 3 – Investigating Health

In every profession, including health, there is the need to evaluate new information, particularly as evidence-based practice has become so important in recent years. However, there is often not enough evidence, or there may even be competing research findings, so the need to evaluate and research constantly remains ever present. This chapter is therefore an essential read for all those studying health, as it will enable them to understand the key components of the research process and therefore interpret research findings. Furthermore, a key stage of completing an undergraduate degree is the completion of an honours project or dissertation; this chapter has been written with this specifically in mind and so is an ideal guide to help students on their journey to complete such undergraduate projects. Indeed, many undergraduate Quality Assurance Agency benchmark statements make clear reference to the importance of research within their programmes, so this chapter is a fundamental read for all health students.

Part II

Chapter 4 – Sociology and Health

Chapter 4 will be useful for all health students because it outlines the focus of the discipline of sociology specifically in relation to health and illness. Readers will gain an insight into the social world from the point of view of sociologists and therefore begin to be able to develop new perspectives, understand various theoretical viewpoints and think critically about social situations in terms of both structure and agency. The focus in this chapter upon health as social and the importance of health inequalities is a central theme for those completing health studies degrees. In addition, this chapter is a useful introductory resource for broader health professionals such as nurses, allied health professionals and those studying health promotion, who are often required to complete sociology modules as part of their degree programmes.

Chapter 5 – Social Anthropology and Health

This chapter gives an insight into the relationship between health and culture, demonstrating the importance of lay beliefs in relation to understanding health and treatment. It is important for those completing health studies programmes because it further enhances their knowledge about the importance of the social in relation to health. The chapter also facilitates the ability of the reader to make comparisons between a range of health contexts. The chapter is again relevant to any health professional because it creates an awareness of different cultural settings and draws attention to the importance of the everyday understandings (lay perspectives) that co-exist alongside medical and professional viewpoints.

Chapter 6 – Health Psychology

This chapter focuses on a discipline that makes a major contribution to health studies. Health psychology is fundamental in many ways and for many reasons, as it is about exploring the ways in which people behave in relation to their health. Underpinning behaviour is a range of complex influences, which this chapter explores, drawing on theory and recent research in the discipline. This chapter will be of interest to students on health-related courses as well as those on health professional courses, such as nursing, and other allied health professions that encourage and facilitate behaviour change at an individual level through one-to-one encounters. Of course, students of psychology, especially health psychology, will find this useful reading for their studies.

Chapter 7 – Health Promotion

This chapter provides the reader with an introduction to health promotion and gives an overview of the frameworks used to underpin health promotion practice. It also outlines the principles and values that underpin health promotion so the chapter is an excellent introduction to all of those interested in learning about health promotion. The chapter is essential for students who are beginning to study health promotion across a range of subject areas such as health studies, health promotion and public health. It is also a useful resource for inter-professional health care students and nurses who are often required to undertake health promotion modules and is internationally relevant because health promotion is practised across the world in a variety of contexts.

Part III

Part III of the book takes the reader on a journey looking at influences on health starting at the individual level and moving on to consider wider structural factors such as the importance of global society. It draws explicitly on Dahlgren and Whitehead's determinants of health model using it as a framework for developing understanding about the determinants of health and the chapters are therefore structured to reflect this.

Chapter 8 – Individual Characteristics and their Influence upon Health

This chapter critically explores a range of individual characteristics that influence health. Some of the topics covered include foetal programming, the influence of age, the influence of biological sex and gender and the influence of personality. The range of subject matter means that it will be of general interest to students on a variety of different health-related courses. This chapter can be read alongside chapter 6, which focuses on behaviour at an individual level. It may be of particular interest to students studying for a range of health professions that consider individual differences and development across the lifespan.

Chapter 9 – Social and Community Characteristics and their Influence upon Health

This chapter explores how social and community networks act as determinants of health. Two major concepts, social support and social capital, are defined and debated and evidence presented of their relationship to health status. The proposed mechanisms of how social support and social capital influence health are explained. In the final section the implications for policy-makers and practitioners of social and community network influences on health are considered. This chapter is useful for all those studying public health, health promotion and health studies, as social capital is increasingly cited as an important health determinant and is used within contemporary policy. The chapter will also be of interest to those working with communities in any context, such as community development workers and community nurses.

Chapter 10 – The Physical Environment and its Influence on Health

This chapter considers a range of factors within our physical environments that impact on health. These include all of the factors appearing in Dahlgren and Whitehead's framework, namely agriculture and food production, education, working environments, water, sanitation and housing. Each factor is considered in critical depth drawing on recent research findings and debate. This chapter may be of particular interest to environmental health students; however, it will also have relevance to a wide variety of health-related courses.

Chapter 11 – Policy Influences upon Health

Social policy permeates all areas of society and is the subject of everyday discussion and daily experiences. It is also controversial and often debated; hence this chapter is essential reading for anyone studying health, because social policy is fundamentally about who is entitled to support from the state in terms of both health and welfare and the kinds of support that can and should be provided. The chapter explores what social policy is, how it is made, the ideological basis of policy and offers an insight into how many policy sectors have an impact upon health. The chapter draws specifically upon UK health policy and so is a useful resource for practitioners, nurses and health studies students as a general introduction to the area.

Chapter 12 – The Global Context of Health

Dahlgren and Whitehead's framework does not make reference to the importance of the global context of health but, given the way in which the world is more closely connected through the processes associated with globalization, it is essential to understand how the global context influences and determines health outcomes. Globalization is a key determinant of health. This chapter uses the concept of globalization specifically to explore health within the global context, examining global health patterns, inequalities, health care and governance. Given that health is global in so many respects, as this chapter demonstrates, this is an essential read for everyone studying health or working in a health profession.

Chapter 13 – Synthesizing Perspectives: Case Studies for Action

Chapter 13 brings everything discussed in previous chapters together. It provides three detailed case studies that consider much of the content of the book in relation to specific and contemporary public health challenges. The individual case studies are about malaria, cervical cancer, neighbourhoods. Each case study introduces the issue in depth and then considers ways in which health might be promoted in relation to it. The chapter then critically considers Dahlgren and Whitehead's determinants of health rainbow framework in some depth, examining its strengths and how it might be improved upon. This chapter will be useful to those working in the public health field because it demonstrates the application of different schools of knowledge to specific health problems. Consequently, readers gain practice related insights here as well as the ability to build upon the theoretical understandings provided across the earlier chapters.

Introduction

The overall aim of this volume is to enable the reader to examine how health is conceptualized in various ways and how it is understood from a variety of disciplinary **perspectives**. Health studies is a distinct **discipline** in its own right that attempts to explore all of the **factors** that can and do influence health, while examining the very meaning of health itself, which is the starting point for this book in chapter 1. As the scope of health studies is extremely large, this book will enable the reader to focus upon the central tenets of health studies by exploring the human experience of health across several contexts; for example, **community** in chapter 9, the **environment** in chapter 10, the policy context in chapter 11 and the global context in chapter 12. The book also critically discusses and analyses the many factors influential in relation to health such as the contemporary threats to health considered in chapter 2 and the individual **characteristic**s considered in chapter 8. Indeed, as there are many diverse **discourse**s that surround health, these are illustrated in detailed case studies throughout the chapters. Health studies is also **interdisciplinary** in its **nature** and so draws upon many different disciplines including sociology (chapter 4), anthropology (chapter 5), psychology (chapter 6) and health promotion (chapter 7). Through the examination of different disciplines and influences, health is shown to be overwhelmingly socially influenced, and is situated within a **multidisciplinary** critical framework. The key strength of health studies as a discipline is its ability to synergize understandings and influences from a variety of fields, as chapter 13 clearly demonstrates. Indeed, another key aspect of the discipline of health studies is the scope of analysis that can be achieved across a variety of fields, aided by the examination of evidence and **research** findings, which are discussed in detail in chapter 3. Through easy to navigate interactive chapters this book also enables the reader to develop and enhance subject specific skills such as the ability to compare health contexts and to understand the range of influences upon health (part III), the ability to draw upon research methodologies and to analyse research findings (chapter 3) and the ability to enhance theoretical understandings (part II).

Detailed outline of the book

The book is divided into three parts to take readers on a journey through several specific areas related to health studies. The first part of the book, Understanding and Promoting Health, begins with three chapters that introduce the reader to key issues within the field of health studies. From the outset these chapters encourage students to begin to think both critically and reflectively about health. Chapter 1 tackles the very complex question: what is health? Readers are encouraged to consider critically and in depth the **concept** of health and to think deeply about a concept that is often taken for granted, by considering **definitions** and conceptions of health. Widespread understandings of health as the absence of disease are challenged through discussions drawing upon both lay and theoretical perspectives. The second chapter in this first part of the book gives a critical overview of the main contemporary threats, issues and challenges in relation to public health within the twenty-first century, considering a range of both **communicable** and **non-communicable** diseases. This chapter also explores the ways in which these problems can be tackled through both prevention and treatment. The third and final chapter in this first part tackles the importance of research in relation to health and health studies. This chapter introduces students to the entire research process, discussing the **methods** and processes by which information about health is gathered, analysed and used. The chapter demonstrates that health can be investigated in a number of different ways, exploring both quantitative and qualitative approaches to researching health. The strengths and weaknesses of these different techniques for gathering data are also considered. Readers are also shown how to formulate questions about health and how to decide upon the most appropriate research approaches.

The second part of the book is called Disciplinary Context and introduces the reader to four specific disciplinary areas that all have relevance and influence within the health studies arena. Hence, this section introduces the reader to the disciplinary context in which health studies itself is located. By understanding the complexity of disciplines underpinning health studies at different levels, readers will be able to conceptualize the importance of a range of factors and influences upon health. Chapter 4 introduces students to the discipline of sociology, demonstrating what sociology as a discipline tells us about health being ultimately socially influenced. **Social** influences upon health are discussed through consideration of different theoretical perspectives and the social **model** of health. Chapter 5 focuses upon anthropological perspectives and concentrates upon the importance of **culture** as an influence upon health. The chapter discusses interesting examples of different cultural practices affecting health from across the world, considering how culture can be both positive and detrimental for health. The next chapter in this section, chapter 6, turns the reader's focus to the discipline of health psychology and, specifically, health behaviour. The chapter concentrates upon what health psychology has to offer in terms of understanding how people behave, the choices that they make and the

Figure 0.1
The Dahlgren
and Whitehead
determinants of
health rainbow.

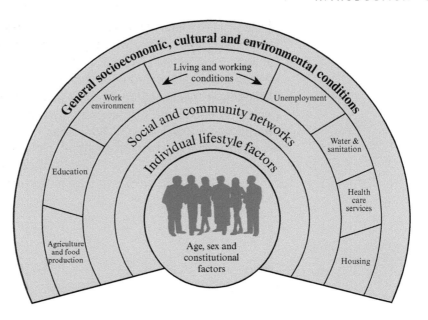

Figure 0.1 The Dahlgren and Whitehead determinants of health rainbow.

risks they take with regard to their health. The reader is also given a critical discussion of why behaviour change is so complex. The final chapter in this section is chapter 7, which defines and illuminates the scope of the field of health promotion. The key **values** and principles of health promotion are illustrated and models of health promotion are both discussed and evaluated to provide a foundation for the final chapter of the book, which considers how to address public health issues in detail.

The third part of this book considers a range of influences upon health, examining a number of **determinants** outlined in Dahlgren and Whitehead's (1991) rainbow model, shown in the figure.

Chapter 8 begins with an exploration of individual characteristics in relation to health, drawing upon Dahlgren and Whitehead's framework. Individual characteristics considered are developmental factors such as foetal experiences and age, constitutional factors such as genetic inheritance and social **constructs** such as **gender** (how concepts of femininity and masculinity influence health). Chapter 9 then examines the importance of social and community networks as determinants of health. Concepts such as social support, **social capital** and social dominance are evaluated in relation to and how they mediate health status. The features of healthy communities are also explored. Chapter 10 explores the physical environment to show how living and working environments influence and impact upon health. Chapter 11 provides the reader with an overview of social policy and then more specifically demonstrates that many facets of policy combine to influence and determine health in a number of ways. The chapter also discusses and evaluates health policy in depth. Chapter 12 examines health determinants within a global context because the global environment is important in determining some aspects of health. Hence, this chapter examines how being part of a global society affects health in both positive and negative ways, particularly in relation to **globalization**. The final chapter, chapter 13, synthesizes the perspectives discussed throughout the book. Three detailed case studies are used to explain how understanding determinants of health can aid the development of public health strategy and action. Detailed discussion and **critique** of the Dahlgren and Whitehead determinants model is also provided to conclude the volume.

Part I

Understanding and Promoting Health

The first part of this book critically examines a range of issues that address the overall question 'what is health?' It is divided into three chapters and, together, these chapters set the scene for the whole book and the general context of the discussion within it. The question 'what is health?' is key to any text about health studies and this is why a substantial part of this book is devoted to addressing it.

Chapter 1 specifically explores the question 'what is health?' This chapter offers an overview and a critical in-depth discussion about the nature of health, how we define it and how we experience it. This chapter facilitates deeper reflection on a term that is used a lot and often taken for granted. It considers how health is defined and the different things that might influence definitions, as well as how we understand and experience health. The chapter challenges the singular, but widely held assumption that health is the absence of disease and offers a variety of different understandings and explanations as alternatives. It draws on both lay and theoretical perspectives illustrating contrasting and competing ideas and constructing a debate about health that moves beyond received wisdom.

After considering what health is in the first chapter, chapter 2 considers the contemporary threats to health and provides an overview of the main issues and challenges in relation to public health within the twenty-first century across the UK and much further afield. The nature of threats is conceptualized and then changing patterns of health threats are analysed. The chapter outlines the contemporary threats to public health including climate change, population growth and poverty. The chapter examines both communicable and non-communicable diseases and evaluates the threat of these to contemporary societies. The chapter also considers issues such as emerging **epidemic**s and the implications of these for public health. Finally, **lifestyle** diseases as a threat to health are critically discussed.

The final chapter in this section, chapter 3, Investigating Health, goes on to discuss how health might be investigated, measured and researched. This chapter gives an overview of the importance of research in relation to health and introduces the research process as a whole. The various methods and processes by which health information is gathered and analysed are presented, illustrating the importance of researching health for health studies. Quantitative and qualitative approaches to researching health are presented and critiqued, highlighting strengths and weaknesses of different data-gathering techniques. The chapter provides a clear outline of the research process for students who can use this to inform the development of their dissertations at undergraduate level.

1 What is Health?

Key learning outcomes

By the end of this chapter you should be able to:

- understand and articulate the complexities of health as a concept

- reflect on, define and defend your own perspective on health

- summarize and critique key debates about the concept of health within the literature drawing on theoretical and lay understandings

Overview

This chapter addresses the key question 'what is health?' There are no easy, straightforward answers to this. Trying to define health relies on developing understanding about a wide range of perspectives, subjectivities and experiences that are, in turn, socially, historically and culturally located. Nevertheless, this chapter will try to uncover some of the inherent complexities in attempting to understand what we mean by 'health'. To do so, an array of different materials will be drawn upon in order to make sense of what it is we are trying to 'capture' (or, in the first instance, 'define').

Definitions of health

Health has been called 'an abstract concept' that people can find difficult to define (Earle, 2007a: 38). You may appreciate this more fully having completed learning task 1.1. Nonetheless different attempts have been made. One of the most frequently referenced definitions of health in the last few decades is the classic one offered by the World

Learning task 1.1

Question

Health is one of those things that most people assume they understand. But if we just stop and consider it for a moment and try to focus on it, it starts to float about in our minds. (Johnson, 2007: 45)

Reflect on your own understanding of what 'health' is. Think about the following:
(a) What does the word 'health' mean to you?
(b) What does it mean to you, to be 'healthy'.
(c) Can you come up with a definition that captures what you mean by 'health'? If you can, try not to focus on this in terms of health as being only the absence of disease (or there being something 'wrong').

Write your ideas down and you can refer back to them as you read this chapter.

Health Organization. Health is defined as 'a state of complete physical, mental and social **well-being** and not merely the absence of disease and infirmity' (WHO, 1948 cited in WHO, 2006). One of the strengths of this definition is its all-encompassing breadth. It moves away from the notion that being healthy is simply about not being ill. In this sense it has a more positive, **holistic** view about what health is. However, the WHO definition, has also been criticized on many counts, for example, as being unattainable and idealistic (see Lucas and Lloyd, 2005). According to this definition, is it possible for anyone ever actually to be healthy? In addition there are other dimensions of health that are not considered in this definition such as sexual, emotional and spiritual health (Ewles and Simnett, 2003)

It is possible to view health as a purchasable commodity.

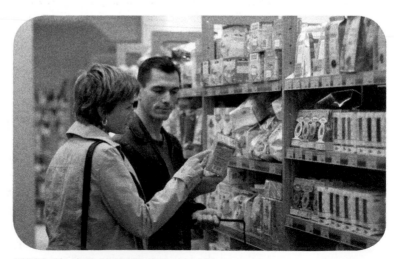

© Voisin/Phanie/Rex Features

Health can be viewed positively or negatively. Tones and Green (2004) refer to this as dichotomous differences in approaches to defining health. On the one hand there are positive approaches to defining health (health as well-being or as an asset) and on the other hand there are more negative definitions of health – those that are illness or disease oriented. When health is viewed in a negative way, then definitions will tend to focus on health as absence of disease. When health is viewed in a more positive way definitions tend to be broader and take into account concepts such 'well-being'. The World Health Organization definition outlined earlier is an example of a more positive definition and marks a shift in understanding away from a more narrow, medical and negative view of health.

'Well-being' is another rather slippery concept and is also difficult to define (Chronin de Chavez et al., 2005). There is a lack of consensus as to what well-being is, although generally theoretical understandings converge around the three major aspects of physical, social and **psychological** well-being. Like the notion of health, this makes it difficult to investigate, as it means different things to different people. However, drawing on the concept of well-being to understand health is important. Laverack (2004) offers a useful way of thinking further about the concept of well-being. He separates well-being into three different types – physical, social and mental. Physical well-being is concerned with healthy functioning, fitness and performance capacity, social well-being is concerned with issues such as involvement in community and inter-personal relationships as well as employability and mental well-being – which involves a range of factors including **self-esteem** and the ability to cope and adapt. The concept of well-being varies between disciplinary perspectives; however, it is receiving increasing attention and it is generally argued that it offers a broader understanding of health than those drawing on a more scientific, medically dominated position (Chronin de Chavez et al., 2005). A further concept that is arguably related to how health may be perceived is **quality of life**. For example, functional perspectives may assume that increased health automatically results in increased quality of life (Lee and McCormick, 2004).

Definitions of health can also focus on different aspects of health. Some are idealistic, as in the WHO definition offered earlier. Some definitions have a more functional view of health, where it is seen as the ability to be able to 'do' things and get on with life. Other definitions centre on the idea of health as a commodity. For example Aggleton (1990) argues that health is something that can be bought (by investment in private health care) or sold (through health food shops), given (by medical intervention) or lost (through disease or injury). The parallels with contemporary **consumerism** are evident in this type of definition.

Other types of definitions draw on the idea that health is about being able to cope and adapt to different circumstances and achieve personal potential and may be more aligned with ideas from **human-ism**. Drawing on humanist ideas, health might also be considered as self-actualization, which links with the idea of **empowerment**, a concept discussed in more detail later in this book. Health might enable the process of self-actualization or the attainment of health might constitute self actualization. Either way, research appears to show that this is an important idea that has implications for health and, specifically, health-promoting behaviours (Acton & Malathum, 2008). Seedhouse (2001) describes health as the 'foundations for achievement'. In keeping with the position of this chapter Seedhouse starts from the point of acknowledging that health is a complex and contested concept. Seedhouse views health as the means by which we achieve our potential, both as individuals and as groups. Seedhouse (1986: 61) therefore describes a person's optimum state of health as being 'equivalent to the set of conditions that enable a person to work to fulfil her realistic chosen and **biological** potentials'. This perspective also broadens understandings of health beyond the absence of disease or 'abnormality' as understood using a medical model (this will be discussed in more detail later in the chapter). Someone may be, for example, encountering disease or be disabled and still lay claim to health, thus challenging assumptions of a 'normality' of health. As Blaxter (1990: 35) argues 'health is not, in the minds of most people, a unitary concept. It is multi-dimensional, and it is quite possible to have "good" health in one respect, but "bad" in another.'

Health can also be conceived of in a number of other ways. Health may be regarded as a value (Downie & Macnaughton, 2001) and, while most people would argue that 'good' health is *of* value too, the degree to which people will strive for, or prioritize, health will, of course, vary according to individual circumstances. Health is also viewed both as a right and as a responsibility. The Constitution of the World Health Organization of 1946 first held up health as a human right in the statement 'the enjoyment of the highest attainable standard of health is one of the fundamental rights of every human being' (cited in WHO, 2008a: 5). Article 25 of the **Universal** Declaration of Human Rights of 1948 references health in relation to the right to an adequate standard of living and many of the other articles are indirectly related to the 'right to health'. 'The right to health was again recognized as a human right in the 1966 International Covenant on Economic, Social and Cultural Rights' (WHO, 2008a: 5). Viewing health as a 'right' can create tension, because with this comes a sense of responsibility for health that in turn generates debate as to who has responsibility for health – the individual or the state? These issues are discussed in more detail later in this book.

The variety and breadth of definitions of health presented here are not exhaustive but they serve to illustrate the many different ways in which health can be conceived and experienced and the problematic

---

Learning task 1.2

Activity

Compare and contrast two different definitions of health as discussed.

(a) What do the definitions have to offer in terms of furthering our understanding about health?

(b) What are the limitations of them? What are their strengths?

(c) How would you alter the definitions? What would you add or remove and why?

(d) How do the definitions compare or contrast with your own definition of health from learning task 1.1?

---

nature of trying to produce a definition that suits everyone. Downie and Macnaughton (2001: 11) argue that 'health does not have a clear **identity** of its own' and therefore we are faced with a real challenge when trying to define what it is. However, what we do know is that health is influenced by a wide range of factors. This will be discussed in more detail throughout this book.

To end this section, a useful framework about definitions of health is included. This is offered by Colin Johnson (2007). He classifies definitions into four main types – dictionary definitions, assumptive definitions, determinist definitions and spiritual definitions. These are further explained and sub-classified in table 1.1.

Essentially the concept of health is not static or stable over time or within different contexts. It is influenced by a plethora of things and means different things to everyone. The meaning of health is also contested and, as has been demonstrated, there is no universally agreed definition (Pridmore & Stephens, 2000: 30). Indeed, the concept of health remains elusive (Johnson, 2007). In his book *Creating Health for Everyone: Principles, Practice and Philosophy*, Colin Johnson (2007) offers a definition of health that extends to nearly four pages, which illustrates the nebulous nature of it and the somewhat impossible task of trying to produce a universally acceptable definition! However, he does state that 'the concept of health is a cluster of sub-concepts, which together constitute a dynamic whole' (p. 91) acknowledging the range of influences on understanding. While the framework Johnson uses provides a valuable contribution to our knowledge about definitions of health, and a useful framework, we are really not that much further forward in terms of concrete understanding (and, indeed, we may never be). The extent to which this actually matters is debatable.

Given the difficulties of trying to produce a satisfactory definition of health, the next section of this chapter will examine different theoretical perspectives on the *nature* of health and consider what these might have to offer to our understanding of 'what health is'.

Table 1.1 Classifications and sub-classifications of 'health' (adapted from Johnson, 2007: 46–60).

Classification and Sub-Classification	
Dictionary Definitions	These describe common everyday ways in which health is defined but, Johnson (2007) argues, are unhelpful!
Assumptive Definitions (including) – the Conceptually Relative – the Aspirational (or Idealistic) – the Descriptive (or Stipulated)	Health is *assumed* to exist if certain conditions can be achieved. Health is defined by reference to other concepts (such as disease). See the WHO definition for a classic example of an aspirational definition of health. Definitions using terms such as 'good' or 'bad' to describe quality of health.
Determinist Definitions (including) – the Statistical – the Functional	Based on a range of determinants that can be measured and recorded. Measuring different phenomena as 'health' (for example, **mortality** rates, Healthy Life Years. Health as the ability to function (produce, act etc).
Spiritual Definitions – Religious – Alternative – Humanist	Based on a degree of faith, a degree of affinity in 'other' existence or any other mantra. These are important to holistic ideas about health. Health linked with the 'moral' and with faith components. Definitions centre on 'holistic' ideas about health or 'wholeness'. Can be highly **subjective** and very personal. A specific approach to human life concerned with development – health is a means to an end.

Theoretical perspectives

This section of the chapter will consider a range of different perspectives on health, including theoretical perspectives, alternative models of health and also lay perspectives versus professional perspectives. Theoretical perspectives on health are distinguishable from lay perspectives on health (we return to these later) as those that are derived from academia. Theoretical perspectives on health inform professional perspectives, which are also distinguishable from lay perspectives.

To begin with, it is useful to consider two fundamental theoretical constructs of health – the medical model of health and the social model of health.

The medical model

The medical model of health is located within a scientific **paradigm** of understanding. It is sometimes also referred to as the 'biomedical' model (see Blaxter, 2004), the 'biological' model or even the 'Western scientific medical model'. The medical model draws on scientific, mechanical, individualistic and **reductionist** understandings of what health is and views health in terms of **pathology**, disease, diagnosis and treatment. The physical body is viewed as being separate from social or psychological processes (Lyons & Chamberlain, 2006). Health is seen as being 'located' in the individual body and the causes of ill-health are viewed as being biological or physiological in origin, requiring expert intervention. Health, according to a medical view, is conceived of as the absence of disease or 'abnormality'. If medically defined illness and disorder are absent then health is assumed to be present. The medical model is, and has been, very influential in terms of understandings of what health is. The dominance of ideas of health as 'the absence of illness' in **mainstream** discourse about health is testimony to this. The medical model does, however, have some distinct advantages and through technological advances in scientific knowledge it has been extremely influential in Western societies within the last two centuries. As a result the medical model of health forms the basis of much health care provision within these contexts.

However, the medical model of health has faced heavy criticism. One of the main criticisms is that the wider context is given little attention and therefore the numerous social, psychological and environmental factors that influence, or determine, health are not considered. It is difficult to account for the complexity of health if we consider it solely in biological terms, using the medical model. Another criticism of the medical model is that its view of health as the absence of disease or abnormality can be seen as being rather negative (Earle, 2007a). Surely health is about more than just this? Are we necessarily healthy simply because we are not ill? However, this is problematic because, as Duncan (2007: 8) argues, one of the main difficulties with arguing that health is about *more* than simply the absence of disease or abnormality is that this can lead to 'muddle and confusion', which may render meaningful description 'impossible'. In addition, the widespread use of the medical model of health has increased perceptions that the responsibility for health, and indeed the control of it, lies with the individual (Jackson, 2007). This is a position that is reflected in more contemporary neo-liberalist stances in the Western world that emphasize personal responsibility for health (Murray et al., 2003).

This position is challenged by other concepts of health such as the social model, which will now be discussed in more detail. Before we move on to the next section take some time to carry out learning task 1.3.

Learning task 1.3

Activity
(a) Take a few minutes to reflect on all of the things that you think impact on, and influence, your health. Write them down.
(b) Can you spot any patterns or group the different influences in any way?

When you have completed this task, see part III of this book and particularly chapter 13 for Dahlgren and Whitehead's (1991) rainbow model of health determinants. Are there influences that you had not thought of?

The social model

In contrast to the medical model of health the social model of health views health as being influenced by a range of different factors, including those that are political, economic, social, psychological, cultural and environmental (as well as biological) (Earle, 2007a). The causes of ill-health are attributed to factors outside the physical body – the wider structural causes, such as inequality and poverty, as well as factors such as social interaction and behaviour. The notion of health is seen as being socially constructed, which is central to the social model of health and this idea is discussed in more detail later in the chapter.

The social model operates from the view that a wide variety of factors need to be taken into account when conceptualizing health – factors such as the environment, influences on lifestyle choices, access to health care services, employment status and gendered identities, for example. The social model recognizes individual differences in health experience as being socially produced. In addition, it seeks to provide explanations for why differences exist. Crucially the social model of health also takes into account lay perspectives about health, which are discussed in more detail later in this chapter.

The social model of health is not without its critiques. It has been criticized for being so broad a model as to render it almost unusable. Kelly and Charlton (1995) argue that the social model cannot necessarily be viewed as superior to the medical model despite criticisms of it. For example, they point out that while health promotion is premised on a social model of health in terms of the way that health is conceived (holistically), the discipline still relies heavily on expert knowledge that can be traced back to scientific origins. Therefore science (and the medical model of health per se) has its part to play in understanding about the nature of health. The social model has also been criticized on the basis that the breadth of understanding it takes into account may lead to practices in health promotion and public health that have different priorities and therefore can only be implemented on a small scale. Earle (2007a: 54) therefore suggests that, rather than being able to pin down the ways that the social model of health may be used to, for example, improve or promote health, the 'rhetoric' of the social model of health has been used in the following ways:

- as a set of underlying values (philosophical approach to health)
- as a set of guiding principles to orientate health work in a specific way
- as a set of practice objectives

In summary, the medical model views health as derived from biology, so ill-health is caused by biological factors that can be identified, diagnosed (as compared with a scientifically defined 'norm') and treated by expert medical knowledge. In contrast, the social model of health views it as socially constructed and influenced, so ill-health is caused by social factors, knowledge about ill-health is not confined to medical expertise and a more holistic, less reductionist view of health is subscribed to. Table 1.2 highlights the key differences between these two models.

The importance of social factors and the social model of health is demonstrated in Dahlgren and Whitehead's (1991) rainbow of determinants (see part III, especially chapter 13).

Table 1.2 The medical model of health compared with the social model of health.

Medical model	Social model
Narrow or simplistic understanding of health. Medically biased definitions focusing on the absence of disease or dis-ability.	Broad or complex understanding of health. More holistic definitions of health taking a wider range of factors into account such as mental and social dimensions of health.
Doesn't take into account the wider influences on health (outside the physical body).	Takes into account wider influences on health such as the environment the impact of inequalities.
Influenced by scientific and expert knowledge.	Takes into account lay knowledge and understandings.
Emphasizes personal, individual responsibility for health.	Emphasizes collective, social responsibility for health.

Salutogenesis   For the most part, in Western cultures at least, when we talk about health we are actually talking about negative health experience or 'ill-health' rather than more positive aspects of health. This has its roots in the medical model of health. **Salutogenesis** turns this idea around. Antonovsky was the instigator of this idea and he has challenged the 'pathogenic' nature of the medical model including its fixation on the elimination of disease constituting 'health'. Antonovsky (1996) argues that the focus should be on 'symptoms of wellness' rather than cases of disease and at-risk groups and that, given that we are 'organisms' we should accept that we will, at time, have things 'wrong' with us. The suggestion is, therefore, that 'none of us can be categorized as being either healthy or diseased, (instead) we are all located somewhere along a continuum' (Sidell, 2010: 27).

The holistic model

The contrasting medical and social models are not the only way to conceptualize health. Another way of looking at health is by taking a 'holistic' view, which takes a more integrated approach (Chronin de Chavez et al., 2005). This takes into account the interaction of biological, psychological and social factors (Earle, 2007a) and also views the person as a 'whole' rather than a sum of their 'parts'. Holistic notions of health may be seen as taking into account mind, body and spirit (see Patterson, 1997 – in Earle 2007a). The difference between the social model and a holistic approach to health is that the holistic approach tends to focus on the individual rather than social structures that influence the individual (Chronin de Chavez et al., 2005 and Earle, 2007a). A holistic approach underpins many complementary (or so called 'alternative') approaches to health. While a strength of an holistic approach is that it takes spiritual health into consideration one of the criticisms of holistic approaches to health is that, similarly to the medical model, it is more individualistic and does not take wider social factors into account.

The biopsychosocial model

The biopsychosocial model of health is very closely aligned to holistic views about health but is nevertheless distinguished from it in the wider literature. Engel (1977, cited in Marks et al., 2005: 75 and Sarafino, 2002: 16) developed the biopyschosocial model of health and illness – an expansion of the (bio)medical model that combines social, psychological and biological aspects of health and accounts for the interaction between these. Biological factors include factors like genetics and our physiological condition and systems. Psychological factors include taking into account how we behave, how and what we think and how we feel. Social factors include consideration of the fact that we are social beings who interact with others within groups, communities and societies. This is a model of health that has influenced research, **theory** and practice in health psychology but arguably has not had as much impact in other disciplinary areas in relation to health.

Different perspectives

Different perspectives offer different contributions to our understanding of health. In the first instance let's consider philosophical perspectives about health. Seedhouse (2001) argues that it is important to consider **philosophy** when trying to answer the question 'what is health?', since philosophy should be employed where competing and conflicting ideas about phenomena exist – health is a very good example of this. Another perspective is offered by psychology. Stephens (2008: 19) argues that psychology views health as 'a matter for individual minds'. Mainstream approaches to health in psychology that focus on the individual in terms of cognitive processes and behaviour are closely aligned to the individualistic medical model of health, and the idea of the body as a machine (Stephens, 2008), which challenges more holistic ideas about health, reflected in more critical psychological perspectives. (See chapter 6, which explores the contribution of psychology in more detail.)

Social construction

One of the key issues when trying to define health that also impacts on perspectives about health is the idea that 'health' is socially constructed. This means that the way we think about health is determined by a range of factors that influence us at any given time, in any given place. As a consequence, the notion of health is seen to be organic and fluid, changing all the time. **Social constructionism** argues that 'meaning' is socially constructed. In terms of health then, we can see that the meaning we give to it, or the way that we understand it is not straightforward or uncomplex. From a social constructionist perspective the meaning of health is created (constructed) through the way that we, as social beings, interact and the language that we use. Through talking about health we draw on different discourses, creating social consensus about what health actually is. We then reproduce and reinforce ideas about health through our talk and use of different discourses. This means that ideas about health are both time-bound and culture-bound – they change and vary across time and place. In addition, many different ways of talking about health (discourses) may (and do), exist at any one time.

A moral phenomenon

It is also worth considering briefly a dominant theoretical idea about health that is concerned with its moral nature. Crossley

(2003) argues that, increasingly, health has become synonymous with ideas to do with being a good and responsible person. The pursuit of health is therefore seen as something virtuous and highly valued. Lupton and Peterson (1996) refer to this as the 'imperative of health'. The extent to which this notion is prevalent is indicated by research findings that demonstrate that people prefer to claim that they are healthy (Blaxter, 2004) or at least are trying to be (Cross et al., 2010). This ties in with neo-liberalist notions about individual responsibility. The notion that individuals have a moral responsibility to look after their own health is echoed through many aspects of health promotion and health service provision. Lawton et al. (2005) highlights the promotion of self-management and self-care in people with type 2 diabetes, for example. The morality of health is strongly linked to ideas of 'good **citizenship**' and the drive to be a fully functioning member of society – one who protects and maintains their own health rather than being a strain on society's finite resources. In contemporary Western societies this can be seen, for example, in the way that people who are overweight or obese are judged and blamed for their size.

So far we have focused on the way that health is theorized, which has largely drawn on professional discourse about health. The next section of this chapter will explore these ideas in more detail in relation to lay understandings about health.

Lay perspectives

This section of the chapter will consider lay perspectives on health and how these can contribute to understanding what health is. First we need to determine the meaning of the term 'lay' in this context. Lay perspectives (or 'lay knowledge', Earle, 2007a; or 'lay expertise' Martin, 2008) are distinguishable from theoretical or professional perspectives in that they are the perspectives of 'ordinary' (or non-professional) people. Essentially lay perspectives are about how non-expert people understand and experience their health and how they perceive it. Bury (2005) refers to lay understandings as 'folk beliefs' and argues that research into lay concepts of health has revealed complex and sophisticated understanding and ideas that go beyond the medical model outlined earlier.

Blaxter (2007) points out that it is not necessarily useful to use the term 'lay' because lay knowledge and understanding is informed, at least in part, by professional knowledge and understanding. So Blaxter (2007: 26) suggests that 'lay understandings can better be defined as commonsense understandings and personal experience, imbued with professional rationalizations'. Nonetheless, since the term 'lay perspectives' is commonly used and understood and is, as such, reflected in much of the literature and research in this area, it will be used in this chapter. From this point on the term 'lay perspectives' will be used as a generic term, which is also seen to encompass the terms 'lay beliefs', 'lay understandings' and 'lay concepts'.

Lay perspectives are central to the social model of health as discussed previously. The importance of paying attention to people's subjective experience of health has been highlighted by many, including Lawton (2003). This is based on the fundamental assumption that people themselves often have the greatest insight into their own experiences of health and that it is therefore important to understand what these are (Earle, 2007a). Most often lay accounts or concepts of health are 'uncovered' through **empirical** research, so it is important to bear in mind the limitations that features such as study design and theoretical assumptions will have on findings and the way in which they are interpreted (see chapter 3 on researching health for further explanation of research methods). When reading research in this area it is also important to make note of whether the research is focused on 'health' rather than illness (as is commonly the case due to the difficulties of defining 'health'). Lawton (2003) and Hughner and Kleine (2004), among others, argue that relatively few studies have actually focused on concepts of health as opposed to illness and Blaxter (2007) argues that different studies use different measures, categories and means of investigation, which is also problematic. Nonetheless there is a body of knowledge that continues to evolve and grow around lay perspectives of health.

Lay perspectives are not homogenous nor are they uncomplex – they have been described as 'multi-factorial' (Popay et al., 2003). They differ across individuals, communities and cultures and evolve over time. They also differ with age, levels of education, **social class** and gender. It is important to consider lay perspectives on health for many reasons. Not least because they tend to challenge theoretical, reductionist notions about what health is and draw on a much wider range of understandings and experiences, which inevitably adds to the debate. Indeed, much of the contemporary health care provision agenda in Western societies is driven by public and user-involvement in which lay perspectives are inevitably key (Martin, 2008).

A study by Calnan (1987) carried out in the 1980s is often referred to in the literature on lay perceptions of health (although it actually focuses on lay understandings of health *inequalities*). Calnan's summary of the findings revealed that 'being healthy' was viewed as such things as being able to get through the day ('functioning'), not being ill, feeling strong, fit and energetic, getting exercise and not being overweight, being able to cope with the stress of life. Being healthy was also viewed as a state of mind. In contrast being unhealthy was viewed as things like being unable to work, being ill or having something wrong – a serious, long-term or incurable illness, not coping with life, being depressed or unhappy, lacking energy and a poor lifestyle.

More recently Blaxter (1990 in Blaxter, 2004) provided a framework of five categories (or ways) of describing health. This was based on the findings of a major UK study in which, among other things, people were asked what it was like to be healthy. The five categories of responses were as follows:

1.   Health as not-ill
2.   Health as physical fitness, vitality
3.   Health as social relationships
4.   Health as function
5.   Health as psychosocial well-being

Blaxter's findings are referred to in more detail throughout the rest of this chapter in relation to different lay understandings. Stainton-Rogers (1991) also studied lay descriptions of health and illness and offers a framework of seven different lay accounts for health as follows:

1.   Body as machine (links with medical model understandings)
2.   Body under siege (external factors influence health, i.e. germs)
3.   Inequality of access (i.e. to medical services)
4.   Cultural critique (linked with ideas about exploitation and oppression)
5.   Health promotion (linked with ideas about responsibility for health as being individual and collective)
6.   Robust individualism (linked with rights to a satisfying life)
7.   Willpower account (linked with ideas about individual control)

In trying to define health lay understandings (and indeed, professional ones) we are constrained by the use of language and for the most part, people tend to draw on mainstream discourse around health in order to articulate their understandings. Changes in knowledge and understanding over time also bring changes in understanding about health. In a study on Eastern Canadian 'baby boomer's' perspectives on health (and illness), Murray et al. (2003) noted several different narratives about the changing nature of health and illness.

Things such as age, class and gender influence how we think about health. In a sense, these different aspects of an individual co-exist and it is not really possible to separate them out. I, for example, am a Caucasian woman, aged 21 years (plus a bit!) and would be described as being middle-class – as defined by my profession. All of these features may influence the way I think about health, in addition to my past experience, my beliefs, my culture and many other things. However, for the purposes of this discussion, lay understandings of health will be considered under some of these different aspects while the problematic nature of using this type of categorization, which is 'very social in nature' (Stephens, 2008: 6) are acknowledged.

Understandings according to culture

One of the major things that has been seen to influence understanding about the nature of health is culture. Cultural perspectives on health offer many different ways of looking at health and the way that we think about health is influenced by our culture (see chapter 5 for more detailed discussion of the relationship between culture and health). Likewise different belief systems, for example, about the origin of life, the existence of a 'higher' being, and the meaning of life, all influence understandings about health. An example of the way that culture impacts on ideas about health is the promotion, in contemporary Western cultures, of the slender body as equated with health. This results in the promotion of the thin ideal through the discourse of 'healthy weight', which equates being slim with being healthy (Burns and Gavey, 2004). This type of discourse suggests that health is achieved by being within certain weight limits (as medically and socially defined). Critics of this position argue that this is more to do with *looking* healthy (as defined by Westernized body ideals) than *being* healthy (see Burns & Gavey, 2004 and Aphramor & Gingras, 2008 for example) and yet this is a very pervasive idea in contemporary culture, which is being seen to have wider influence globally (chapter 12 explores global influences upon health).

With regard to mental health research in Zambia, Aidoo and Harpham (2001) explored the ways in which urban women in low-income groups explained mental ill-health as compared with local health care practitioners and found that the women tended to speak of 'problems of the mind' while the practitioners used terms such as 'stress' and 'depression'. This illustrates two points about the influence of culture on understanding of health. Firstly, that the practitioners were likely to have been influenced by more Westernized ideas about mental health through their training and secondly that the 'culture' of the practitioners contrasted with the culture of the non-practitioners in terms of understanding and experiencing mental ill-health. The practitioners used different definitions of ill-health, viewing depression as an indication that something was wrong, while the non-practitioners – the women – only defined physical symptoms as ill-health (note again that the focus here was on negative (or ill-) health rather than positive health). 'Problems of the mind' were not necessarily viewed as ill-health (Aidoo & Harpham, 2001).

Understandings vary according to social class and level of formal education   Several authors (see Bury, 2005; Blaxter, 2004; Duncan, 2007 and Marks et al., 2005 for example) reference a substantial, seminal piece of published work examining beliefs about health by Herzlich in 1973. Herzlich carried out one of the earliest studies that looked at lay concepts of health in middle-class French people and she found that ideas about health were closely linked with the 'way of life' in urban living. The way of life was seen to mitigate against good health (by causing stress and fatigue) and to generate illness. In contrast, positive health was viewed as being something inherent within the individual – health as existing in a vacuum (acknowledged only by its absence or being ill), as a 'reserve of strength' and as 'equilibrium' (Duncan,

2007: 19). Ill-health resulted from the impact of environmental factors when there were not enough 'reserves'. Blaxter (2004: 49) states that these three representations are also sometimes discussed as health being to do with '*having, doing and being*'.

Blaxter is an influential writer and researcher in the area of concepts of heath (see Blaxter, 1990 and 2004). Her research has focused on exploring lay beliefs about health within the UK. An early study by Blaxter and Paterson (1982, cited in Blaxter, 2004) found that middle-aged women, and their daughters, in poor socio-economic situations defined health as 'not being ill' first and foremost. Blaxter's (1990) *Health and Lifestyles* study found that the better educated and those with higher incomes used the 'health as not-ill' definition more frequently as well as the 'health as psychosocial well-being'. This draws on a medical perspective viewing health as absence of illness.

Understandings across the lifespan

Children and young people's perceptions of health Many studies have explored how children and young people talk about health.

When asking children about their health Brannen and Storey (1996) found that relatively few felt that their health was good (34% good, 48% fairly good, 9% not good and 9% unsure: Brannen & Storey, 1996: 25). The children in the study frequently linked their health status with eating habits. In a different study Brynin and Scott (1996) asked children if they thought that health was a 'matter of luck'. They found while younger children are more likely to accept this, older children are more likely to believe that health is under their own control and less a matter of luck.

Ideas about health appear to change with age during childhood and adolescence. Chapman et al. (2000) examined how children and young people define health. The younger children (aged 5 –11 years) defined health in terms of diet, exercise and rest, hygiene and dental hygiene. They described health in more negative terms such as illness, smoking and the environment. The younger children also referred to emotions and mental health. The older children (over the age of 12 years) included things like smoking and drinking behaviours, having a healthy mind, feeling happy and confident and self-acceptance. Interestingly the older children also linked looking good, being happy and feeling confident with being healthy.

A more recent study, carried out in New Zealand, also explored children's understandings of health and found that these were wide-ranging (Burrows and Wright, 2004). Being healthy was seen to be about being happy, thinking positively about yourself and being kind. In addition the children linked health with physical bodies, morality and character and also took into account mental, social, spiritual and environmental factors.

The effects of smoking are well publicized; however it still remains a major health issue for people of all ages.

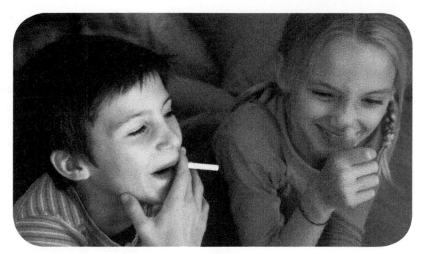

© Voisin/Phanie/Rex Features

Older people's perceptions of health   In terms of age, research shows that understandings about health become more complex and develop 'multi-layers' of understanding over a person's **lifespan** (Hardey, 1998). Blaxter's (1990) *Health and Lifestyles* study found that older people tended to define health more in terms of being able to function and do things or care for themselves. Much of the research claiming to focus on lay perspectives in older age actually examines illness experience rather than concepts of health or well-being (in common with other research into 'health' across the lifespan). What it tends to reveal is that the onset of chronic diseases is viewed as being inevitable in older age and part of normal transition through this specific life-stage, as such challenges to 'health' in older age are more or less anticipated (see Lawton, 2003 for an overview). In addition being 'independent' is strongly linked to ideas about being healthy (Lloyd, 2000).

Understandings of health vary according to gender   Among others, Emslie and Hunt (2008) contend that gender has a major part to play in lay perceptions of health. Again we can draw on Blaxter's work here to illustrate the fact that ideas about health may vary according to gender. Blaxter (2004) claimed to find clear gender differences, particularly in the way that men and women responded to questions about health. Women seemed to be more interested in talking about health and generally gave more detailed answers. Specifically she found that young women's ideas about health included the importance of social relationships and being able to look after the family (drawing on functionalist notions of health). Emslie and Hunt (2008) likewise found that, with regard to perspectives on differences in life expectancy between males and females (on average women live longer), women's accounts were more likely to focus on reproductive and caring roles and men's accounts more on the disadvantages of their 'provider' roles.

Gendered assumptions about health tend to portray that women are interested in health and men are not. However, Smith et al. (2008), in their research on Australian men, found that the men self-monitored their health status to determine whether to seek professional help and they argue that this shows a higher degree of interest in health than has previously been assumed of men as compared with women generally. Robertson (2006) carried out a study exploring men's concepts of health, including sub-samples of gay and disabled men. He found that many of the men's narratives about health involved notions of control and release that were associated with issues of risk and responsibility. While these themes are echoed in research focusing solely on women, ideas about the nature of risk and responsibility in health do differ with gender.

Learning task 1.4

Activity
Consider what health might mean to a range of different types of people in different contexts.

For example:
(a) What do the definitions have to offer in terms of furthering our understanding about health?
(b) What are the limitations of them? What are their strengths?
(c) How would you alter the definitions? What would you add or remove and why?
(d) How do the definitions compare or contrast with your own definition of health from learning task 1.1?

Perspectives and theoretical (professional) understandings about health can be very different from one another. While lay accounts undoubtedly draw on expert and professional understandings, to some extent they can, and do, offer alternative and increased understandings about the nature of health. A substantial amount of research has been done in this area and, as Robertson (2006) argues, this has shown the extent to which lay perspectives understand health as something that is integrated with daily life rather than being a separate entity. The importance of lay perspectives to how health is defined and theorized is therefore apparent.

Nevertheless, some criticisms have been levelled at taking lay perspectives into account in terms of the legitimacy of them and the value that they bring to general understandings of health (Entwistle et al., 1998). Entwistle et al. (1998: 465) argue that lay perspectives may be biased, unrepresentative and, it can be argued, they are 'rarely typical'. In addition there are assumptions of mutual understandings, which may be problematic. Are 'expert' interpretations of 'lay' opinion accurate and reliable? Are we using the same language to mean different things or different language to mean the same things? With regard to 'beliefs' Shaw, in his 2002 paper 'How lay are lay beliefs?', problematizes the concept and examines the inherent difficulties with using this term. He argues that it is virtually impossible to study lay beliefs because they are intertwined with a number of things including medical rationality. Even 'commonsense' views, he argues, are 'based upon understandings within expert paradigms' (Shaw, 2002: 287). Given the problematic nature of lay concepts of health Shaw contends that what we should be focusing on are lay 'accounts' – specifically lay accounts of illness. Kangas (2002) contests this position however and warns against juxtaposing lay and expert perspectives on health arguing that this can 'blur the analysis of their complex relationship' (Kangas 2002: 302). So this is something that is worth bearing in mind – despite the distinctions the majority of the literature makes between 'lay' and 'expert' (or professional) perspectives, in reality the boundaries between the two are often less clear cut. With respect to terminology Prior (2003) notes a change over the last twenty or so years in the academic literature from a focus on lay health beliefs and understandings to a focus on lay knowledge and expertise, which is worth noting, since it may affect the way we attempt to 'understand', account for and incorporate non-professional definitions (and concepts) of health. Prior (2003: 45) criticizes those who use the term 'lay expert' as failing to be specific about 'how exactly lay people might be expert' but later in her paper argues that lay people do have information and knowledge to share.

In summary, health means different things to different people. Notions of health may differ between groups and between different contexts. Perceptions of health will vary across the lifespan and are influenced by a range of factors including individual experiences and socialization. Personal experience and subjectivities mould our understandings of what health is and the meanings that we attach to it. These are, in turn, influenced by a range of things such as our social and physical environment and culture.

Why is this important for understanding health?

There are several reasons why it is important to look at different perspectives about health – both theoretical perspectives and lay perspectives. Firstly, appreciating different understandings of health may help towards understanding why people behave in certain ways when it comes to their health (Hughner & Kleine, 2004). This, in turn, can influence the way in which interventions intended to improve health are designed, communicated and implemented. As Earle (2007a) argues, anyone concerned with trying to change or influence health needs to understand what people mean when they talk about health. Secondly, in terms of health promotion we need to be clear about what it is we are actually trying to promote (health promotion is explained and analysed in chapter 7).

Thirdly, it is important because, as Entwistle et al. (1998) argues, lay perspectives can complement 'expert' perspectives and add to knowledge and understandings. As such they should be incorporated into, for example, health care provision and also research into health. Understanding what health is about is crucial to researching it (Earle, 2007a). If we don't know what we mean by the term 'health' how can we investigate its existence and meaning? Parallels between lay and expert understandings do exist with regard to some things; for example, in terms of how stress is conceived and understood (Clark, 2003) but this is not always the case. Differences in understandings have been found in relation to a range of health-related phenomena such as, for example, the body (Nettleton & Watson, 1998). Finally Schoenberg et al. (2005) points out the need to take people's views into account in terms of influencing policy and programmes (in health) that are appropriately designed and sustainable.

As Duncan (2007: 93) argues, 'we can assume nothing about the nature of health' – it is contested, varied and changing. In addition, in order to understand health we need to take into consideration a variety of different perspectives to avoid having a narrow, constrained idea about what health is. Drawing on different disciplines and giving due consideration to lay perspectives can aid and enhance our understandings about health. In addition Tones and Green (2004) argue that trying to come up with a working definition of health can provide a basis for practice in promoting health – after all, as pointed out earlier, we need to have at least an idea of what it is we are trying to promote! Definitions of health therefore have implications for a range of things including theory, practice, policy and promoting public health (Marks et al., 2000). In a special issue of the *Journal of Health Psychology* published in 2003 on the topic of health concepts, the editor at the time, Flick, argued that there were still a lot of 'open questions and unresolved problems' when it came to addressing the main issues (Flick, 2003: 484). Flick summarized these as the variety of health concepts that are encountered in everyday life and through professional practice. Now, a few years later, it seems that the same challenges remain. Lawton (2003: 32) argues that more work needs to be done, the reason being that the 'contexts within which health (is) defined and experienced are constantly shifting and changing'.

Case study

Conflicting perspectives on the phenomenon of 'binge-drinking'.

Binge-drinking is a good example in contemporary UK society of how expert and lay perspectives can differ with regard to understanding about health.

In the last few years or so a substantial amount of research has focused on professional and non-professional discourse around binge-drinking. From a professional point of view binge-drinking is seen to be harmful, risky behaviour that needs to be brought under control. The 'binge-drinker' is almost viewed as being deviant. Binge-drinking is seen as being bad for your health (Courtney & Polich, 2009).

Drawing on lay perspectives, binge-drinking is often viewed as being much less problematic. Rather than framing this practice as detrimental, lay perspectives (particularly among young people among whom binge-drinking is almost portrayed as being 'epidemic') highlight the use of alcohol as a social lubricant, something that they use to increase confidence and cement social relationships. In addition the practice is viewed as a way of 'letting your hair down' and creating space to be free from inhibitions and the stresses of modern day life (Cross, forthcoming). Binge-drinking can therefore be seen as almost being 'good' for health, a way of managing or coping with stress for example. The benefits of the practice are seen to outweigh the negatives.

So, as Szmigin et al. (2008) argues, experts in public health and health promotion need to work to find ways in which messages about binge-drinking can be framed to take account of lay understandings and perspectives rather than focusing on the issue from a more expert viewpoint – one that is likely to be rejected or ignored by the very people it is trying to 'target'.

Summary

- Health is a complex concept and is difficult to define. Many different definitions and understandings exist.

- Understandings of health differ according to experience and expertise. Factors such as age, social class and gender impact on these. Theoretical perspectives about health can aid our understandings of subjective health experience.

- Lay and expert understandings of health may differ but both are central to developing understandings about what health is, how it may be explored and how it may be maintained.

Questions

1. Health means different things to different people. Consider what health might mean to other people in different contexts for example – a person who uses a wheelchair, a person in a country experiencing conflict, a person who is experiencing a mental health problem or some other person of your choice. How might their understanding of health differ from yours and why?

2. Drawing on the material in this chapter, compare and contrast theoretical (or professional) understandings/concepts of health with lay understandings/concepts. Take time to reflect on why it is important to take both types of perspectives into consideration.

3. What factors do you think impact on, and influence, your understandings about health and what health means to you? Which of these are most significant and why?

Further reading

Blaxter, M. (2004) Health. Cambridge, Polity.
This book is one of the most useful, readable texts around on lay perspectives and health. Readers should note that it focuses mainly on understandings of health within a 'global north' (or 'Western') context. However, it explores the meaning of health in some depth, drawing on a range of literature and research so it is a very good introduction to the key issues.

Duncan, P. (2007) Critical Perspectives on Health. Basingstoke, Palgrave Macmillan.
This book addresses the question 'what is health?' and critically examines a range of diverse perspectives. It is a useful follow-up to this chapter and explores a number of issues in greater analytical depth than can be achieved here. See Part III, Critical Perspectives on Health, for a more in-depth critical discussion about the nature of health.

Seedhouse, D. (2001) Health: The Foundations for Achievement. 2nd edn. Chichester, Wiley.
This is another useful text in terms of exploring, in more detail, the nature of health and its complexities. David Seedhouse has a very specific, philosophic perspective about health that contributes to contemporary understanding and debate. This book focuses on two key issues – 'what is health?' and 'how can health be achieved?'

2 Contemporary Threats to Health

Overview

This chapter aims to give an overview of the main issues and challenges in relation to public health within the twenty-first century and explore the key health 'issues' within the current public health agenda in the UK and beyond. Firstly, the nature of threats and factors that influence societal decisions about what are public health threats are discussed. Secondly, the changing patterns of health threats and experience are outlined and epidemiological transitions are discussed. Thirdly, current key threats to public health including both communicable and non-communicable diseases are examined. Finally, the chapter critically discusses current threats to health such as lifestyle diseases that are inherently socially influenced. For example, illnesses associated with the over-consumption of food and alcohol, the problems of inactivity and sedentary lifestyles and risky behaviours such as unprotected sexual encounters. These issues are also discussed in more depth in chapters 6 and 8. Complete the following learning task, which will help you to think about how you personally perceive and rate health threats.

Learning task 2.1

The significance of health threats.
Place in rank order which you think are the most significant threats
to health at the current time, where 1 is the most significant and 10
the least significant.
Obesity
Poverty
Drought and its associated famine
Flooding
HIV
Malaria
Global recession caused by the 'credit crunch'
Cutting health care expenditure
Unequal societies
Mental illness
What kind of things influenced your ranking order and decision-
making?

You should have seen from the above learning task that deciding what
are the most important threats to health is not easy and there are a
numbers of factors that can and do influence our decisions. You may
have decided to rank topics higher up the scale that affected most
people, or based your decisions upon the seriousness or importance
of the threats from the list. You could have been influenced by what
you read and see in the media on a daily basis when making your decision. A number of factors that can influence both our perceptions and
conceptualization of contemporary health threats are outlined in the
next section.

Conceptualizing the identifying of threats

Nature and determinants of health

As we have seen in chapter 1, defining what we may see as a threat
to health will be intrinsically linked to how we define health. Even
the word 'threat' is linked to negative, commodity, pathogenic and
biomedical concepts of health. Implicit in this discussion is that full
health is compromised by a threat and that it can be restored by preventive, treatment and curative interventions. If, however, we consider
health under more positive and salutogenic (what generates health
and well-being, as discussed in chapter 1) conceptual frameworks,
then the word 'threat' is not as appropriate, as we are concerned with
the creation of health not the avoidance of disease, illness and disability (Antonovsky, 1996). Often an understanding of the word health

Obesity is an increasingly important health threat in higher-income countries.

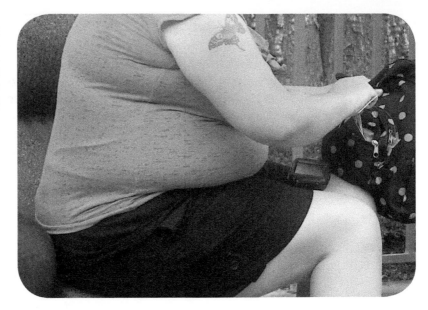

© Zoran mircetic

in the popular sense is limited to notions of physical health, with increasing recognition of mental illness, although social and community health is relatively neglected in popular discourses of health (see chapter 9 for a discussion of community as a determinant of health). This can shape what are defined as threats to health.

Similarly if we define the influences on our health as ultimately biological in nature, leading to ill-health and malfunctioning of the healthy physiological state of the body, then the threats will be conceived as factors influencing our biological states. For example eating too much saturated fat in our diet leads to increased plasma cholesterol resulting in atherosclerosis and an increased risk of coronary heart disease (Hu, Manson & Willett, 2001).

However, if we subscribe to the social model of health and acknowledge the importance of socio-economic factors in determining well-being and disease, then we will view threats more broadly and shaped by the social world in which we live (see chapter 4 for a more detailed discussion of how society influences health). Continuing with the previous example and applying the social model of health, we should recognize that the influences on eating high levels of saturated fats are shaped by societal demands for inexpensive, tasty and convenient patterns of eating (Glanz et al., 1998). Similarly, levels of activity are influenced by town planning, the configuration of leisure space and the organization of transport systems, which are all analysed within the scope of the social model of health.

Examining the causal pathways for health and illness can aid our understanding of the diversity of threats to health. Bhopal (2008) provides a useful model for analysing the complexity of causal pathways called a web of causation, which visualizes the interconnected-

Learning task 2.2

Diabetes and health.

Consider type 2 diabetes as a threat to health. Outline as many influences as you can think of in relation to what determines the development of type 2 diabetes among individuals. Use the internet to help you explore the causes of type 2 diabetes. Represent these influences in a diagram, for example a 'spider's web of causation'.

Finally, think about how you conceptualize these influences. Do you see the influences that you listed as threats?

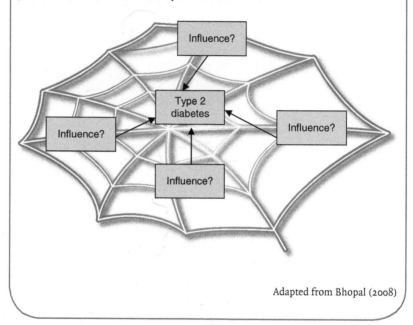

Adapted from Bhopal (2008)

ness of factors that influences health and illness. Bhopal's (2008) diagram represents a complex group of health determinants such as the environment, behaviour and the workplace. It also shows the inter-relatedness of these factors in terms of how they contribute to the occurrence and spread of disease. Now complete learning task 2.2, which demonstrates the complexity of health determinants in relation to a specific illness.

The dominant contemporary discourse for health is one of threats and disease. Giddens (2009) argues that the societal focus upon health risks leaves both governments and individuals debating the outcomes of such risks because there are no definitive answers. This is not entirely surprising as generating positive health appears for many to be a less important priority than preventing and reducing mortality and **morbidity**. Indeed most supposed 'health' targets that underpin practice are framed around reducing illness. However, a good example of an integrative framework of action in relation to desired health outcomes are the Millennium Development Goals (see chapter 12 for a description of these), which consider the wider determinants of health.

This book demonstrates throughout part III in particular that there are a large range of determinants of health. Consequently, the threats to health discussed here are conceptualized as broad in scope to encapsulate the broad nature of determinants of health outlined in Dahlgren and Whitehead's 1991 rainbow model. In this way seemingly non-related health factors such as climate change, war and conflict and poverty can be considered to be threats to health. This has important implications for who is defined as a health workforce and the types of initiatives and programmes that are considered to impact upon the health of populations.

Magnitude and severity

Other factors that can influence what issues are seen as threats to health are the number of people affected and the seriousness of the threat. Large and visible dangers tend to receive more attention and are therefore more likely to be categorized as threats to health. For example, if the rate of consultations for flu-like symptoms in a sample of reporting by general practitioners exceeds 400 per 100,000 population in one week, then this increases the perceived and actual risk of the threat (Fleming, 1999). **Pandemics** can be classified as stronger threats because of their scope being across continents and the world. Notions of mortality (death), morbidity (burden of diseases), impact on quality of life and chronic and acute disease can also be brought to bear on how threats are conceptualized. For example head lice **incidence** rates within the UK can be as high as 37% (Harris et al., 2003) and can affect children across the world but very few people would suggest that head lice are a major threat to health as they do not lead to death. Whereas HIV-related illness does lead to death, has high incidence rates, is associated with **stigma** and discrimination, results in reductions in quality of life and is therefore a significant contemporary threat to public health, particularly in sub-Saharan Africa and Asia.

However, conceptualizing health threats using this approach can mean that marginalized sub-populations or hidden health issues can be neglected. For example issues that are perceived by society as stigmatized or shameful can go under-reported, under-investigated and unrecognized; for example, disability.

Media construction and moral panics

The way that health issues are reported within the media influences how both lay people and policy-makers understand the nature of these threats and interpret their subsequent risk to health. In most countries, there are now many health scares reported in the media. These scares often emphasize both physical and emotional threats that are posed by everyday occurrences such as sunbathing, using a mobile phone and vaccinations like measles, mumps and rubella (the combination of three vaccines into a single injection known as **MMR**). The media play a key role in this process, headlining stories about health scares despite the lack of science behind many of the claims that are made (Wainwright, 2009a). The availability of information via the media can lead to the social amplification of risk, where risks categorized as minor by scientific experts actually elicit strong public concerns and even reactions, resulting in large-scale impacts. Despite the fact that physical health and general life expectancy have improved massively over the last century, perceptions of threats to our health are increasing. The health scares reported in the media arguably give rise to a heightened sense of public panic, creating more physical and mental vulnerability (Buckingham, 2009).

The media have certainly been influential in enhancing our fear of risk by over-reporting health scares and by advising the public to change their behaviour, be vigilant and to take precautions despite the actual risks to us being small. However, the government can also contribute to our fear of illness and disease, when it launches campaigns about looming epidemics. A good example of this was the expected influenza A H1N1 epidemic of 2009. Boseley (2009) argues that the first flu pandemic of the twenty-first century was far less lethal than expected as it only killed 26 out of every 100,000 people who became ill. However, it can be argued that the government had to stock-pile vaccinations (despite the vested interests of the pharmaceutical industry) in case the pandemic did become as lethal as the others have been historically.

Science has also been blamed for playing a role in the generation of fear and heightened perceptions of risk because many studies are methodologically flawed but this is not recognized, despite the findings often being used as the basis of both media (mis)reporting and government campaigns. Consequently people often have higher levels of fear than are necessary (Buckingham, 2009). Even when research is dismissed by a large number of scientists, as in the case of the study claiming to find an **association** between the MMR vaccination and childhood autism, the conflicting views discussed by experts were enough for many members of the public to see a threat (Burgess, 2009) and to change their behaviour for example, by refusing vaccinations. This was due to the perceptions of bad science being associated with the vaccination. Moreover it took time for the truth to emerge about the safety of the MMR.

Now complete learning task 2.3. This will help you to think about how the UK media influences perceptions of risk.

Although we have outlined separate factors that influence how public health issues are identified and can reach the public conscious-

Box 2.1   Example – Moral panic: global perspectives of HIV.

Media and lay network discourses have sought to raise moral panic about HIV. As patterns of transmission have emerged differently in Western and African contexts, the associated moral panics have been constructed differently.

Moral panic can be thought of as anxiety and fear generated by moral judgements about people and behaviour that poses risks to social order.

In both Western and African contexts HIV has been conceptualized as retribution and a plague on individuals that engage in 'deviant' behaviour. For example in the US the '4-H risk groups' were initially used to describe at risk groups namely homosexuals, Haitians, haemophiliacs and heroin addicts. A further classification identified different groups of individuals as either guilty or innocent (i.e. haemophiliacs and children respectively).

This moral panic is especially prevalent in evangelical communities when minority groups have been blamed for society's ills, and used to create a 'climate of fear' that somehow society will break down if the threat is not countered.

The implications of this moral panic are huge, leading to further stigmatization of vulnerable people and increasing barriers for practitioners lobbying for less victim-blaming approaches and more open policies for tackling HIV.

Accoron & Watson (2006)

ness and policy and practice agenda for action, in reality the factors all act in concert to create notions of threats to health.

Communicable and non-communicable diseases

In general the types of diseases that affect populations change as countries develop, so risks shift from infectious diseases such as cholera in poorer countries to non-communicable and lifestyle associated health problems such as cancers and heart disease in richer countries. Indeed, the risks for non-communicable diseases are also higher for richer individuals living within poorer countries. Therefore identifying threats ultimately depends upon the context in which the population is based.

Wainwright (2009a) labels this as an 'epidemiological transition' (p. 5) whereby the traditional diseases of poverty, such as infectious diseases and malnutrition, are replaced by diseases of affluence, such as cancers and heart disease. The WHO (2009) labels this as a 'risk transition' caused by improvements in medical care, the ageing of the population and successful public health interventions such as vaccina-

Learning task 2.3

Contraceptive use and media reports.

Examine the excerpts from a newspaper article about Implanon, a long lasting contraceptive implant embedded in the arm.

Hope, 2011 Contraceptive implant alert: Hundreds of women fall pregnant after birth control fails (*Daily Mail* 5 January 2011)

Hundreds of women have become pregnant after a long-term contraceptive implant failed, it emerged last night.

Even more have complained that they were left injured or scarred by the rod inserted into their arm, which was supposed to protect them against conceiving for three years. The NHS has had to pay compensation to women hurt when the implants were inserted and seven women who were left traumatized by unexpectedly becoming pregnant have received payouts totalling more than £200,000 – an average of more than £28,000 each. In total 584 women who had the hormone-filled rod inserted in their arms have reported unwanted pregnancies to the Medicines and Health Care Regulatory Agency – the government's drugs and medical devices watchdog. But the total could be far higher, as many women may not have complained after becoming pregnant, either undergoing abortions or giving birth.

The MHRA received 1,607 complaints about the implant going wrong, some from doctors deeply concerned that the devices are difficult to insert and that it is impossible to check if they are correctly installed because they are invisible to X-rays. One in four women who go to family planning clinics gets a long-term contraceptive implant. They are especially popular with teenagers, with 10 per cent of 16 to 19-year-olds saying they prefer an implant because they do not have to remember to take a pill. Around 80,000 women use implants of the same type as Implanon.

A lawyer revealed that many of the women affected had suffered 'psychological difficulties', had miscarriages or decided to undergo abortions after the implants went wrong.

One woman who became pregnant and underwent an abortion said the trauma had led to her marriage ending. Last night a woman who had the implant, named only as Lara to protect her identity, told of her trauma when she later discovered she was pregnant. 'I feel very, very disturbed – hitting my head on the table,' she told Channel 4 News. 'Weeping like a young child. My mind was so disturbed – thinking why is this happening to me?'

The fiasco involving the implant is one of the worst mass contraceptive failures to hit the NHS in living memory.

Identify the differing viewpoints in this narrative.

Which viewpoints did you trust and why?

If you, or your partner, were using this implant how would you evaluate your risk of
(i)   pregnancy?
(ii)   side effects?
How realistic do you think your assessments would be?

tions and sanitation. Therefore, the impact of risks to health varies at different levels of socio-economic development. So although new and infectious diseases can occur anywhere in the world, risks do indeed vary according to where people live. Put simply there are 'hot spots' that favour the emergence and spread of specific conditions. Evidence for this is given in table 2.1, which describes changing patterns of disease, health and illness.

Data in the table utilizes childhood mortality rates, which are considered to be one of the most sensitive indicators of the health of a population, as they are intrinsically related to the whole scope of determinants of health. In a comparison between England and Wales and Botswana it is evident that the industrialization and improvements in working and living conditions have impacted on life expectancy and the patterns of ill-health, although life expectancy has increased proportionally more in the UK, largely due to the industrial revolution taking place prior to 1900. In Botswana gains in life expectancy have been limited mainly as a result of high childhood mortality and adult deaths related to infectious diseases, particularly HIV and AIDS, malaria and cholera.

Kaufmann (2009) identifies a number of factors that favour epidemics such as poverty, catastrophes and conflicts because people often have to live in unhygienic and crowded conditions in such situations. The incorrect use of antibiotics, which leads to the development of resistant microbes, is also an issue (think about Western concerns with MRSA). He argues that it has never been so easy for epidemics to spiral into pandemics because of diseases travelling across the world via the global movement of both people and animals, for example, the SARs epidemic was spread in this way. All of these threats combine differently according to location. Indeed, countries historically show different trends in relation to changing life expectancy because of the inter-relationship of these threats to health and other social determinants. Learning task 2.4 will help you to explore changing trends in life expectancy.

In the next section we begin to analyse the nature of specific health threats.

Table 2.1. Changing patterns of disease, health and illness.

Timeline	Life expectancy at birth (England and Wales) no.1	Life expectancy at birth Botswana, Southern Africa no.3	Key events influencing mortality, morbidity and health	Causes of death	
				UK no.2	Botswana
1900	50.5	34.1	1900 British Rule of Botswana 1900 First mission hospital in Makoulane, Botswana	In 1900 Infectious and parasitic diseases caused 33% of all deaths.	Data not available
1920	57.6	34.1	1901 Trans-Atlantic radio message	Cancers less than 2%	
1940	68.8	34	1913 Asylums built in UK for mentally ill patients 1914–1918 World War I	Childhood mortality 140 per 1000 births.	
1960	71.2	51.2	1918 Influenza pandemic		1960 Infant mortality 118 per 1000 births no.4
1980	73.5	50.6	1929 Great Depression discovery of penicillin		
2000	78.0	52.4	1939–1945 World War II		
2009	80.0	52.3	1946 Inception of NHS service in England and Wales 1950–1970 Botswana place of asylum for refugees from neighbouring conflicts in Angola 1952 First Open Heart Surgery Baby boom in UK 1966 Botswana Independence from Britain 1981 The term 'AIDS' first used	In 1997 Infectious diseases account for 17% of deaths. Cancers accounts for 44% of deaths. Childhood mortality 5.8 per 1000 births.	In 2001 infectious and parasitic diseases caused 33% of all deaths. Cancers less than 4.2% no.5 In 2000 Infant mortality 75 per 1000 births no.4

no.1 Office of Health Economics @ http://www.ohe.org/page/knowledge/schools/appendix/life_expectancy.cfm (2007)
no.2 Hicks & Allen (1999)
no.3 World Bank Indicators (2008)
no.4 United Nations Statistics Division (nd)
no.5 WHO (2007b)

The World Health Organization statistics of probable SARs cases from November 2002 to July 2003 show that there were a total of 8,096 cases resulting in 774 deaths worldwide.

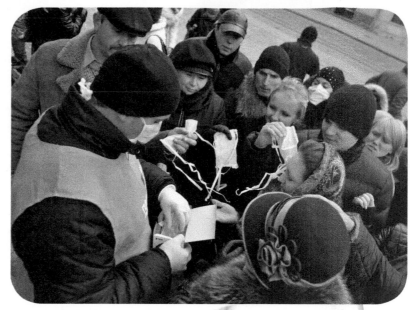

© Martin Purmensky

Learning task 2.4

Analysing trends in life expectancy.
Visit the website – http://www.gapminder.org/
    Click on the second tab at the top of the page called gap-minder world where you will see a graph that compares life-expectancy to levels of income. From the right-hand side of the page choose the following three countries,

- Australia
- Cuba
- The Democratic Republic of Congo

Then go back in time to 1800 using the toolbar at the bottom of the graph and click on play. You will now have a graphical representation of changing life expectancy across the three countries.

1. Describe the different trends between income and life expectancy shown in the graph for all three countries and why this is the case.
2. Think about what might influence these trends and list possible factors.

Contemporary threats

It is not possible to consider all health risks within the scope of this chapter; therefore in this next section we aim to give a sense of the threats drawing on the conceptual framework outlined earlier, rather than producing a definitive list of the major threats to health. More comprehensive reading about **risk factors** and diseases can be found in the suggestions for further reading at the end of this chapter. This section is organized into a discussion of key global threats to health starting with a description of broader threats and then moving to a focus upon more direct health issues.

Climate change   Climate change is now receiving both media and political attention and is certainly a health threat based upon the evidence that has been gathered about how potential changes in the climate might impact upon health. Table 2.2 outlines different categories of the different key impacts on health.

Table 2.2. Effects of climate change upon health.

Main impact of climate change	Effect on health
Extreme weather events	Increased – • Typhoons • Cyclonic events • Torrential rains • Extended hot dry periods • High winds • Hail storms
Water	↑ water in high latitudes ↓ water and drought in mid and low latitudes
Food	Cereal production reduced in some regions negative impacts on small holders, subsistence farmers and fishers
Coasts	Increased damage from floods and storms e.g. Brisbane and Brazil, in January 2011
Ecosystems	Increasing species shifts and extinctions may lead to collapse of food chains
Summary Projected impact on **health indicators**	Increasing burden from malnutrition, diarrhoeal, cardio-respiratory, and infectious diseases Increased morbidity and mortality from heat waves, floods, and droughts Changed distribution of some disease vectors e.g. mosquitoes transmitting malaria Risks from populations on the move resulting in homelessness and overcrowded conditions Substantial burden on health services

Adapted from Summerhayes, 2010.

Rao (2009) suggests that impacts within the UK may include increased deaths, injuries and disease because of heat waves, floods and storms, poorer air quality, increased pollens, and reduced food safety. Extreme weather events are certainly happening more often and when these do occur they result in deaths, disease and injuries because people drown and sanitation and clean water supplies becomes a problem. Rao (2009) also argues that we can expect to see changes in the pattern and distribution of vector-borne diseases as a result of climate change. Consequently, globally there will be higher risks of people being infected with often labelled tropical diseases such as malaria and dengue fever. Heavy rains and more flooding may lead to the further spread of diseases carried by rodents too. The depletion of the ozone layer is also a related health issue because of increased exposure to ultra-violet radiation (UVR). This is not specifically associated with climate change, rather with air pollution, but too much exposure to UVR can result in many detrimental health effects; sunburn, heatstroke, skin cancers, cataracts and weakened responses to immunizations. The environment is also likely to be affected negatively by climate change and the health impact may again be detrimental.

Our health is linked to the environment and the destruction of the natural environment is therefore a threat to our health. In destroying our environment, we threaten our basic needs such as food, shelter and clean air and water (Stone, 2009). Degraded environments are associated with health problems, and high levels of mortality. Evidence gathered by the WHO tells us that each year 800,000 people die from causes related to air pollution, 3.5 million from malnutrition and 1.8 million from lack of clean water (WHO, 2005b; 2008). These numbers are likely to increase as current damage to our environment continues. All of these physical health problems certainly may impact upon mental health too and the effects of climate change upon mental health have not yet been estimated. For example, post-traumatic stress rates are likely to soar after events like flash floods, typhoons and torrential rains.

In the year 2000, climate change was estimated to have caused over 150,000 deaths worldwide (WHO, 2005a) and its health-related impact is likely to continue because the climate takes time to respond to change (Pope, 2008). So even if we begin to tackle some aspects of climate change, and its effects are stopped or even reversed, the impact upon our health still remains a threat. Hence, climate change remains a risk to health for the immediate, as well as the long-term future.

Population growth   An issue intrinsically linked to climate change is the growing population of the world and movements of people from rural to urban areas in search of better and more affluent lives. All continents are predicted to increase in population size in the twenty-first century and globally, while the rate of population growth has slowed over the past few decades, the absolute number of people continues to

Figure 2.1.
Population
pyramids and
projected growth.

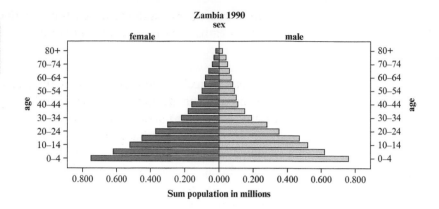

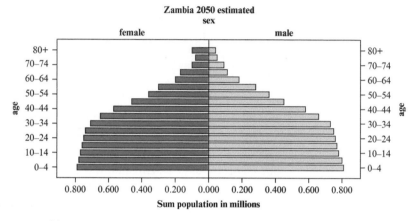

Source of data: US Census Bureau

increase by about one billion every thirteen years, and the environment continues to deteriorate. (Hinrichsen & Robey, 2000).

Above are two population pyramids from Zambia in sub-Saharan Africa indicating the population structure by **sex** and age categories. The second pyramid is an estimate for 2050, which shows projected increases in total population size, as people live longer.

Population growth is generally argued to be problematic for health because of increased demands for scarce resources including food, shelter, fuel, water and all types of service provision (for example education and health care). These factors will not only impact on physical health but will also threaten social and mental health as a consequence of overcrowded living conditions. However, an alternative argument is that having a healthy population of working age can serve to enhance economic development which in turn promotes better health (Bloom & Canning, 2001).

One way to address population growth is to deliver effective family planning services. However some cultural, moral and religious objections to contraception can pose practical barriers in the development of these services. Hinrichsen and Robey (2000) note that the number of people in lower-income countries who want family planning services has risen, but annual global spending on family planning programmes is less than half the US$17 billion agreed to for 2000 at the UN International Conference on Population and Development in Cairo in 1994.

Ageing populations   Viewing the population pyramids for Zambia, it is evident that most societies are projected to have higher life expectancy and have larger proportions of the population who live to much older ages. The WHO (2007a) predicts that the world's elderly population (by which they mean people aged 60 years and over) will reach two billion by 2050. To some degree this should be seen as the success of health improvement programmes and an economically developed world. However it does require a revision of what may be needed to provide healthy older age. This is influenced by two main factors:

- The changing patterns of illness and disease to conditions associated with fragility, chronic diseases and disorders such as dementia.
- Universal state pension schemes to keep older people out of extreme poverty may not be able support the increased growth in over 65s.

Preparing health providers and societies to meet the needs of elderly people is essential: training for health professionals on old-age care; preventing and managing age-associated chronic diseases; designing sustainable policies on long-term care; and developing age-friendly services and settings. Work around promoting positive images of older people may be also be crucial to reduce older age discrimination.

Safety, security and fear   A whole range of related issues can be considered under the terms 'safety and security'. These all impact upon health, and are summarized in table 2.3.

The above issues are commonly not perceived as being public health threats in their own right but are seen superficially in terms of how public health should be providing health care responses (Geiger 2001). Crime and terrorism are constructed as media/moral panics that potentially exaggerate the risks and create a culture of fear but in some areas of conflict there is great evidence that fear impacts upon holistic health, while the direct effects also have a large health impact (Bleich, Gelkopf & Soloman, 2003).

War and conflict pose a major threat to health, not only in direct ways as we may expect, but also as economic and social development are impeded. Basic infrastructure such as roads, sanitation and commercial settings can be devastated, affecting the ability for basic human needs (e.g. food and shelter) to be satisfied. Displaced persons who have been fleeing their homes in order to avoid the effects of armed conflict and violations of human rights experience much poorer health as a result of this displacement, which can exist for generations. The Saharawi people who have lived in a state of transition since 1973 when there were territory disputes in the Western Sahara in Northern Africa are a good example of this (Spector, 2009).

Table 2.3. The impact of safety and security upon health.

Issue	Potential effects	Reference
Conflict and war	Deaths and injuries on the battlefield Displacement of populations Breakdown of health and social services Sexual violence Heightened risk of disease transmission Psychosocial impact of living with conflict Reduction on development and maintenance of infrastructure Disruption of subsistence agriculture	Murray et al. (2002)
Domestic Violence	Physical injuries and death Living in pain Depression and post-traumatic stress disorder Poor esteem	Campbell (2002)
Crime	Death and injury Emotional impact long-term stress Loss of work earning Property destruction	Dubourg et al. (2005)

Terrorism
  Bombing
  Bioterrorism
  Kidnapping
	Direct death and injury
	Rape as an instrument of war
	Direct effect of psychological impact of trauma and fear
	Indirect effect on society living in fear of terrorism even if the actual threat is low
		Bleich, Gelkopf & Soloman (2003)

Poverty and inequality   There is a large amount of evidence to show that among all threats to health risks, it is poverty and inequality that are much more likely to limit the achievement of full health. As a result of poverty individuals experience under-nutrition, unsafe sex and poor sanitation (WHO, 2009), thereby increasing their health risks significantly. This is discussed more fully in chapters 10 and 12.

In recent years, evidence has been used to demonstrate that material deprivation plays a huge role in the causation of disease (see chapter 4 for further discussion of health inequalities). This social determinants of health model shows a strong social gradient for most diseases, with those who are poorer experiencing higher rates of disease than those who are richer (Wainwright, 2009a). The WHO (2000) demonstrates this when discussing the global burden of disease based upon 2004 data, showing that

- Africa accounts for 90% of childhood deaths from malaria, 90% of deaths due to Aids and for 50% of the world's deaths due to diarrhoeal diseases and pneumonia.

Box 2.2	Examples of wide-ranging health inequalities.

- Gender health inequalities, e.g. risk behaviours such as drinking alcohol, are more prevalent among men
- Social class inequalities, e.g. people in high social classes having better health compared to lower social classes
- Geographical inequalities, e.g. health is generally poorer in the North of England compared to the South of England
- Ethnic inequalities, e.g. suicide rates in young Asian women are more than double those for young white women in the UK
- Age inequalities, e.g. many risk factors for poor health, such as obesity, hypertension, disability and poverty increase with age

(Raleigh & Polato, 2004)

- In high-income countries the leading cause of death is heart disease, followed by stroke, lung cancer, pneumonia and asthma/bronchitis.
- In low-income countries, the leading cause of death is pneumonia, then heart disease, diarrhoea, HIV/AIDS and stroke.

Health inequality refers to the differences in health status between people and/or places and manifests in many ways, as box 2.2 demonstrates.

Health inequity refers to those differences that are perceived to be unfair and unjust (Graham & Kelly, 2004). For example, it can be argued that everyone has the right to health care; however, despite the presence of health care in many countries, not everyone is able access it, which results in health inequity.

Mental health Mental health issues are often neglected in a world that tends to prioritize physical health. However, separating mental, social and physical health contradicts our understanding of the holistic nature of health. As a whole person, the domains of health are inextricably linked and influence each other. Achieving good mental health is fundamentally important in daily functioning, quality of life and integral to the health of individuals and communities (Brundtland, 2001)

The WHO (2001) suggests that approximately 450 million people worldwide are suffering from some form of mental disorder. This means that one in four people will be mentally ill at some point in their life, representing 13% of the global burden or morbidity (WHO, 2001). This is likely to be a significant underestimation as it only captures data about people who are classified as 'disordered'. Many people experience anxiety and poor mental health without ever receiving a diagnosis of illness or disorder. A major issue for mental health sufferers is the serious stigma and discrimination associated with poor psychological and psychiatric status. Indeed, stigma is a major barrier to both mental health treatment and recovery (Pinto-Foltz & Logsdon, 2009).

Infectious diseases   The media are forever drawing our attention to the problem of infectious diseases. In 2009 there were concerns about the possibility of a swine flu pandemic, with many countries stockpiling vaccinations, implementing vaccination programmes, offering health advice and developing emergency plans. Here a **political economy** perspective would critically examine the role of the pharmaceutical industry as part of the construction of this health threat (see chapter 4 for further discussion of Marxist understandings of health and illness). This is interesting given that it is the case that at least once a year an epidemic occurs somewhere in the world. There are many infectious diseases that threaten the health of humans such as rotavirus, ebola, HIV and the more recently discovered SARs and H5N1, bird flu (Kaufmann, 2009). These epidemics are transnational, having no boundaries and being increasingly hard to control. As a consequence they instil fear in many people. However, our experience of infectious diseases varies according to where we live in the world.

In higher-income countries, we all experience coughs, colds and sore throats, generally for a few days and then we feel restored back to normal health. These minor illnesses are often the result of contact with viruses and are experienced as inconveniences rather than as a major threat to health. However, about four million people die annually from respiratory infections, mostly in lower-income countries. This is also true of diarrhoeal diseases. In high-income countries bouts of diarrhoea are unpleasant but generally do not cause a major health impact or result in death (this can happen in rare cases of cholera or e-coli infection when prompt medical attention is not sought) whereas in lower-income countries death is not an uncommon result (Kaufmann 2009), especially in the under fives. This issue of the disproportionate burden is the same story for lower-income countries for most infectious diseases including measles, HIV and Aids, dysentery, cholera, typhoid and polio, to name but a few.

HIV as an infectious disease is often seen as being a major contemporary threat to health and, as highlighted earlier, has received much media attention. Since the disease was first identified over twenty-five years ago, it has killed over twenty-five million victims and in 2006, between four and five million people became infected with the virus. Again, the worst of the infection is found in lower-income countries with sub-Saharan African being disproportionately affected (Kaufmann, 2009). The major problem with the prevention of HIV lies in the relationship between prevention and behaviour change (see chapter 6 for an in-depth discussion of behaviour change). Currently an effective vaccination has yet to be developed, therefore prevention via condom use and behaviour change (such as abstinence from sexual encounters) is advocated. However, some individuals find themselves powerless to negotiate safe sex and strong cultural traditions also serve to influence individual perceptions of risk.

The re-emergence of old infectious diseases   On some occasions, a number of infectious diseases has been declared to have been 'defeated' and eradicated, only later to reappear and pose a threat to the health of humans. Tuberculosis is one such example within contemporary society (Kaufmann, 2009). This is because of TB's close relationship with those infected with the HIV virus, so people often develop TB as a result of their weakened immune systems. In addition the situation has been made worse by the bacterium that causes TB becoming increasingly resistant to drugs and treatment. TB is still treatable, especially if caught in its early stages, and there is a global programme organized by the WHO to try and control the epidemic. This is known as DOTs, the 'directly observed treatment short course', where patients have to take their medication under the watchful gaze of professionals to ensure that they adhere to the regime and therefore do not increase the risk of further TB strains becoming drug resistant. There is a vaccination available for TB, but this only protects against a specific strain of the disease more common among children. Hence the disease remains a problem in that outbreaks continue to occur within specific populations, once again especially among those living in poverty because this is an ideal breeding ground for such an infectious disease. The principal reasons for the re-emergence of the disease are overcrowded housing, increasing homelessness, rising immigration rates, poor urban living conditions and rising levels of HIV infection (Kaufmann, 2009).

Lifestyle diseases   Whereas the social determinants of health approach emphasizes the larger structural influences that affect our health (chapter 4 discusses both structure and agency in relation to health), in recent years threats to our health are also seen to be related to our own illness behaviour and the lifestyle choices that we make. The way in which we all live our lives is argued to have a huge impact upon our health. Lupton (1993) argues that risk discourse is used to blame the victim and to displace the real reasons for ill-health. Risks are located at the level of the individual, which serves to avoid people from examining broader, structural determinants. Perceptions of health risks are indeed changing (Giddens 2009) and are numerous, as this chapter tells us; populations are generally ageing and patterns of physical activity, alcohol and tobacco consumption are also shifting, leaving many countries facing a burden of increasing chronic and non-communicable diseases (WHO, 2009), often labelled as lifestyle diseases.

The types of food we choose to consume, levels of inactivity, our sexual behaviour, **attitudes** to alcohol and recreational drug use as well as attitudes to risk are all having a huge impact on our health, and this is borne out in evidence of changing social trends. For example, the **prevalence** of obesity in England is the highest in the European Union. So in 2005, 24.3% of UK females were obese and 22.1% of men were.

In addition, in the same year only 25% of females were physically active and just 37% of men (*Health Survey for England*, DOH, 2007a). Changing lifestyles are cited as a significant causal factor in relation to obesity, as well as in relation to a number of different health problems. These lifestyle theories are used to explain the social variations and gradients that exist between the different social classes. Thus, the lower social classes arguably smoke more, consume more alcohol and dietary fat, and exercise less and as a consequence these factors are used to explain their higher rates of cancers and heart disease by some commentators. However, the evidence between lifestyle choices and disease is incredibly complex and much research has been criticized for lacking scientific rigour (Skrabenek & McCormick, 1989). There is also the issue of moral judgements being made here in relation to lifestyle choices, about people who make 'wrong' and unhealthy choices, with personal volition increasingly used as a mechanism to label the deserving and undeserving sick. Therefore, the idea of lifestyle choices as a threat to our health has been associated with victim blaming and in some instances the treatment of individuals with lifestyle diseases has become highly politicized in the media. For example, there have been debates about the refusal of treatment for smokers, those who are obese and individuals who are seen to 'refuse' to change their behaviour without broader recognition of the structural factors underpinning the causation of lifestyle diseases.

In conclusion, the population of the world faces some large health risks and lower-income countries face even more of a risk because populations living there are exposed to multiple risk factors and face the more risky conditions associated with poverty. Indeed, there are some commentators who argue that we are living in a 'risk society' (Beck, 1992), where the main risks that we produce are the result of our own activity, for example, pollution and terrorism. However, the measurement of risk, now possible as a result of increased technology, the availability of large data sets, and improved computer capacity allows perhaps too many risks to be highlighted. Wainwright (2009a) argues that although many identified risks are genuine, the evidence for others are 'weak' and based upon spurious relationships such as the links between some lifestyle choices and specific conditions. Thus, risk ratios often used to demonstrate specific threats to health can be misleading and misreported in the media, affecting our perception of the actual risks that we face. On a positive note, we do have the capability to measure these threats and to try to control them within modern society (Giddens, 1999).

Why and how is all this important ?

In order fully to understand health within contemporary society, it is essential to be able to identify what the key health issues and challenges are. As this chapter shows, the conceptualization of key threats to health is a complex process, and health threats also evolve over time. What are considered as key health threats are influenced by the context in which we live and our social position, which also determine our levels of risk. Indeed, key health threats can also be contested (e.g. climate change is still being debated, so for those who hold the view that it is not happening, then it will not be conceptualized as a health threat). As this chapter shows, there are many threats to public health and therefore it is essential that these are identified in order to prioritize strategies for action in relation to managing and dealing with them. Interventions intended to improve health can be designed, communicated and implemented in relation to many of these key health threats – for example, vaccination programmes can very effectively tackle infectious diseases.

Case study

Bovine Spongiform Encephalopathy (BSE) and variant Creutzfelt-Jakob Disease (vCJD) 'Mad cow disease panic of 1990s'.

In 1986 a new infectious disease in cattle was identified called BSE, which produced sponge-like holes and degeneration in the brain of cattle. There was great fear at that time that the infective agent (a prion) could be transmitted to humans who had eaten infected meat. Subsequent restrictions on the export of UK cattle and beef led to enormous losses to farmers and associated industries. The UK media constructed links between transmission from infected meat to humans contracting vCJD (Henderson & Oldfield, 1993). The actual reported number of cases to this day remains incredibly low, despite the panic of the time and the large-scale media attention directed at vCJD.

Parsons (1995) cited in King and Street (2005) developed a framework to explain the process leading to public panic and lobbying to policy-makers.

- An incident e.g. new disease identified in cattle
- Media uptake of a story
- Incident reconceptualized as wider social issue e.g. threat to public health and devastation of cattle farming
- Stereotypes identified e.g. uncaring government only concerned with economic issues rather than public safety
- Distortion of issues e.g. misreporting of scientific evidence
- Overblown media coverage e.g. daily reporting and scary images
- Public panic
- Demands for policy action by state

Summary

- Identifying substantive health threats is constructed by definitions of health, considerations of determinants of health, magnitude and seriousness and media and moral panics about health threats.

- Epidemiological transition has changed global patterns from infectious diseases at the start of the twentieth century to chronic diseases in the twenty-first century and this pattern is predicted to continue.

- Health threats in the twenty-first century will require global action around the major determinants of health such as poverty, inequity, climate change and population growth.

Questions

1. This chapter shows that risk is a complex and multi-faceted concept. Can you identify all of the factors that influence the construction of health-related risk perceptions?

2. Identify one area of risk to public health, for example, pandemic flu. Now think about all of the consequences of risk perceptions in relation to this. Reflect upon the likely political, economic and health consequences of risk perceptions in relation to this area.

3. Consider the role of science in relation to the conceptualization and management of health risks. How important is science within this process?

Further reading

World Health Organization (2009) Global Health Risks: Mortality and Burden of Disease Attributable to Selected Major Risks. Geneva, WHO.

This is an excellent summary of the complex issues presented in a structured easy-to-read format. The report highlights the major health risks for mortality, measured in disability adjusted life years (**DALY**s). The report uses a specific framework for studying health risks and gives a chapter by chapter description of specific threats.

Bennett, P. & Calman, K., eds (2010) Risk Communication and Public Health. 2nd edn. Oxford, Oxford Medical Publications.

This book discusses public responses to risk as well as a variety of responses to risk in relation to food, vaccinations and pandemic flu. It provides both theoretical discussion and uses research findings to illustrate key aspects of risk communication within the public health field. It also gives the reader a number of case studies through which to analyse key issues.

Elbe, S. (2010) Security and Global Health. Cambridge, Polity.

This book analyses the international context of global health issues as well as considering the rise of the notion of 'health security'. Global health threats are discussed as an 'epidemic of epidemics', no longer characterized by a single disease threat. The book examines the conceptualization of the relationship between health and security and discusses its likely impact.

3 Investigating Health

Overview

This chapter gives an overview of the importance of research in relation to health and an introduction to the research process as a whole, introducing students to both the methods and processes by which information about health is gathered, analysed and used, showing the importance of research for health studies throughout. This chapter examines how health can be investigated in a number of different ways. It explores both quantitative and qualitative approaches to researching health and evaluates the strengths and weaknesses of different techniques for gathering data. Finally a brief discussion of evidence-based practice in health completes the chapter. This chapter provides the reader with an overview of the research process in its entirety, detailed in a linear fashion. It cannot describe the research process in depth or discuss the entire field, as the scope of the chapter is too small to achieve this. It is however important for students to be aware of the basics of research in order to complete research projects, which are usually required as part of undergraduate degree programmes.

Hence, this is what the chapter provides as well as some useful signposting to more detailed discussions. It is also crucial for students to be aware of the importance of the research within the field of health; hence this is demonstrated throughout this chapter through the exercises, examples and the detailed case study.

What is research?

Research is an active and systematic process of inquiry in order to discover, interpret or revise facts, events, behaviours, or theories. Part of the research process is also making practical applications with the help of the information gathered through the research process. So research is a process by which questions can be both explored and answered. Research is therefore a tool to explore, describe, understand, explain, predict, intervene (change), evaluate and assess impact. This may already sound difficult, especially when you are faced with completing a research project, but as a starting point research interests often emerge from an area in which we enjoy working and find fascinating. Complete the following learning task, which will help you to explore your own research ideas.

The literature in your subject area is also a good starting point. Researchers read relevant literature to help them understand what has been studied and what gaps exist too. In completing your project you will need to write a literature review explaining how the literature is

---

Learning task 3.1

Where do I begin in thinking about my research project?

Ask yourself the following questions and make notes about your answers.

1. What really interests you in terms of a topic?
2. What interests you in terms of media reports? Are there frequent reports and discussions about an area that you find interesting?
3. Have you studied a particular module that interested you more than others? If so, what was the most interesting aspect? Perhaps this may be an area in which you could develop some research questions?
4. Who are the people involved in your topic area and can you get access to them?

These questions are starting points to stimulate your thoughts about potential areas that you might want to explore in your project.

relevant to your area of research and contextualizing your study within existing research. There are some useful guides to help you to do this such as

1. Hart, C. (2001) *Doing a Literature Search. A Comprehensive Guide for the Social Sciences*. London, Sage – a book dedicated to searching for literature.
2. Moule, P. & Hek, G. (2011) *Making Sense of Research. An Introduction for Health and Social Care Practitioners*. London, Sage – see chapter 5, which explains how to search and review the literature.
3. O'Dochartaigh, N. (2007). *Internet Research Skills: How to do your Literature Search and Find Information Online*. London, Sage – a book that takes you through using the internet for finding relevant literature.
4. Saks, M. & Allsop, J., eds (2007) *Researching Health. Qualitative, Quantitative and Mixed Methods*. London, Sage – see chapter 3 – Doing a literature review in health.

These are all good resources. You will also find that most comprehensive research methods textbooks will also include a section about dealing with the literature, so do explore other texts. When you have an idea to investigate, the next issue that you need to consider is how to explore and research the issue. How researchers begin to study the social world is informed by philosophical frameworks.

Philosophical frameworks

Research is underpinned by models of understanding known as paradigms. A paradigm is a perspective and a way of examining and understanding (therefore researching) reality (Hennick et al. 2011). There are two distinct paradigms and philosophical traditions that underpin research. **Positivism** is associated with **quantitative research** while **interpretivism** is used within qualitative approaches (Seale, 2004). The main ideas that inform these two different paradigms are listed in box 3.1.

Box 3.1 separates these approaches to outline their differences but in practice they are interrelated and overlapping. This may be sounding very complex to you already but here are the key points that you need to understand about the philosophy of research,

- Researchers can use a specific paradigm and therefore apply its associated techniques in practice. If you are trained in a positivist position then you will use quantitative methods. Comparatively, if you are trained in an interpretivist tradition then you will apply qualitative tools of data collection.
- So there are different views of what social reality looks like. The term to describe this is **ontology**. Ontology is defined as 'the study of the nature of reality' (Broom & Willis, 2007: 25). There are a range of

> **Box 3.1.**
>
> **Assumptions of positivism**
>
> - Reality exists beyond our perceptions. This can be meaningfully conceptualized and is therefore measurable.
> - Deals with facts not values. There is a single 'truth' or reality.
> - It is possible to observe and measure phenomena in an objective, reliable and valid manner.
> - The research process is neutral and value free (adapted from Bryman, 2001).
>
> **Assumptions of interpretivism**
>
> - Understands things from people's point of view (insider's perspective).
> - Places emphasis on lived, subjective experiences and acknowledges that there can be multiple equally valid realities which coexist.
> - Reality is constructed by the social world in which we live.
> - Importance placed on understanding the social context in which data are generated and how social actors including researchers influence this process
>
> (adapted from Hennick et al., 2011).

ontological understandings each discussing the nature of the social world in a different way.

- There are also different views about what represents knowledge, how it is produced and how it can therefore be measured. These are epistemological considerations, or 'the study of the nature of knowledge' (Schwandt, 2001: 71).

Figure 3.1 provides a hierarchical schema to help you to frame health research according to these different philosophical traditions.

Figure 3.1 has been simplified to outline different philosophical traditions but in practice many health researchers use mixed method approaches in which they combine these understandings in a variety of ways. Quantitative (positivist) and qualitative (interpretivist) research can be used within a single study. For example **qualitative research** can be used to explore and develop hypotheses for quantitative testing. So how does all of this relate to your research project? You will need to consider which approach is best suited to answering your research questions.

Research question/s

All research starts with a question/s and this is an essential part of the research process, with the aims and purpose of the research needing to be clearly defined at the outset of the process. The research question/s

Figure 3.1. Schema outlining the philosophical underpinnings of research.

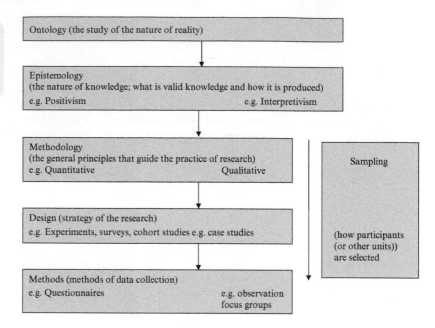

Ontology (the study of the nature of reality)

Epistemology
(the nature of knowledge; what is valid knowledge and how it is produced)
e.g. Positivism   e.g. Interpretivism

Methodology
(the general principles that guide the practice of research)
e.g. Quantitative   Qualitative

Sampling

Design (strategy of the research)
e.g. Experiments, surveys, cohort studies e.g. case studies

(how participants
(or other units))
are selected

Methods (methods of data collection)
e.g. Questionnaires   e.g. observation
                                             focus groups

Table 3.1. Generating research questions.

Emerge from	Examples
Literature – are there gaps in our knowledge i.e. what don't we know?	Why is eating processed food associated with a higher risk of depression? Has junk food become a social norm?
What is needed in a practice-based context?	How can we encourage families to come to healthy eating classes in the local community?
Strengthening evidence for practice	Does the delivery of healthy eating classes lead to any alteration in family eating habits?

helps the researcher to clarify what they are investigating and guides the researcher towards the most appropriate methods to address the question. Research questions arise in a number of ways as table 3.1 demonstrates.

All research has limitations in answering questions so when a research question is posed a researcher has to be aware of what they can realistically achieve within the time-frame available and the resources at their disposal. So if a researcher asks the question, 'what do cancer patients prefer in terms of support services?', they have to acknowledge that it would not be possible to include all cancer patients in the UK in their data collection. It is much more realistic to focus upon a smaller sample, perhaps a specific type of cancer and to conduct the study within a region rather than a country. Putting limits onto data collection does not mean that research questions cannot be answered fully; the important point in any research is to ensure that the questions are answered in an appropriate way. There are some

Table 3.2. Example research questions and methodological approaches.

Overall research aim	Detailed research questions	Methodology
To explore the knowledge and attitudes of students to chlamydia.	1. Are students aware of the risks posed by chlamydia? 2. Does knowledge and awareness differ between male and female students? 3. Do attitudes affect the level of risk a participant may perceive themselves at? Is there a male/female difference?	• This study adopted a quantitative/positivist approach. • A self-completed questionnaire was administered.
To explore levels of understanding of the causes and risks of type 2 diabetes of some young Asian people.	1. Are young people aware of the causes and risks associated with type 2 diabetes? 2. Are there differences between males and females with respect to their knowledge about type 2 diabetes?	• This study adopted a qualitative / interpretivist approach. • Face-to-face in-depth interviews.
A study to explore the different attitudes between men and women towards healthy eating.	1. Do men and women understand the concept of healthy eating in the same way? 2. Are there differences of opinion between men and women in relation to healthy eating? 3. Are there gender differences in terms of the practice of healthy eating?	• This study adopted a mixed method approach using quantitative (positivist) and qualitative (interpretivist) methods. • Use of a questionnaire to examine dietary habits and practices. • Follow up semi-structured interviews to explore participants' views in more depth.

really good books that can help you with the development of your research questions:

- See White, P. (2008) *Developing Research Questions. A Guide for Social Scientists*. Basingstoke, Palgrave, for a step-by-step approach.

An essential part of the process of answering research questions is choosing a research design and method that is suitable and feasible. Table 3.2 provides some examples of student research questions and the methods that were used to answer them.

Table 3.2 highlights example research questions and shows how they were answered using different research paradigms as well as a mixed method approach. There are many ways in which a researcher can investigate their areas of interest and address research questions. Again there are several good books that can offer you advice and suggestions in terms of research design.

- See Blakie, N. (2000) *Designing Social Research*, Cambridge, Polity, for a comprehensive overview of research design, the development of research questions, discussion of strategies to answer questions, methods and sample research designs.

Before you begin to think about your methodological approach, read the next section, which discusses quantitative and qualitative research in more depth.

Quantitative research

Nature of quantitative research

Put simply, quantitative research refers to a collection of techniques that seek to quantify and measure phenomena. The data generated is numerical in nature and quantitative researchers are concerned with four main preoccupations.

1. The valid measurement of concepts and constructs.
2. (a) Causality e.g. does smoking cigarettes lead to development of lung cancer?
    (b) consistency and association of strength between **variables** e.g. is there a relationship between a lack of exercise, unhealthy eating and the development of coronary heart disease?
3. Generalizability e.g. can the reported associations among variables be generalized to populations similar to the ones from which the variables were drawn?
4. Replication e.g. can the research process be repeated and similar findings obtained (Bryman, 2004)?

Deduction underpins quantitative research. This is a process that starts with theories and hypotheses; these are tested through data collection leading to either the confirmation or rejection of them (Trochim, 2006). For example as a lecturer I may have a **hypothesis** that students achieve higher marks when they attend more teaching sessions. Data (observations) can be collected from registers and performance marks in order to test and ultimately reject or confirm this hypothesis.

Quantitative methods

There are a number of data collection tools available for those wishing to use a quantitative approach as box 3.2 shows.

The main data collection method used for quantitative research is the questionnaire and this is likely to be the most appropriate tool for you to use in your project. Table 3.3 outlines surveys and experiments, both of which are used within health research.

Table 3.3 gives you an introduction to the key aspects of these methods and signposts you to further reading so that you can explore these methods in more detail if they are suitable for addressing your

Box 3.2 **Sources of quantitative data**

- Biochemical assessment e.g. CD4 cell count in the blood which is an indicator of immune suppression in HIV+ patients).
- Documents e.g. death certificates and GP notes.
- Routinely collected data e.g. hospital records and registers of disease.
- Secondary analysis of survey data e.g. Census and British Household Survey.
- Quantitative diaries in which numbers of events and behaviour are recorded e.g. food diaries.

research questions. Once you have selected a method, you then need to consider how you will select a sample.

Quantitative sampling

Sampling is the process of selecting units (e.g. people, organizations) from a population of interest. The goals of quantitative sampling are different from those of qualitative sampling in line with the overall differences in the nature of quantitative and qualitative research. Generalizability is the most common goal in quantitative sampling, meaning that findings existing in the sample will also be similar in the population from which the sample was drawn. Figure 3.2 (p. 62) is a diagram of how representative sampling operates by drawing upon the general population to select 'representative' elements (e.g. people, organizations) for inclusion in the sample of the study.

Steps in quantitative sampling

1. *Identifying the population of interest* In the example below the theoretical population of interest is women aged over 16 in Ireland but this is a difficult to access as a whole, so the accessible population is women aged over 16 attending general practice (although these are not likely to be representative of all women as they will be attending the GP for specific reasons).

2. *Deciding on type of sampling strategy* There are two main types of quantitative sampling: non-probability and probability (also known as random sampling). The latter relies on the principle that every sampling unit has the same theoretical chance of being selected from the population into the sample. In order to undertake random sampling a list of population members (units) known as a sampling frame is needed to select members into the sample. In the example below a sampling frame was used, namely the faculties of the Irish

Table 3.3. An overview of quantitative data collection techniques.

Method	Key features of the methods	Things for you to consider	Examples of its use	Further help when designing your project

Surveys (these often involve question-naires)	• Can gather data from large numbers of people.
	• Designed to study variables, attitudes, values and demographic details of a population.
	• Structured, closed questions used such as 'what is your sex, male or female?'
	• Some open ended questions can be used with predetermined categories such as 'how can we improve this service?'
	• Has 5 clear stages
	  1. Deciding a research question and design
	  2. Developing the questionnaire and thinking about ethical issues
	  3. Sampling
	  4. Collecting data
	  5. Analysis.
		• Closed questions are quick to answer.
		• Open ended questions allow respondents more freedom.
		• How will you administer this, via the post, face to face, online, via the telephone etc? This will affect your response rates.
		• Think about convenience for your responders.
		• Think about the language that you use and the types of questions you are asking.
		• You would need to test your questionnaire first to remove any ambiguities. This is called a pilot.
			1. See www.statistics.gov.uk for examples of various surveys with different designs such as
			  • Census
			  • British Crime Survey
			2. See www.understandignsociety.org.uk for an example of a longitudinal survey with some health related questions.
			3. See www.dh.gov.uk for information about the health survey for England.
				• There are excellent guides by Trochim (2006) and Bowling (2009a).
				• See chapter 6 in Whittaker, A. & Williamson, G.R. (2011), *Succeeding in Research Project Plans and Literature Reviews for Nursing Students*, Dorset, Learning Matters for an excellent overview of surveys.
				• There are many validated, high quality instruments already developed. Our advice is to find existing instruments and questions that address your research question/s rather than trying to design an instrument yourself. A good review of instruments can be found in Bowling (2001) and the internet based survey question bank available at UK Data Archive at the University of Essex, see www.data-archive.ac.uk.

Experiments		
• The key purpose of experimental design is to determine if causal relationships exist and at the heart of their design are interventions that are thought to cause effects. • Classically drugs are tested to examine if they produce positive health effects, for example testing whether statins reduce cholesterol levels. • In social science research we may also wish to determine the effect of social interventions in community settings for example by posing questions such as 'do peer sex education programmes reduce incidences of unprotected sex in young people?' (Stephenson et al., 2004) • These include the randomized control trial, the gold standard of quantitative research.	• There are many different types of experimental designs. • There are quasi experimental designs too. • Experiments have limitations such as the non-compliance of patients with treatment and dropout rates. • Whilst experiments can establish effectiveness of treatments they are unable to provide data about patients' experiences.	• See www.thelancet. com for discussion of results from a range of randomised control trials. • See www.bmj.com for discussions of randomised control trials and issues with their use. • See chapters 12 and 13 in Saks, M. & Allsop, J. (2007) *Researching Health. Qualitative, Quantitative and Mixed Methods* (eds) London, Sage which give a clear overview of randomised control trials and experimental methods. • See Trochim, WM. *Research Methods Knowledge Base*, 2nd Edition available at http://www. socialresearchmethods. net/kb/ This gives an easy to understand description of quasi-experimental research methods.

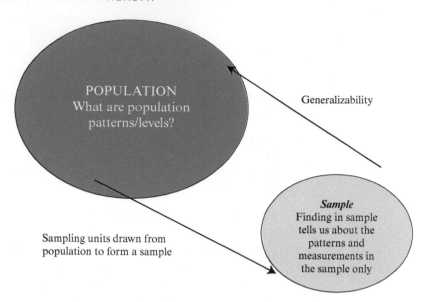

College of General Practitioners. Random sampling enhances the possibility of obtaining a representative sample that is very similar to the population from which the sample is drawn, therefore increasing the generalizability of the findings. However, random sampling can be difficult to achieve because of the lack of accurate sampling frames available to researchers, ethical limitations and data protection issues. Therefore non-probability sampling methods are often utilized.

Non probability sampling methods do not rely on the random selection of units into a sample but can still provide a mechanism to produce a representative sample. One of the main approaches used is 'proportional quota sampling'. For example, suppose the population of interest is students attending a Northern university. The major characteristics that you would want to represent are gender, faculty, full-time/part-time, age and ethnicity. You are unlikely to obtain a sampling frame of the names and addresses of all students attending the university because of data protection, but could set quotas in order to achieve a representative sample. The registrar may give you information about each of the major characteristics of the population so you can mirror them in your sample. For example in the gender category the university has 60% women and 40% men attending. If you require a total sample size of 200, you will continue sampling until you achieve these percentages and then stop. So, if you've already got the 120 women for your sample, but not the 80 men, you will continue to sample men, and even if legitimate women respondents come along, you will not include them in your sample because you have already fulfilled your quota.

3. Difficulties in gaining access and recruitment of participants   A neglected but fundamental area of sampling is gaining access to participants and

Box 3.3   **A practical example of quantitative multi-stage sampling.**

Main objective: To determine the extent of exposure to violence by a partner or spouse among women attending general practice

Sampling procedures
Initially the research team reviewed literature to estimate prevalence rates of domestic violence in order to determine the required sample size.

Multi-stage sampling procedure
First sampling unit – six geographically based faculties of the Irish College of General Practitioners (four urban, two rural).

Second sampling unit – all general practitioners and their associated practices in these faculties were invited to take part. Thirty-four practices agreed to participate. Twenty-two practices were then selected on the basis of maximum diversity in terms of the sex of the general practitioners, singlehanded/group practices and location.

Third sampling unit – women respondents attending general practice. Receptionists were asked to hand a patient pack (a consent form with study briefing, a questionnaire for self completion, and a return envelope) to each consecutive female patient over the age of 16 years, over a data collection period of two weeks.

Source: Bradley et al. (2002).

encouraging them to take part in the research. In the example below general practitioners acted as gatekeepers to access women and receptionists recruited women to take part in the study. In order to encourage participation, information was provided about the usefulness of the research.

4. How to improve response rates   The final issue to be considered is trying to boost response rates. If participants do not take part in research then it can be difficult to obtain a representative sample, which limits the research findings in relation to determining probability. In the example below a pre-paid return envelope was used to ensure completion and return of the questionnaire. For a fuller discussion about enhancing response rates see Bowling (2009b). In addition Trochim (2006) provides a fuller treatise of quantitative sampling procedures.

So after sampling and then data collection you will have data that needs to be analysed. The next section gives an overview of how you can begin to think about this for your own project.

Quantitative analysis

This section will cover important conceptual issues and steps involved in analysing quantitative data. Quantitative data involves the analysis of numerical data and is best undertaken using statistical packages. The most commonly used package PASW (formerly SPSS) is user-friendly and there are excellent manuals of its use.

- See Pallant, J. (2010) *SPSS Survival Manual: A Step by Step Guide to Data Analysis Using SPSS*. Maidenhead, McGraw-Hill, for really clear guidance and instructions.

Quantitative research is concerned with measurement. Measurement is simply assigning values to outcomes. There are different levels and scales of measurement, which helps researchers to decide upon the most appropriate mathematical manipulations to undertake on their data and to choose appropriate statistical tests. The different levels of measurement are outlined in table 3.4; you can compare your data with these to determine what levels you are using in your analysis.

Nominal data is the least sophisticated and few mathematical calculations can be performed on it. Categories of housing type are just coded with numbers but they are not numbers in the true sense of units. Presentation of nominal data is generally in the form of frequency counts and percentages. For example 234 (23%) people lived in council rented accommodation.

Ordinal data are more sophisticated than nominal data but are still not a 'true' number and it is therefore difficult to produce meaningful mathematical manipulations on the data, as the numbers act as codes for categories. However, what distinguishes ordinal from nominal data is that the numbers are in a rank order. For example, using the Registrar General's classification of social class, we know that some classes have a higher status than others because there is a rank order of categories from high to low. Ordinal data also ranks from better to worse (the winners of a race to the losers). This data is presented in a similar way to nominal data in the form of frequency counts and percentages. Nominal and ordinal data are referred to as categorical data because numerical codes are applied to these levels of measurement. This limits the type of statistical tests that can be performed on this type of data. Interval and ratio data are 'true' numbers and therefore can be subjected to the usual mathematical manipulations. Data can be presented in the form of means and standard deviations. Parametric statistical tests can be performed on both interval and numerical data.

You will also need to give consideration to how you will present the data that you have gathered. Descriptive data analysis involves presenting data about the findings within samples and does not make inferences or claims about patterns or associations. Descriptive data can take the form of frequency counts, percentages, means (the average calculated by adding up the numbers in a sample and dividing that

Table 3.4. Levels of measurement.

Level	Characteristics of data	Example
Nominal	Nominal level variables are names, so data is organized into categories according to how it is named. Nominal data is a classification. Numerical codes can also be given to categories but no numerical significance is given to these codes, so the numbers are not ordered in rank. There are no overlapping categories, so data has to fit into one category; for example, you can't be both a Conservative Party Supporter and a Labour Party Supporter.	Housing type: for example, detached, semi-detached, terrace. Ethnicity is often given a numerical code. White 1 Mixed 2 Asian 3 Black 4 Gender can be a category, male or female. Such categorizations are often used in questionnaires as part of surveys.
Ordinal	This level of measurement is concerned with order. Variables in this category are sorted by ordered rank. Variables in this category can also be included when the distance between each category can't be measured precisely so we know that Sally got the job when she was interviewed and that David came second, but we are not able to measure the precise distance between these levels.	For example finishing positions in a race such as first, second and third are ordinal data. Another example is the categorization of social class (Registrar General's Scale) based upon occupations and employment. I = 5 highest status V = 1 least status.
Interval	This is where the distances between intervals are equal on the scale being used for the measurement of variables.	The time between years is interval level data. So the time between 1992 and 1993 is the same as that between 1995 and 1996 (365 days, assuming it is not a leap year of course!) Temperature measurements are interval level data.
Ratio	This level of measurement is the same as the interval level but it has an absolute zero point on the scale being used.	The specific weight of a respondent in kg is an example.

answer by the sample size), mode (this is the value that occurs most frequently), medians (this is also an average but is defined as the mid-point of a set of scores) and standard deviations. The standard deviation is more complex. It is a statistic that describes the relationship between all of the cases in a sample and the mean (average). This is often represented in the form of a graph. If all of the cases are clustered around the mean then the standard deviation is small. However, if the cases within the sample are further apart then there is a large standard deviation. For example, if you are comparing the results that students achieve in a specific A-level subject, the standard deviation would be a useful tool to tell you how diverse their marks were across a region or the entire country.

Box 3.4   **Help for the development of your project.**

- The website www.neighbourhoodstatistics.gov.uk has some discussion and examples of the use of different levels of measurement.
- See www.ats.ucla.edu/stat/mult-pkg/whatsta/default.htm for the University of California's guide to which statistics to use and how to run them in various computer packages.
- An excellent book that can help to guide you with exploring appropriate statistical tests is Salkind, N. (2011) Statistics for People Who (Think They) Hate Statistics. 4th edn. LA, Sage.
- The website www.neighbourhoodstatistics.gov.uk has some discussion and examples of the use of different levels of measurement.
- See www.ats.ucla.edu/stat/mult-pkg/whatsta/default.htm for the University of California's guide to which statistics to use and how to run them in various computer packages.

Inferential statistics allow us to make judgements of the probability that an observed difference between groups is a dependable one, or one that might have happened by chance or to infer from the sample data what the population might think. Thus, we use inferential statistics to make inferences from our data to more general conditions (Trochim, 2006).

Inferential statistical tests are used to determine differences between groups, for example, 'are the birth weights of babies whose mothers who are classified in manual occupations different from those of mothers who are classified in non-manual occupations?' Or to assess correlations between variables, for example, 'does health status decline with age?' In conducting your analysis it is important to understand that certain tests are used upon particular data and to answer particular analytical questions. For example, chi-squared tests are designed to be used on nominal data and examine whether factors are related.

When statistical tests are performed a P value is presented, which allows judgements to be made about the results occurring by chance. The P value simply represents the probability of a result (a given sequence) happening by chance. When running statistical tests we write hypotheses that state what alternatives we may expect to find as outlined by the following.
For example

- Ho (null hypothesis)

There is no statistically significant difference between exercise levels between men and women.
- Hi (alternative hypothesis)

Men have higher exercise rates than women.

Inferential statistical tests enable us to determine what factors influence the birth weight of babies.

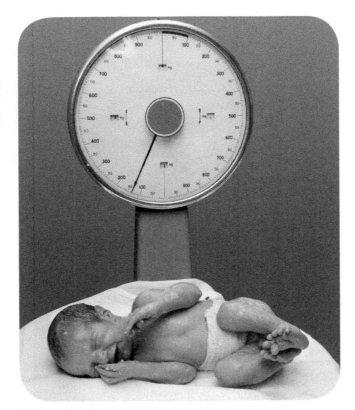

© Zoran mircetic

The P value allows us to either reject or accept the null hypothesis. The P value is the probability of rejecting the null hypothesis (Ho) of a study question when that hypothesis is actually true. Using a significance level of 0.05 this means that the probability of a correct decision about acceptance or rejection is 95%, i.e. that in 95 out of one hundred cases we will make the correct decision.

This next section now turns to giving you an overview of qualitative research, another approach that you may consider when thinking about developing your research project.

Qualitative research

Nature of qualitative research

Qualitative research has a long and distinguished history, and is often considered as originating from the work of anthropologists who developed the fieldwork method. This work was then extended further by the Chicago School of Sociology during the 1920s, when sociologists became interested in studying the urban environment by using both theory and fieldwork to explore issues such as poverty, family, immigration and race relations in depth.

So what is qualitative research? Herein is the first difficulty as there

Box 3.5   Example interpretation of quantitative analysis

- Ho (null hypothesis)
  There is no statistically significant difference between exercise levels between men and women.
- Hi (alternative hypothesis)
  Men have higher exercise rates than women.

In a practical example from the above hypotheses the mean (average) exercise rates per week for men are 65 minutes compared to women at 58 minutes.

An independent t-test can be used to compare the difference between the 2 groups (men and women) and a P value of 0.024 was obtained. If the p-value is less than the significance level set (i.e. 0.05) then this means that we reject the null hypothesis and conclude that there is a statistically significance difference between women and men's exercise rates. The P value in this case is 0.024 and so is less than 0.05 and therefore we can conclude that the exercise rates for men are statistically higher than women. This finding is therefore not likely to be a result of chance.

However it is important to recognize that although there is a statistically significant difference this does not infer any clinical or meaningful difference in exercise rates. There is a mean difference of 7 minutes. How important is this for health?

is no consensus in defining qualitative research as an approach, largely because it does not represent a unified set of techniques or philosophies. So underneath the umbrella of 'qualitative research' there are several different qualitative schools operating with distinctive views about what makes the social world go around (Mason, 1996). However, it is possible to succinctly articulate what qualitative research is generally about in the sense that as an approach the word qualitative implies an emphasis on processes and meanings that are not rigorously examined, measured and counted in terms of quantity.

Mason (1996) identifies a loose working definition of qualitative research based around three key points.

1. Qualitative research is concerned with how the social world is interpreted, understood, experienced and produced.
2. Secondly, data generation is completed in a flexible way and this data is sensitive to the social context in which is produced.
3. Finally, it is based upon methods of analysis and explanation building that demonstrate understandings of complexity, detail and context.

Denzin and Lincoln (1998: 3) also attempt to deal with defining qualitative research as an approach and in doing so argue that it is

. . . multi-method in focus, involving an interpretive, naturalistic approach to its subject matter.

So overall, the nature of qualitative research as an approach simply means that researchers study things in their own settings, try to make sense of them and interpret them in terms of people's meanings, perceptions and views.

Qualitative methods

So how is it done? How can we make sense of the social world and the people within it from their viewpoint? We can use several empirical methods to gather qualitative data; for example, interviews, focus groups and observations. Often researchers employ a range of interconnected methods when they are doing qualitative research, so they may well combine all of these approaches within one research study. Table 3.5 provides an overview of qualitative methods.

This table gives an overview of the main methods used by qualitative researchers. Now complete learning task 3.2, which will help you to think about choosing an appropriate method to address your research questions.

Irrespective of the method that you chose, you will have to sample participants to conduct your research. Quantitative approaches have already been discussed so now the chapter considers qualitative sampling.

Qualitative sampling

Qualitative research is fundamentally concerned with the meanings and interpretations held by social actors. So to achieve this qualitative samples are mostly made up of people, characteristics, experiences, documents, images and settings (Mason, 1996). Unlike quantitative research there is no set rule for having a specific sample size within qualitative research. As a rule of thumb, when researchers are trying to gain an idea of the experiences of a single population a sample of about ten participants has been suggested as adequate (see Morse, 2000). When the aim of the research is to gain a comparison across different people or experiences then samples do need to be larger (Polit & Beck, 2006). Ultimately the nature of the research question, the scope of the study and the length of time available will influence the size of any qualitative sample. A good measure of adequate sample size is when the research reaches a point of theoretical saturation. Put simply, this is the stage of the research at which no new data is emerging and it is at this point that no further sampling is needed.

Qualitative samples do not aim to be representative in the quantitative sense as more often than not sampling relationships are designed to give a meticulous view of particular areas of social life such as a specific organization or group of people. Thus, qualitative samples are

Table 3.5. An overview of qualitative data collection techniques.

Method	Key features of the methods	Things for you to consider	Examples of its use	Further help when designing your project
Inter-views	• In-depth, semi-structured or loosely structured forms of interviewing. • They can be conversations with a purpose (Burgess 1988). • Useful to access people's knowledge, experience, perceptions and everyday accounts (Ackroyd and Hughes 1992). They are a mechanism for interacting with people and gaining access to their everyday accounts. • Can be used creatively – they can be about life histories, narratives and may use a range of techniques to stimulate conversations. • Asking open-ended questions during the interview process, one on one is a good way to achieve comparable responses between participants (Wisker 2001).	• You will need to focus the conversation. • The use of an interview schedule or an aide-memoire is common. • Interviews allow participant to discuss what they feel as well as their experiences as part of the process. • They involve interaction so you may be asked about your opinion. • You need to be careful not to lead respondents and to avoid bias. • You will need to be sensitive to participants and to create a relaxed and comfortable atmosphere.	• See the journal Sociology of Health and Illness at http:// blackwell publishing.com to find several examples of how interviews are used in health-related research.	• See chapter 4 in Whittaker, A. & Williamson, G.R. (2011) Succeeding in Research Project Plans and Literature Reviews for Nursing Students Dorset, Learning Matters for an excellent overview of both interviews and focus groups. • See Opdenakker, R. (2006) 'Advantages and disadvantages of four interview techniques in qualitative research' Qualitative Social Research 7,4 article 11 at http://www.qualitative-research.net/index.php/fqs/article/view/175/392 • See Hennick, M., Hutter, I., Bailey, A. (2011) Qualitative Research Methods London, Sage, chapter 6 for an overview of in-depth interviewing.

Focus Groups	• These are qualitative group interviews. • Conversing within a group setting is normal, so focus groups can be seen to be a more natural reflection of the social world.	• Focus groups are cost effective and time-saving because they access a number of participants at a single time. • Less useful for sensitive topics. For example participants may find discussing bodily functions embarrassing in a group setting. • Ethical issues arise as you often cannot fully anonymise participants. • You will need clear rules about contributions to the discussion, such as no interruptions, to manage group dynamics. • You will need to be sensitive to participants and to create a relaxed and comfortable atmosphere.	• Go to http://www.ncbi.nlm.nih.gov/pubmed/ and enter focus group in the search box. The search results will list a range of studies that you can look at that have used focus groups.	• See chapter 7 in Saks, M. & Allsop, J. (2007) *Researching Health. Qualitative, Quantitative and Mixed Methods* (Eds) London, Sage which gives a clear overview of focus groups. • See Kreuger, R. & Casey, M.A. (2000) *Focus Groups: A Practical Guide for Applied Research* London, Sage for lots of practical advice about all stages of focus groups.
Obser-vation	• This involves immersing yourself in a research setting to systematically observe aspects of it. • Researcher roles vary in relation to how far researchers participate. • Observations can be overt (where participants are aware of the presence of the researcher) or covert (where the researcher is not identified).	• This is a positive method for allowing researchers to view interactions, relationships, actions and behaviours in situ because context can be fundamental in assisting the researchers understanding social behaviour. • Think about how you will develop relationships in the setting, what you are looking for, can you determine categories for observation before you go into the field? How will you generate data? How will you keep and use field-notes?	• See http://www.uk.sagepub.com/saks_allsop/s_chapter6.htm the companion web-site to the book listed in the next column; this gives clear links to several examples.	• See chapter 6 in Saks, M. & Allsop, J. (Eds) (2007) *Researching Health. Qualitative, Quantitative and Mixed Methods* London, Sage which gives a clear overview of participant observation in health research. • See Kawulich, B.B. (2005) 'Participant observation as a data collection method' *Qualitative Social Research*, 6 at http://www.qualitative-research.net/index.php/fqs/article/view/466/996 for an overview of this method and some useful tips on how to train yourself as an observer.

Qualitative interviews have been described as 'conversations with a purpose'.

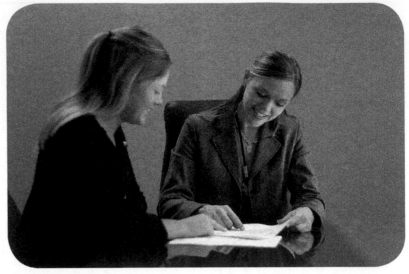

© Martin Purmensky

Learning task 3.2

Choosing an appropriate method for your project.
Think about your topic and make some notes on the following questions. How would you conduct your investigation

(a) Quantitatively?
(b) Qualitatively?

1. Think about what these different approaches would mean for your data collection and results. Do you want a broad picture or a more detailed in-depth view of your topic area?
2. So what tools would you use as a quantitative researcher? How would these be different to the tools you would use as a qualitative researcher?
3. What types of data would you have from the quantitative project and how would this differ from the qualitative project?

Now read your notes and think about which approach is best suited to addressing your research questions. You will need to justify your choice of methods, so give this task careful consideration.

concerned with including a relevant range of units such as types, cases, categories and examples (Mason 1996). These can be drawn from a sampling frame. However, the relevance of sampling frames to qualitative research has been questioned because qualitative research uses

Table 3.6. Overview of qualitative sampling approaches.

Sampling approach	Features of the method	Examples
Convenience sampling	Gathering information from who is available at a specific moment in time. The biases associated with this particular approach to sampling are greater than in any other sampling technique.	Often used by market researchers who stand in the street and ask those who pass by to answer questions. Other examples of convenience samples could include students in the library on a Thursday morning or patients attending a GP surgery on a Wednesday morning.
Quota Sampling	Participants are selected according to criteria or a pre-determined quota, which aims to ensure that a range of criteria are included in a study. Criteria are often based upon social characteristics such as age, gender, ethnicity, specific experiences of an illness. This technique is an attempt to reduce **bias** within the sample.	For example, when studying how vaccinations are perceived by the public, a researcher using a quota sample would want to include both genders, a range of ethnic groups, a range of ages, people in different locations, those who have had vaccinations and those who have opted out.
Purposive Sampling	Samples are created with a purpose in mind. Central to this approach is the selection of the type of participants needed to address the research question. Researchers can also select successful cases or contrasting cases within this approach. An excellent piece on purposive sampling is contained in Patton (2002).	For example, to investigate the experiences of teenage girls accessing family planning services, a research creating a purposive sample could include teenage girls who have accessed and used services, as these individuals have the necessary experience to answer the research question.
Network/Snowball sampling	A researcher starts with respondents who meet the criteria for inclusion in their study, and then asks the first participant to recommend others who they may know who also meet the criteria, and this continues with each participant included, so snowballing into a larger sample. This is an especially useful approach when you are trying to reach populations that are inaccessible or hard to find. Does raise issues of bias in that these networks are made up of people who know each other.	For example, a researcher investigating the health needs of homeless respondents could employ this strategy to gain access to a local network of homeless people.

> **Learning task 3.3**
>
> **Sampling for your project**
> In relation to your topic of interest answer the following questions about sampling:
> - What characteristics will your sample have? So who will you include?
> - What size will your sample be?
> - What is your sampling logic? For example, why those characteristics? Why that size? How does this strategy relate to answering the research question?
> - How will you gain access to your sample?

non-random methods to sample in a non-probability manner. Table 3.6 gives an overview of qualitative sampling approaches.

All of the above methods are deemed as qualitative approaches but it is worth mentioning that they can be used as part of quantitative approaches too, when there are no data available to allow researchers to sample in a random manner too. Now complete learning task 2.3, which encourages you to think about sample selection in relation to your research project.

Qualitative analysis

One of the defining characteristics of qualitative data is in the form of words. Interviews result in transcripts, observations in field-notes and recorded conversations. As a result of the data being in the form of words, qualitative researchers do not have a specific set of formulae to analyse their data. Instead the process of analysing qualitative data usually involves the identification of themes.

The initial starting point is always reading the data and then beginning to organize it; this is called indexing or coding. So as a starting point for analysis, the qualitative researcher needs to gain a descriptive sense of what the data is about and then to label it into codes and categories. This is not a 'neat' procedure in the sense that data do not fit neatly into one category; they can often overlap into a number of codes. The process can be done by hand by the researcher but there are also computer programmes that offer assistance. This process of qualitative analysis is structured. Miles and Huberman's (1994) framework for qualitative analysis is that data is reduced, then displayed and finally the researcher then draws and verifies conclusions.

So, in order to reduce data, researchers begin by indexing and coding their data. Coding data can also be part of quantitative analysis. For qualitative researchers this is a helpful process in relation to getting a systematic overview of the data and it allows the researcher

Box 3.6   **Help for the development of your project.**

- See Miles, M.B., & Huberman, A.M. (1994) *Qualitative Data Analysis. An Expanded Source-Book*, 2nd Edition, London, Sage is a classic text that gives a good overview of qualitative analysis.
- See http://caqdas.soc.surrey.ac.uk. CAQDAS, computer assisted qualitative data analysis software website gives training, information and support in the use of a range of computer program for qualitative analysis.
- See Mason, J. (2002) *Qualitative Researching*, London, Sage for a detailed overview of the entire qualitative research process.

to begin to gain analytical distance and a more measured perspective. Data can also be indexed according to the research question as this will give the researcher an idea of whether the data are beginning to address your questions. So, when qualitative researchers begin to look at data, they begin to explore what their categories and codes represent; for example, are they just text or are they emotions, accounts, attitudes and discourses? The data may also be on different levels, so individual, organizational or even institutional. Data may also be organized according to case studies, stories, narratives and biographies. Qualitative researchers also look at the relationships between their categories of data; however this is not necessarily linked to causation. Qualitative analysis can also include counting to determine how frequently codes and categories appear.

During this process of analysis it is important always to remember context of data collection as this allows the researcher to analyse the attitudes, values and beliefs of participants within broader contextual influences such as organizational influences; structures, power and rules. Furthermore, the beauty of qualitative research means that researchers often find emergent data and are able to highlight areas not encompassed within the research questions. Indeed, there is also a large array of possibilities available to researchers when they are presenting qualitative data, with the dominant mode of presentation being the illustration of key findings and themes supported by quotations from research participants. However, diagrams, tables and charts can all be used too, to display comparisons or summaries of key points.

Differences between quantitative and qualitative research

Many discussions of quantitative and qualitative research show that they are different approaches and so far this chapter has discussed them distinctly. Certainly, each method has its own way of understanding and investigating the social world because they each adopt different epistemological and ontological viewpoints (see box 3.1 at the beginning of this chapter). There have also been many discussions in the literature about which approach is more scientific, but there are limitations with both approaches. The methodologies do demonstrate clear differences as table 3.7 demonstrates.

Table 3.7. Differences between quantitative and qualitative research

Approach to research	Quantitative	Qualitative
Relationship between researcher and subject	Distant	Close
Researchers stance	Outsider	Insider
How theory and concepts are used differently within the research approaches	Confirmation (a theory is confirmed when a hypothesis is tested and proved)	Emergent (theories emerge from the data once the research has been carried out)
Scope of findings	Generalizable	Non-generalizable
Image of social reality (the social world is understood differently within these paradigms)	Static and external to actor	Processual and socially constructed by the actor
Nature of data	Hard, reliable	Soft, rich and deep
Research strategy	Structured	Unstructured
Research tools	Experiments, RCTs, surveys	Interviews, focus groups, observations

Despite these differences between quantitative and qualitative approaches there are also many similarities. Indeed, the debate about quantitative and qualitative research exaggerates their differences, with the literature treating them as mutually antagonistic when this is not the case in many instances. So there are many overlaps; for example, qualitative research can allow the investigator to discuss causal processes similar to causal statements made within quantitative research. Quantitative research can also explore meaning and collect qualitative data, for example via social surveys. Participant observation can be used to test theories as well as generate them. Finally, developments in grounded theory mean that qualitative data collection can be more structured, reliable and replicable, despite all of these being used as quantitative indicators. Both approaches also share common problems in that they both have to deal with the issue of reactivity, that is, the reaction on the part of those being investigated to the investigator and research instruments. Indeed, the selection of people who are the focus of research, called representativeness, is an issue for both traditions.

It is also possible to combine these different forms of research within a single study. Increasingly mixed methods are used to study aspects of the social world. Accessing multiple sources of information,

Box 3.7 An example of a mixed method approach.

Yount and Gittelsohn (2008) conducted an investigation into child morbidity and mortality within poor countries. They simultaneously collected both quantitative and qualitative data about perceptions of illness, the order in which illness events happened and when care was sought. These researchers developed a tool, a survey instrument that included both quantitative and qualitative responses and analysis techniques. The researchers argue that in using this mixed method approach they were able to gather more complete information about the perceived cause of illness, the symptoms of the illness (both biomedical and lay) and the seeking of health care.

using a range of different tools is likely to provide the researcher with a much more comprehensive picture of the area that they are investigating. So mixed methods are generally used to compare different findings, to investigate different perspectives on issues and to generate different types of data from both methodological traditions, quantitative and qualitative. Combining research techniques in this way is commonly called methodological **triangulation**.

You may consider using a mixed method approach in your project. There are some good books that can offer advice about combining research methods.

- See chapter 17 in Bowling, A (2009) *Research Methods in Health: Investigating Health and Health Services.* 3rd edn. Maidenhead, McGraw-Hill Open University Press. This discusses a variety of mixed research approaches.
- You will also need to give consideration to research ethics when planning your project.

Ethics of research

There are key principles relating to ethics that should underpin all research projects and some of these are of particular concern in relation to health research, as the areas investigated may be personal or could involve using confidential records and medical information. Research projects often require ethical approval and are expected to adhere to specific codes of ethics. There are many ethical codes available for researchers but they are all concerned with respecting the **autonomy** of those being researched, ensuring confidentiality, adhering to the principle of informed consent and ensuring that harm to participants is both considered and minimized.

So what do these ethical principles mean in terms of conducting

Box 3.8   Principles of research ethics.

- Protection from harm – harm to both participants and researchers.
- Informed consent – participants should be fully aware of the research process and be able to consent freely. This is achieved by the use of information sheets and consent forms.
- Anonymity – participants should not be able to be identified.
- Confidentiality – participants should be aware of what happens to the data they provide and who will see it.
- Right to withdraw – from the research process up to a clearly identified point if they choose to.

Box 3.9   Example ethics codes.

The Economics and Social Research Council
http://www.esrc.ac.uk/ERSCInfoCentre/Images/ESRC_Re_Ethics_
Frame_tcm6-11291.pdf

The College of Occupational Therapists
http://www.cot.uk/members/publications/ethics/pdf/codeo6o5.pdf

The Chartered Society of Physiotherapists
http://www.csp.org.uk/uploads/documents/csp_effecprac_reso7.
pdf

research? All researchers should adopt a clear ethics policy in terms of informed consent, anonymity and confidentiality. This means that any participants in research can not be identified, their identity is protected and they understand fully what they are involved in as a research project. So participants should be given a description of what the research is about, what their involvement means and how the information that they provide will be both used and stored.

The final part of this chapter gives consideration to the importance of research and evidence for practice within the health field.

Evidence-based practice

Research is essential within the field of health for practitioners to acquire an evidence base. Evidence-based practice is simply the application of research findings to practice situations. Such evidence can be drawn from a variety of methodologies, several already discussed in this chapter for example, **randomized control trials**, surveys and interviews. For example, research has helped develop and improve practice in a number of ways:

- By evaluating services and their effectiveness.
- By evaluating the clinical effectiveness of interventions and treatments.
- By determining the cost effectiveness of treatments.
- By examining improvements for patients undergoing treatment using quality of life measures.

A useful definition of evidence-based practice is 'The process of systematically reviewing, appraising and using scientific evidence to underpin health practice' (Gray, 1997 p 24). Gray suggests three stages that practitioners and students will need to go through in order to draw on evidence to inform their practice.

Finding evidence

This is a first crucial element as it is important to find the whole body of evidence in order to make judgements. Imagine if in a criminal case half the evidence was missing or could not be found. The jury would not be able to make a fully informed decision about the outcomes for the defendant. The same is true for acquisition of evidence in health practice. Imagine you are trying to find evidence of the most effective strategies to encourage behaviour change and good self care practice in type 2 diabetic patients. You find some material but much of it you have not been able to locate. How could you make an accurate decision about what you may want to act on in your practice?

A useful tutorial for you to develop your searching skills can be found at the Internet for Allied Health website @ http://www.vts. intute.ac.uk/tutorial/alliedhealth/

Appraising evidence

Once the available evidence has been acquired the next stage is to appraise the quality of the evidence. This process is contingent on the principle that the findings in poor methodological quality research are not credible and may not be trustworthy. Just because authors of research make statements in their discussion and conclusion does not mean that they should be accepted by the reader. The purpose of the appraisal is to unpick the methodological strengths and weaknesses of the methodology, design, methods and sampling.

The criteria used to judge the methodological quality of each study vary depending on the types of design used. Criteria to assess the quality of an RCT cannot be applied to an appraisal of a qualitative research study. Several tools are available at the Critical Appraisal Skills Programme based in Oxford available at http:// www.sph.nhs.uk/what-we-do/public-health-workforce/resources/criti cal-appraisals-skills-programme.

Learning task 3.4

Appraising evidence for your project

Thinking about your chosen topic, find a relevant academic article that reports and discusses findings from a research study. Now read the article and make notes, answering the following questions

1. What is the source? Is it a good source and how can you make a judgement about this?
2. Is the article credible? For example, is it in a peer reviewed, high quality journal?
3. What is the key argument of the article? Is it clear?
4. Are the arguments made based upon evidence?
5. Are there any weaknesses in the study? Here you should pay attention to the methods, the sampling approach and size, the way in which the data was analysed as well as any author-acknowledged problems and limitations.

These questions are a useful starting point to guide your reading and to develop your critical appraisal skills. You will also need to think about how the literature that you appraise relates to your specific research focus.

Once judgements have been made about the quality of the articles that have been appraised the overall findings are synthesized to make simple conclusions. When you are examining the literature in relation to your chosen research topic, you will also need to appraise the evidence. Complete learning task 3.4 to develop your skills in this area.

Applying evidence to practice

Drawing on the conclusions from the appraisal of evidence, practitioners now need to consider two questions. What do the results mean for my clients and are the findings applicable in my setting? This is largely a subjective assessment based on practitioners' judgements about their clients and their setting. Wang, Moss and Hiller (2005) provide a useful framework for strengthening this decision-making.

Irrespective of the methodological approach used to answer research questions, research can never give answers that can be categorically stated as the truth. Furthermore, problems arise with evidence-based practice such as knowledge translation, knowledge diffusion and the knowledge-based transformation of practice. For example, evidence-based clinical guidelines are not always implemented in practice even when they are widely published and supported

Table 3.8. Types of research question and associated methodological design.

Question	Methodology and design
Cause and effects questions Do higher levels social capital lead to reductions in health inequalities?	Quantitative RCTs, quasi RCTS Cohort studies Case control studies
Is this intervention effective? Does providing early intervention in at risk children protect against poor educational achievement?	Quantitative Systematic review RCTs, quasi RCTS
Are factors associated? Is discrimination related to poor mental health outcomes?	Cohort studies Case control studies Surveys
How does something work? Explanatory	Qualitative research Survey
Why does something happen? Explanatory and exploratory	Qualitative research
Descriptions of how much, how often, how many Quantification	Quantitative research Surveys

by sanctions. So despite the function of any research to accumulate good quality evidence to provide practitioners with hypotheses of what is currently the best approach available, this is not always easily applied in practice. There are also ongoing debates about the nature of evidence.

In **biomedicine** and allied professions the dominant type of epistemological standpoint is positivism and the associated experimental design particularly randomized control trials. This has shaped ideas about which types of design should be trusted, creating a hierarchy of evidence. More recently the idea that some designs are intrinsically better than others has been challenged. Petticrew and Roberts (2003) produced a **typology** of evidence and suggested that different designs should be used to address different research questions. This relates to the notion of how research questions relate to methodologies (see table 3.1 at the beginning of this chapter).

The process of choosing the most appropriate methodology, design and methods should all be ultimately driven by the research questions posed.

The chapter ends by presenting a case study that synthesizes many of the conceptual issues already discussed by applying a research framework to the study of pain. This will help you to see how the same topic can be explored in different ways to produce interesting and varied research findings.

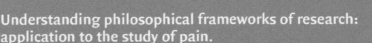

Case study

Understanding philosophical frameworks of research: application to the study of pain.

The issue of pain will be used as an example to explain the relationships outlined in figure 3.1. Ontologically, we know that people experience pain and therefore it can be said to exist. It can be observed, as individuals exhibit signs and symptoms. In addition observations can be made in biological neural systems associated with the sensation of pain. These biological systems have to some degree been elucidated, and questionnaires have been developed that attempt to quantify pain. These points are all allied to positivist notions of understanding pain and therefore quantitative methodology. We can consider studies where different countries can be compared to produce a league table of pain or we can measure pain levels through time in response to treatment, using a longitudinal survey approach.

However, objective measurements of pain are difficult to achieve as pain is a sensation that is experienced and expressed differently by individuals and therefore pain is difficult to quantify. Consider a parent's reaction to a child when they have injured themselves. Parents' reactions can influence how a child expresses pain and it may appear that one child is in greater pain than another, demonstrating that notions of pain are socially constructed. Consider reactions to pain that are not biological in origin, such as the pain of bereavement. Does that type of pain exist, as it is not transmitted in the neural pain systems? Some types of pain are socially constructed to be public or private depending upon the types of community or culture in which they are exhibited (see chapter 5 for an example of different cultural expressions of pain). People may also hide their pain in order not to be perceived as attention seeking or as someone who cannot cope.

These latter ideas are much more closely linked to ideas about interpretivism where measuring amounts of pain are not emphasized but understanding the experience and expression of pain is of more interest. We can see that people have multiple realities of pain rather than a single numerical score (single reality or truth) that measures their pain. To tease out these issues more exploratory methods need to be employed such as focus groups where the dynamic interaction of participants may reveal a richer representation of pain.

Why is understanding research important?

We hope that after reading this chapter and indeed every other chapter in this book you can see how health research is used in a whole variety of ways. Health-related qualitative research has provided a wealth of data about people's experiences, how people experience pain, how they feel about treatment and what is important from a patient's perspective. Qualitative approaches have enabled the voices of social actors to be heard so that they can articulate their own stories and narratives in relation to their health. Such approaches have also provided insights into interactions between health care professionals and patients, so demonstrating the process and power within them. Qualitative approaches have also been used to empower participants for example, getting patients to think positively about cancer while allowing researchers to explore patients' talk (Wilkinson & Kitzinger 2000). Quantitative approaches have also provided large data sets that document changing health trends across the UK and further afield, demonstrating which areas should be of priority for practitioners. For example, the *Health Survey for England* (2008) shows changing UK trends such as increasing rates of obesity and rates of death from alcohol associated diseases. Indeed, as you read through the chapters you will see that the findings from health research have shaped our own ideas about what health is and how it is understood by lay people (see chapter 1). As practitioners working with clients, understanding issues from a lay perspective is vital so that we can try and put ourselves in the position of our clients. Researching health has also led to a greater understanding of social **justice** and how and why people experience health inequalities (see chapters 4, 9, 11 and 12). An understanding of research epistemology and methodology also underpins evidence-based practice. Practitioners need to make judgements about the quality of information that they read in order to make sound decision about how to improve practice, meet the needs of their clients and provide efficient, effective services.

Summary

- Research is a systematic process drawing on philosophical and theoretical concepts about design and methods.

- In order to provide a rich understanding of health-related issues both quantitative and qualitative research methodologies need to be utilized.

- Different research questions can be addressed by differing research designs and methods.

Questions

1. This chapter has given you an introduction to the research process and the importance of evidence within the field of health. Think about the way in which the media draw upon research evidence to report health issues and concerns and consider some of the consequences of this.

2. Write an overall plan for your research project focusing upon the key stages of the research process. Choose a topic, develop a research aim and some associated research questions. Think about your overall approach to investigating these questions; what will your method of data collection be, how will you sample and analyse your data? Do not forget to think about research ethics too. Finally think about how long the project will take you and draft a time-table including time for writing up the project too.

3. Thinking about the use of evidence to inform health-related practice, how would you know that a study was of good quality? You will already have some ideas after completing learning task 3.4 but have you thought about using specific criteria as part of this process? For example, is research reliable, valid (for quantitative projects), or credible and transparent (for qualitative projects)?

Further reading

Bell, J. (2000) Doing Your Research Project. A Guide for First-Time Researchers in Education, Health and Social Science. 5th edn. Maidenhead, McGraw-Hill, Open University Press.

This is an excellent book that is a user-friendly simple guide to completing a research project step-by-step. The first part is called preparing the ground and covers approaches to research, planning the project and ethics. The second part discusses selecting methods of data collection. The third and final part covers interpreting the evidence and reporting the findings.

Bowling, A. (2009) Research Methods in Health: Investigating Health and Health Services. 3rd edn. Maidenhead, McGraw-Hill, Open University Press.

A good all round book that is specifically concerned with health-related research. The book describes theoretical concepts, a range of research methods, sampling and analysis, illustrating points with clear examples throughout. The book has seventeen chapters and so is a comprehensive discussion of all of the key aspects of the research process.

Robson, C. (2007) How to do a Research Project. A Guide for Undergraduate Students. Oxford, Blackwell.

This is an introductory book divided into three broad sections: making preparations, doing it and making something of it. The book discusses potential pitfalls of the process and gives the reader things to consider in terms of issues that are likely to happen in the research process. The chapters are concluded with tasks to help the reader to navigate the research process, research topics to avoid and useful reference tools.

Part II

The Disciplinary Context of Health Studies

Multi-disciplinary public health is a concept that has emerged recently and it is therefore still developing (Jones & Earle, 2010). Despite this recent emergence, it is clear there are many disciplines contributing to our knowledge and understanding of health. These disciplines also offer a range of different perspectives and interpretations about what is important in relation to health. So this part of the book will explore four different disciplinary notions of health, introducing you to the disciplinary context in which health studies itself is located. Health studies draws upon the contributions of many different understandings and interpretations of health allowing those studying the subject area to build a broad understanding of health (Yuill et al., 2010). Health studies is both multi-disciplinary and inter-disciplinary because it draws upon various disciplines to understand health and while these are independent, they also have an often critical relationship with each other. Each discipline has a different viewpoint and focus and no single discipline can be used to fully interpret and explain health thus cementing our understandings of health as complex (see chapter 1).

This part of the book contains four chapters that cover the key disciplinary contributions to health within the subject area of health studies. Each chapter also ends with a useful section that discusses why these disciplinary perspectives are important in helping us to understand health and health studies. Each chapter introduces you to a specific discipline and then clearly outlines what its contribution to health is. Chapter 4 provides an insight into how examining structural, macro-level factors contribute to knowledge. Chapter 5 examines culture and so shows the importance of the context of our health at a different level. Chapter 6 turns to health psychology, which focuses upon the individual level and explaining behaviour. Finally, chapter 7 gives a useful insight into the importance of models of practice within health promotion. These disciplines have been chosen as they give insight into the variety of disciplines that inform health studies, so reading these four chapters will further enhance your understanding of the complex nature of health and health studies.

The first chapter in this part, chapter 4, introduces you to the discipline of sociology, taking you on a journey to demonstrate clearly its relevance to studying and understanding health. The chapter uses a Sociological lens to view aspects of health and health-related behaviour in a critical manner, delivering the key message that health is overwhelmingly socially influenced. Chapter 5 then introduces you to the discipline of social anthropology, concentrating upon culture as a focus through which to begin to explore health, showing that the social location of culture has large implications for health and health-related behaviour. The chapter discusses interesting examples of different cultural practices affecting health from across the world. Chapter 6 then moves onto the discipline of health psychology concentrating upon what health psychology has to offer in terms of understanding how people behave, and the choices that they make, as well as the risks that they take with regard to their health. It will also provide a critical discussion of why behaviour change is so complex, examining a range of mainstream behaviour change theories as part of this process. The final chapter in this part of the book, chapter 7 examines the discipline of health promotion, its key values, ethical underpinnings and a number of models of how health promotion works. The chapter also provides an analysis of the strengths and weaknesses of particular approaches used as part of health promotion practice.

This part of the book will develop your knowledge and understanding of the complexity of disciplines underpinning health studies. Therefore, after reading this part you will be able to conceptualize the importance of a range of factors and influences upon health. This breadth of knowledge is what is important within health studies, as it allows you to see how different disciplines relate to health, as well as allowing you to identify a number of key determinants of health.

Sociology and Health

Key learning outcomes

By the end of this chapter you should be able to:

- understand what social anthropology as a discipline is
- identify how social anthropology contributes to understanding of health and illness
- identify how society and social influences relate to and affect health

Overview

This chapter will introduce you to the discipline of sociology and demonstrate its relevance to studying and understanding health. The chapter will demonstrate how sociology as a discipline contributes to our understanding of health as primarily socially influenced. The chapter outlines what sociology is as a discipline and analyses how different theoretical perspectives contribute to understanding health and illness. The chapter discusses the social model of health, looking critically at the medical model of health in relation to health inequalities. The chapter uses a sociological lens through which to view aspects of health and health-related behaviour, showing that by using such a mechanism we can begin to view health and health-related interactions and behaviour both differently and more critically. Finally, the chapter uses the theory of social construction to explore disability and offers the reader a case study to discuss the gendering of mental health.

What is sociology?

Sociology is the study of interaction between groups and individuals in human society and involves the critical examination of everyday aspects of human life. Sociology as a discipline examines both the macro and the **micro-level**, examining large organizations and institutions such as the economy, education and work, as well as looking at individual behaviour such as the interactions that take place between people. Sociology does not just look at the macro and micro-level separately, rather it attempts to explore the relationships and interactions between the two; how does society influence individuals and conversely how do individuals influence society? So sociology is interested in social processes and how society is structured and works. A key lesson that can be drawn from sociological theory and research is that social structures can often exert more influence over our behaviour than we would expect and this is certainly true in relation to health (see the chapters in part III of this book for a more detailed discussion of determinants). Sociology then in relation to health explores many dimensions of health, illness and health care. Sociological research has also been crucial in drawing attention to the experiential aspects of health and illness. For example, examining doctor–patient relationships and lay perspectives about health and illness (these are discussed in depth in chapter 5, research related to health is also discussed in depth in chapter 3).

Sociology has been described as the science of society and theorists attempt to use their sociological imagination when examining aspects of society such as health and illness. Using the sociological imagination (Mills, 1970) simply invites us to think beyond our own subjective perceptions; this is a mechanism for moving away from commonsense understandings of society. Put simply, to think in a sociological way is thinking beyond personal experience and beginning to challenge any obvious explanations of human actions. Jenkins (1996) argues that thinking sociologically is the result of systematic inquiry; it is carried out objectively and finally involves generalization, analysis and theory. Sociologists therefore think about society in a specific way by distancing themselves analytically from what are considered the usual and normal practices of everyday life. This process has been described as defamiliarizing the situation (Bauman and May 2001) and can be used to explore aspects of health and experiences associated with health. The following learning task will help you to defamiliarize a health-related situation.

This task should help you to understand how defamiliarizing is the process by which sociologists are able to study the normal and usual functions of society and to begin to interpret them theoretically. There are a number of theoretical interpretations within the discipline and so understandings of health vary according to the theoretical viewpoint held (differential definitions and understanding of health are explored in chapter 1).

Learning task 4.1

Developing your sociological thinking about health.
Think about what it is like to stay in hospital. Rather than thinking about this in a commonsense way, begin to think about how might this look from a sociological point of view.

In thinking more objectively about this you may wish to consider issues such as power, regulation, routine and symbolization as starting points.

1. Think about the key concept of power in relation to a hospital stay. Who holds the power, how is this demonstrated and maintained? How does power permeate the hospital routine?
2. Think about how patients are regulated while staying in hospital. For example, how do interactions with professionals serve to regulate health-related behaviour?
3. Now consider the routine associated with a hospital stay, such as the order of events occurring on a daily basis and the scheduling of check-ups and meal times. Are patients simply expected to adhere to these routines? What happens if routines are ignored?
4. Finally think about symbolization within a hospital context. Symbolization is the process by which symbols represent something other than themselves. Such symbols can include accents, dress, words, etc. For example, the white coat traditionally worn by doctors has been argued to be symbolic of power. How do symbols express the values of the medical profession within a hospital? What might symbolize good health?

Sociology of health and illness

Each sociological theory explains society in a different way and therefore health too. Theories that adopt a consensus approach tend to be more positive in their analyses of society whereas conflict theories are more critical of the processes and organizations found within the social world. For example, Marxist theorists are critical of the power of medicine. Such critiques of the power of medicine are also associated with other writers and other perspectives too. Indeed, there are often overlapping critiques from different theoretical positions. Theorists also examine power and how it functions within society from different perspectives, so feminists are critical of male-dominated medical power. Theories also differ in terms of the level at which they discuss society; macro (large scale), versus micro (small scale). Interactionists are, for example, concerned with doctor–patient relationships at the micro-level.

Central to all theories within the discipline of sociology are debates about structure and agency. Some sociologists focus upon the structures of society, so they are concerned with the features of the social world that constrain people or indeed force them into an action. Others investigate the meanings that people attach to their actions (agency) and the events that occur in their lives. Structure refers to factors that help determine our experiences through the establishment of expected ways of behaving. In contrast, the concept of 'agency' reminds us that individuals do not simply act out predetermined roles but 'interpret' those roles in a way that is unique to them. For example, socio-economic status relates to a societal health gradient in the UK but neither structure nor agency is able to fully explain such health differences.

These different theoretical perspectives also demonstrate a range of understandings about the experience of illness and illness behaviour. The way we behave when we are sick is influenced by a variety of factors and therefore illness behaviour is social, it can be explained and understood specifically in relation to the social context in which it is located. Sociologists therefore focus upon examining and analysing social context via theory. Different theoretical approaches provide us with interpretations of what people do, looking at context and what drives them and determines their action. Some theories look at human actions; others look at economics, organizations and society in general. There are several key theories in sociology and so these will be considered now, particularly in relation to what they tell us about health.

Functionalist theory

Functionalist theory explains society as a functioning biological organism in which individuals make up the necessary organs to contribute to its smooth running. In this theoretical framework individuals are like parts and organs of the body in that they all have a role and function to perform. Furthermore, society is seen as consensual, with everyone 'doing their bit' to keep society running. This analogy applies when explaining sickness within society.

However, not all sociologists agree with this concept of the sick role because Parsons (1951) suggests that the doctor–patient relationship is unproblematic. For example, it does not account for gender differences, cultural influences or differential power relationships in relation to the adoption of the role. Others have argued that it is often characterized by conflict and negotiation rather than patients simply accepting the doctor's authority without question (Wainwright, 2009a). Moreover, the sick role is not an adequate explanation for those who are suffering from long-term chronic illness or indeed terminal illnesses. It also does not offer an interpretation of illness as experienced from the perspective of the ill as it is more concerned with analysing how the medical profession manages illness.

Box 4.1   Example of Sociological theory – Parsons's sick role.

Parsons's (1951) sick role concept is a functionalist explanation of how the medical profession manage the societal disruption associated with illness and return individuals to their usual function. Doctors have the power to decide if a patient should be allowed to adopt the sick role. If a patient does adopt the role then they are allowed

- exemption and abstinence from usual responsibilities such as work, housework and looking after dependents,
- Exoneration of responsibility associated with illness; the sick person is not blamed in any way for being ill.

Those who adopt the sick role are accountable to broader social norms and rules on a societal level so the patient is expected to adhere to certain rules and obligations. They must

- have the desire to get better and to return to full health,
- seek appropriate help to achieve better health via the medical profession as soon as possible.

The medical profession here then are part of a controlling apparatus within society, functioning to maintain social order.

Symbolic interactionism

This theoretical perspective explains social phenomena from the perspective of its participants and so is a micro-analysis of individuals, examining behaviour on a smaller scale than functionalism. Sociologists adopting an interactionist perspective have consequently attempted to understand these experiences from the perspective of those experiencing them. An insider's perspective concentrates upon the subjective experiences of living with and in spite of illness, focusing and examining the perspective of people with illness (this links to the lay perspective discussed in chapters 1 and 4). Interactionists are also interested in looking at how people interact with each other in different situations. An essential element of the interactionist perspective is the understanding of the unique nature of the social world as made up of the actions of participants. For interactionist theorists all encounters with others are what creates both meaning and significance within the social world. Human action cannot therefore be observed or assumed, but must be 'interpreted' by studying the meanings that people attach to their behaviour. So what meanings are attached to illness behaviour within society? The answer to this question depends upon the very illness being experienced as some illnesses have more negative meanings attached to them. The work of Goffman

(1963) is crucial here in explaining stigma, which is depicted as an attribute or reputation that is socially unacceptable. This consequently results in an individual being rejected or discredited by other members of society.

However, this perspective has been criticized for limiting its focus to those experiencing ill-health rather than focusing upon why discrimination occurs on a societal level in relation to specific illnesses. This perspective is useful however for highlighting how the experience of illness can affect human identity. This is an important area for the sociology of health and illness because patterns of health and illness are changing within society and consequently people are more likely to experience long-term ill-health. Furthermore, chronic illness and disability impact upon individuals in many ways, affecting experiences of daily living, social relationships, identity (how they are seen) and sense of self (their own view). Indeed, more recently it has been suggested that the chronically sick and disabled themselves shape the social world, for example through **new social movements** campaigning to effect change. The social model of disability offers an interesting challenge to experiential analyses of disablement found within some sociological discussions.

Bury (1982) describes chronic illness as biographical disruption in which the experience of illness on an individual basis becomes disruptive to the life experience of the sufferer. The chronic illness disrupts the structures and taken-for-granted assumptions of everyday life for those who are experiencing it. This is particularly the case because sufferers often face uncertainty about their condition in terms of its likely impact. They may experience periods of remission, symptoms can change and are often unpredictable and there may be a longer term prognosis that is difficult to deal with. Sufferers also have to deal with the uncertain reaction of others. Chronic illness therefore can be understood as a critical situation, as it involves pain, suffering and even death. This process also involves several different stages. Firstly, the sufferer has to cope by sustaining a sense of self-worth. Secondly, the sufferer has to develop strategies to manage the condition and the impact it might have upon their interactions and life chances. Finally, the sufferer has to develop a style of adjustment for fitting in with wider society, for example disclosing the illness to others, disguising it so that it becomes hidden or alternatively normalizing the illness in the sense that they distance the illness's effects from themselves.

The notion of biographical disruption then describes the individual patient's lived experience of questioning through the illness, often saying why me and why now? Patients have to deal with the consequences of this biographical disruption, the disruption that their illness brings for everyday life such as limiting their ability to work and participate in 'normal' activities such as family and social events. Patients also have to deal with how others under-

---

Box 4.2   **Example of sociological theory – Goffman and the concept of stigma.**

- Many groups within society have their identity negatively affected by illness and so experience stigma.
- Judgments about health and illness, both physical and mental, are value laden and reflect specific norms within a given time and place (Pilgrim & Rogers, 1994), hence some illnesses are stigmatizing for sufferers.
- Goffman (1963) notes different types of stigma; some stigma are associated with physical deformities such as disablement but social stigma can also be a problem; people become labelled as a result of stereotypes. For example, in the UK in recent years there has been significant stigmatization of poorer people, now often derogatorily labelled as CHAVs (Jones, 2011).
- In terms of illness stigma, the attitudes of others and wider society greatly affect the well-being of those experiencing ill-health.
- Many illnesses are associated with social stigma; HIV/AIDS, mental illnesses such as schizophrenia and depression, genetic conditions such as Down's Syndrome and degenerative mental ageing illnesses such as Alzheimer's.

---

stand their specific illnesses and this relates to the sociological concept of stigma (see the discussion of Goffman in box 4.2) as some conditions are more stigmatizing than others. Finally patients have to cope with and manage the impact of treatment regimes. All of these changes result in the destabilization and questioning of identity after the onset of chronic illness (Bury, 1991). The next learning task will help you to think about the impact of illness upon identity.

However, this interpretation of the experience of ill-health as crucial to identity is not applicable to all. Identity changes are not inevitable for all sufferers of chronic and long-term illnesses. There may be biographical reinforcement rather than disruption. In some cases the experience of ill-health does not lead to changes in self-conception and therefore identity is not necessarily reconstructed. In contrast, the illness is interpreted by the individual more positively and is then used to reinforce some aspects of identity (Carricaburu & Pierret, 1995). Thus, illness is not always understood as having a negative impact, although this depends upon the theoretical perspective being used to interpret the experience, as some understandings construe both health services and illness experiences much more critically, for example Marxist theorists.

Learning task 4.2

Stigma and health: biographical disruption.

Hugo was diagnosed with Tourettes Syndrome around the time that he was seven years old. The condition means that he twitches uncontrollably and spits and swears regularly. Hugo always found it difficult to fit in at school. His condition disrupted the usual classroom sessions and later he had to sit exams alone so as not to disturb his peers. After finishing school, Hugo found many careers off limits as they involved working with the public who are often ignorant of his condition and do not understand that he is unable to control his twitching and verbal outbursts.

- Think about how you might apply the concept of 'biographical disruption' to Hugo's experiences.
- Reflect upon how this condition may have affected Hugo's identity.

Marxist theory

Marxist theory is a conflict theory that focuses upon the power of economics within society. Marxist theory is a political economy theory that focuses upon class inequalities, within an economic framework as being fundamental to understanding society. Marxist theory analyses the way in which capitalism works within society as a social system based upon both inequalities and exploitation. The social class system is of crucial importance for Marxists who suggest that the working classes are essential for the benefit of the owners of the means of production. Hence, power is absolutely fundamental in any Marxist analysis, as capitalists hold the most power within society. Within this framework capitalism is viewed as detrimental to health per se (Navarro, 1979) and health services exist to maintain the health of people to work so that they can continue to contribute to the capitalist system and be further exploited for the benefit of capital. Further to this view of health services as a tool to maintain social order, Marxists have also argued that medicine is a commodity, a product that is bought and sold. Motivation for new drug development is not need, it is profit. Capitalist medicine is seen as increasingly consumerist, creating the desire to purchase both goods and services related to health.

Indeed, this focus upon new health problems has been accompanied by an increasing number of treatments, health expenditure and drugs to deal with them. Consequently, much more has been written in recent years about the power of the pharmaceutical industry in creating a modern dependence upon drugs and treatment for an ever increasing array of medical problems. Busfield (2010) discusses the notion of 'a pill for every ill', whereby the pharmaceutical industry continues to

Box 4.3   Example of Sociological theory – Medicine for profit and control.

- The medical profession effectively disease-monger and create new conditions such as ADHD, attention deficit hyperactivity disorder (Phillips 2006), female sexual dysfunction (Tiefer 2006) and bipolar disorder (Healy 2006).
- In contemporary society a growing range of conditions are now treated medically, including shyness and lack of concentration (Furedi 2008).
- Some lifestyle conditions are also being encompassed under the umbrella of medical surveillance and treatment such as obesity which can now be tackled via a number of drugs that prevent fat absorption or reduce appetites, or much more radical treatments such as bariatric surgical procedures including gastric bypasses or gastric bands. Critics of the medical profession argue that obesity is a social rather than medical problem.

develop and produce a range of medicines for an increasing number of medical 'problems', upon which the general public are becoming more reliant. Much has also been written about the focus of the medical profession and pharmaceutical industry on treating the health problems of the global North (higher-income countries) because of the potential for profit within these areas. Indeed, at an individual level the consumers of health care and drugs within these countries hold expectations about the achievements of modern treatment options and, as Busfield suggests, expect the industry and the medical profession to keep producing solutions for problems. These arguments are part of broader sociological discussions about **medicalization.**

Sociologists refer to medicalization as the process by which usual occurrences from everyday life become understood and defined as medical problems. Illich (1976) suggests that life is generally becoming more medicalized as increasing aspects of daily life are brought into the biomedical sphere of understanding and influence. Zola (1972) argues that within the context of medicalization almost anything can lead to a medical condition such as driving, certain types of clothes and specific activities, if done too much. Medicalization is therefore defined as the ever-increasing influence and control of the medical profession over more areas of our life (Zola, 1972). Sociological discussions of the notion of medicalization are related to how illness and disease are both constructed and treated (Williams et al., 2009), with certain conditions holding as much cultural significance as they have medical importance (Furedi, 2008). For example, chronic fatigue syndrome as a condition is not globally recognized as a health problem. The importance of the role that medicine plays within society is also a crucial part of the medicalization thesis and medical dominance is ever increasing, with medical boundaries expanding and including new conditions and problems. Medicalization is also part of changing societal attitudes associated with understanding of risk that may well change across time (see chapter 2 for a more detailed discussion of risk).

Medicalization and the changing role of the pharmaceutical companies can be understood from a Marxist perspective as part of profiteering and maintaining the health of workers (although evidencing this is problematic). Yet Marxist perspectives have received criticism for limiting their focus to how the capitalist system affects health, while ignoring other social trends and social divisions, such as gender. Indeed, feminist theorists have also written extensively and critically about the medical profession and medicalization.

Feminist theory

Broadly, feminism as a theory is an approach that explains social structures as being fundamentally based on inequalities between women and men. Men are seen to have greater power in both the public and the private spheres. Indeed, even sociology itself has been criticized for being gender blind by feminist theorists. In the context of health, feminist theory has been critical of male dominance within the medical profession, arguing that women's perspectives have been silenced and only understood from a male point of view. Medicalization, it has been argued, has affected some groups more than others. Feminists have argued that on women, the impact of the growth of medical influence has been considerable, highlighting the medical focus upon psychiatric problems, the medicalization of biological processes and the intervention of health practitioners within childcare and the family. It is within this context that the increasing influence of medicine has impacted greatly upon women's lives and most specifically upon their reproductive capabilities (Miles, 1991). Counter criticisms suggest that such perspectives fail to take account of the medical profession successfully dealing with maternal mortality, which was once a leading cause of death for women.

Feminist research such as this has brought attention to the different experiences and treatment of men and women within the health care system. Gender itself has been much explored as a social construction.

Social constructionism

The final theoretical lens considered in this chapter is that of social constructionism, defined earlier in chapter 1. The idea of social construction is fundamental to modern Sociology, with the expression deriving from Berger and Luckman's (1967) book, *The Social Construction of Reality*. For social constructionists, every aspect of the social world has meaning and significance within society. Ultimately there are no universal truths. To say that something is socially

Box 4.4   Example of sociological theory – the medicalization of childbirth.

- Feminist theorists argue that the medicalization of childbirth is part of a wider goal of social control as it has been separated from other social events and reconstituted as a specialist, technical subject under the jurisdiction of an expert authority (Oakley 1984).
- The medicalization of childbirth has removed control from female practitioners within the home environment and now located it under the realms of scientific medicine; a male dominated, hospital-based practice.
- The history of medical care and the surveillance of women is not one of proven and tested effectiveness (Oakley 1993) and some procedures used during childbirth are not based upon evidence proving their effectiveness.

Hysteria, as treated in the nineteenth century by doctors such as Charcot, is a prime example of a socially constructed medical condition.

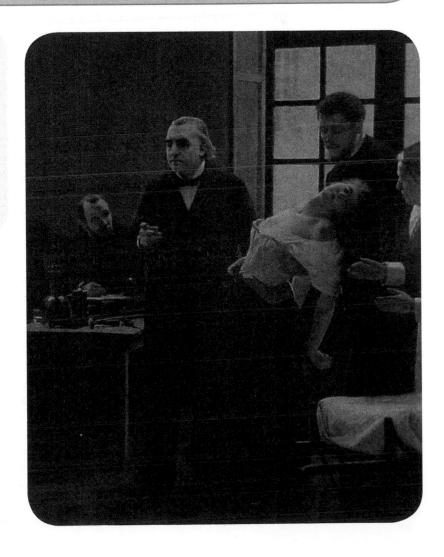

constructed means that it has been fashioned by society and made by humans. The idea of the social construction of health and illness can be supported by changing interpretations and knowledge over time. Homosexuality is no longer seen as an illness, hysteria is no longer diagnosed as a medical condition and new illnesses are now being diagnosed such as ADHD, and Seasonal Affective Disorder (SAD). Thus, social constructionism acts as a useful tool for demonstrating that notions of health and illness change over time and are very much contingent upon broader societal understandings at any given point in time. In relation to health and illness sociologists have argued that the body is often the site of social construction and analyses of lay perspectives have demonstrated this. Social constructionism can be used therefore to analyse disability and societal attitudes and understandings in relation to this. The work of Foucault (1976, 1979) is useful here in analysing the gaze of the medical profession and the control exerted via medical practitioners. Disability is gazed upon by the medical profession as it often involves bodies that are seen to be outside the realm of normality. Research into the experience of disability demonstrates that those who are severely disabled, who seem to have a poor quality of life to outsiders actually report that their quality of life is excellent or good (Albrecht & Devlieger, 1999). There may be many reasons for this; however, the key point here is how society generally perceives and constructs the experience of disability as different from an 'insider's' perspective and construction. There has also been a body of research showing how dependency is constructed by society not adapting itself to the needs of specific groups of people, making it more difficult for them to get out of their homes (Grundy and Bowling 1991).

Post structuralism

The importance of such social constructions are analysed within **post structural** theorists. Post structural sociological theorists argue that scientific knowledge is contaminated by human interpretation as a result of discourse. Bilton et al. (1996) explain discourse as the process by which meanings are imposed upon subjects by the languages that they use to think and attach meaning with. So as humans we experience reality and then interpret this via discourse. In order to understand the meanings that individuals impose upon social reality, individual interpretations have to be **deconstructed**. This perspective is particularly associated with the work of Foucault (1926–84), who analysed the emergence of modern institutions, including hospitals, to demonstrate the role that they played in both monitoring and controlling the population. For Foucault the medical profession was concerned with discipline and surveillance. In his writings about madness, Foucault illustrated how understandings of madness have changed significantly over time to become framed within a medical

Learning task 4.3

The social construction of disability.
The following exercise will helped you to reflect upon the complex interactions that occur between societal and medical understandings in relation to health and certain bodily conditions.

Imagine that you have to debate the following question: is disability the product of society rather than a bodily condition? Think about how disability is socially constructed.

1. Reflect upon whether the able-bodied exclude the less able through their attitudes and the overall accessibility of society.
2. List arguments for and against the idea that disability is the product of society rather than a distinct medical condition.

discourse about illness and treatment. So power works via discourse and in the case of madness is perpetuated by the medical profession. Post structuralist analyses of health and illness, then, are useful for exploring the assumptions upon which beliefs and practices are based (Giddens, 2009).

All of these different theoretical perspectives demonstrate that society and how it works is absolutely fundamental to understanding health and illness. Indeed, sociology has shown this by researching and discussing the impact that society has upon our health and it is to this that the chapter now turns.

Society as a determinant of health

Sociology has also shown how social factors can and do influence health behaviours and how the structure of society is detrimental to some people's health. In this context, Sociology has shown that health and society are closely related; learning about society tells us about health and learning about health tells us about society (Wilkinson, 1996). There is now a huge body of evidence that demonstrates that our health is ultimately determined by our position within the social structure; society determines our health in many ways. The final learning task will help you to explore this further.

Social divisions such as age, gender, class and disability all affect health. The existence of health inequalities within society has been of huge interest to sociologists. The publication of the Black Report (Townsend & Davidson, 1982) detailed a social gradient in terms of health outcomes within the UK, showing that large differences exist between the social classes, genders and ethnic groups in terms of health outcomes (see Graham, 2000). For example, those in the

> ## Learning task 4.4
>
> ### Thinking about social influences upon health.
> Reflect upon the social influences that can and do affect health.
>
> Think about the social influences in your own life. How are the circumstances that you find yourself in likely to affect your health in both positive and negative ways?
>
> List all the influences that you can think of and now consider which are within your control and which are determined by broader structural factors (such as the economy and government policy) that you cannot control.

lowest social class are far more likely to die at a younger age irrespective of gender, ethnicity and at all ages too. So the risk of mortality increases in relation to moving down the class scale. Furthermore, the lower social classes are also more likely to experience higher levels of morbidity, which is greater ill-health during their lifespan. The Black Report also reported the existence of inequalities in relation to the utilization of health services so, despite the existence of the NHS within the UK, a service free at the point of delivery, allowing everyone equal access, it remains the case that those positioned in the lowest social classes actually make less use of the service than those located higher up the class scale. It is also important to note that even when worse-off individuals do use health services at the same rates as better-off ones, the health of the poorer still remains worse, demonstrating that health service usage is not the key to addressing health inequalities.

Since the publication of the Black Report, there has been a plethora of research and related policy documents investigating health inequalities such as *The Health Divide* (1988), *The Health of the Nation* (1992), and the *Acheson Report* (1998). The WHO also held a Commission on the Social Determinants of Health (2008). There is therefore an overwhelming amount of evidence to support the argument that health outcomes and life chances are heavily influenced by our societal position. The social divisions of class, gender and ethnicity all impact upon both morbidity and mortality.

- 2002 figures show that average life expectancy in the UK for women was 80.4 years, whereas men had a life expectancy of just 75.7. So there was a gender difference of 4.7 years (Gjonca et al., 2005).
- 2007 figures show that South Asian men were 50% more likely to have a heart attack or to experience angina than men in the general population. Caribbean men were also 50% more likely to die of a stroke when compared to men within the general population (Parliamentary Office of Science and Technology, 2007).

- 2010 National Statistics show that professional males live an average of 12.5 years longer than those found in manual occupations. For women the average gap was 11.4 years (National Statistics, 2010).

These figures are examples drawn from a massive bank of evidence to demonstrate that health inequalities exist within the UK. Indeed, health inequalities also exist on a much broader global scale (these are discussed in chapter 12). Despite the marshalling of large amounts of evidence to demonstrate health inequalities, explaining why this is the case is much more complicated territory. So why do these inequalities in health exist? Sociologists have not only explored and highlighted these trends but they have also attempted to theorize and explain these very different health outcomes based upon the societal position of individuals. The Black Report itself began to debate explanations for health inequalities and offers the reader four potential answers to why inequalities exist. These are the artefact explanation, the idea of social selection, the notion of cultural differences and finally the influence of material and structural factors that impact upon individuals, which is encompassed under the umbrella of the social model of health. Table 4.1 offers a summary of all of the explanations for the existence of health inequalities, including the four given in the Black Report.

The first two explanations detailed in table 4.1 have been largely discounted. The remaining explanations are still being researched and debated. The importance of place has also been brought into the debate. Popay et al. (1998) argue that lay knowledge about social context and the experience of health are important too as determining health outcomes. Indeed, part III of this book discusses the determinants of health in much more depth.

For sociologists, it is the social factors that remain interesting and the focus of much research in relation to explaining health inequalities. The relationship between social factors and health is considered under the umbrella of the social model of health. The social model of health is seen as crucial by many sociologists in explaining health inequalities as it is seen as a significant determinant of health (for a fuller definition of the social model refer to chapter 1). The traditional biomedical model, focusing upon the **aetiology** and causation of ill-health has been criticized from a sociological perspective for failing to take into account all of the factors that can and do affect individual health. Illness does not necessarily have a clear biomedical indicator as some people can feel ill without any biomedical evidence of causation. Health and illness are seen as existing upon a continuum that individuals move along rather than being clear cut diagnostically as the biomedical model suggests (see Ogden, 1996). However there is no single social model of health and again this explanation is complex because the model is a broad umbrella concept that covers several different areas such as the existence of social divisions and inequalities, lifestyle

Table 4.1. Summary and critique of explanations of health inequalities.

Explanation for health inequalities	Key points	Critique
Artefact explanation	The measurement of class differences in determining morbidity and mortality are flawed methodologically.	• Health and differing health outcomes have been measured in a variety of ways. • Overwhelming evidence exists to demonstrate social class differences in relation to health outcomes.
Social selection as a mechanism	This is tied to the notion of social mobility – those who experience ill-health have downward mobility in terms of the overall class structure, leaving those with better health higher up the social scale.	• Research has shown that the relationship between ill-health and class position is much more complicated than this explanation suggests.
Cultural argument as a mechanism	Class differences in ill-health are caused by broader behaviour patterns – those in the lower social classes experience more ill-health because they smoke more, drink more, exercise less and eat less healthily when compared to others in higher social class positions.	• Such explanations ignore the overall context in which behaviour takes place. • There is a wealth of evidence to show that even when risk factors such as smoking and poor diet are controlled for, social class differences in health outcomes still remain. Thus, individualistic behavioural explanations are simply not the entire story. • This explanation is also 'victim blaming'.
Material and structural factors as mechanisms.	Inequalities are determined by differences in the material circumstances in people's lives, such as unemployment and poor housing.	• The debate about these is ongoing largely because many complexities exist in explaining inequalities.
Psychosocial factors	Inequalities are determined by certain psychological and social factors that pre-dispose people to higher risks in relation to their health.	• Again the debate is ongoing, with some commentators asking questions about the evidence base for the psychosocial hypotheses in leading to physical ill-health.

actors, psycho-social determinants and the social constructions of illness and disease. Busfield (2000) in the book *Health and Health Care in Modern Britain* demonstrates the complexity of social determinants in relation to health. She developed a four-part typology in an attempt to begin to explain health inequalities (also discussed in chapter 10). She contrasts individual behaviour with attributes and circumstances. Then, on societal level, she discusses the material environment and the distribution of resources 'mediated directly on the body' (p. 33), while distinguishing them from social relations and **subjectivity**. Busfield's main argument is that there has been too little attention paid to material and environmental resource distribution as causes of health inequalities. This position is supported by the social determinants of health explanation.

Social determinants   The social determinants of health explanation is that which strongly suggests that material deprivation is absolutely fundamental in leading to disease and ill-health because the poorest sections of society are those who are denied what they need for good health (Wainwright, 2009b). Material deprivation is crucial then in determining health outcomes. Richard Wilkinson and Kate Pickett in their book, *The Spirit Level* (2009), clearly outline the implications of the existence of inequality within society. Inequality is ultimately bad for health as it causes shorter, unhealthier and unhappier lives; it increases the rate of teenage pregnancy, obesity and addiction. Wilkinson and Pickett marshal a range of international evidence to demonstrate clearly that inequality has more detrimental health effects for those found within the lower social classes. The mechanisms by which this occurs are complex indeed and are partly explained by lifestyle factors and psychosocial determinants of health. Marmot's (2010) recent work here is also crucial at the policy level as his report, *Fair Society, Healthy Lives* calls for action across all social gradients, not just in relation to health. Thus to address health inequalities, social inequality across society must also be tackled.

Lifestyle factors   The lifestyle factors approach places more emphasis upon individual choices and responsibility in determining health outcomes by examining the way in which we make unhealthy lifestyle choices and how these relate to health outcomes. Thus, higher mortality and morbidity within the lower social classes are explained by individuals making unhealthy choices: smoking more, drinking higher levels of alcohol, eating less healthy food and exercising less (Fuchs, 1974). However this approach has received much criticism for being victim blaming and not recognizing the broader structural factors influencing the daily decisions people make regarding smoking, drinking and dietary choices. Many lifestyle choices are partly determined by the financial situation in which individuals find themselves. This explanation also pays too little attention to the psycho-social factors that influence our lifestyles.

Psycho-social factors   This explanation is concerned with the relativity of inequality within any given society. Wilkinson (1996) argues that when there are greater levels of inequality, society has lower levels of social cohesion, which lead to more insecurity and social isolation, experienced disproportionately by those in the lower social classes. These experiences cause chronic stress, which in turn affects biological pathways and impact negatively upon health. Psychological health is an important component of this process as those at the lower end

Unhealthy lifestyle choices, such as binge drinking, are often determined by socio-economic factors.

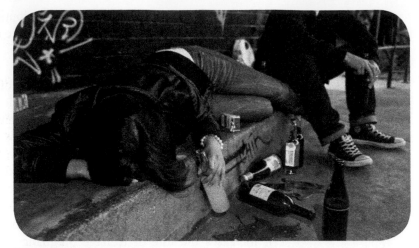

© Action Press/Rex Features

of the class spectrum have less control and power in their daily lives and work environments, a situation that is critical for health (Marmot, 2004). Position in society and its relationship to ill-health is a very complicated matter yet it is widely argued that those in higher social classes can compensate for their experiences of illness and the effects of any disability because of their better access to resources and support networks.

Clearly the social model of health and illness is complex and multi-faceted. The social model despite its complexities does offer insight into how society influences our health and provides us with a different insight into health and illness. This critical interpretation and discussion of the social world and the way in which we understand it is at the heart of the discipline of sociology. Sociologists have also turned their critical gaze to disciplines that aim to improve health and tackle health inequalities, such as health promotion.

Sociological critique of health promotion

Chapter 7 provides a detailed discussion of the discipline of health promotion. The sociology of health promotion has explored health promotion critically as a discipline, discussing its role. Sociologists have also investigated the norms and values that underpin health promotion, analysed power dynamics within health promotion work and critically questioned the effectiveness of health promotion inter-ventions. Ultimately, sociology has opened up debates within health promotion in a number of areas.

Critical sociological discussion has therefore been used to explore the practice of health promotion, leading Thorogood (2002) to argue that, rather than just getting on with their jobs, health promotion prac-titioners need to ask themselves key sociological questions about the nature of their work.

Box 4.5   Key Sociological questions about health promotion.

- What are the norms and values underpinning health promotion? Do these take into account the reality of people's lives enough to be effective (see Graham's 1987 work)?
- Can people always make a healthy choice? Are choices equally available to all people? The idea of knowledge leading to action and ultimately behaviour change is limited by material and structural factors (Tones 1986). Social position may lead to health compromises (Graham & Power 2004).
- Is health promotion simply part of a broader trend of social regulation, in which judgements are made about the value of some choices made by individuals (Tones 1986)?
- Does health promotion increase perceptions of risk related to health and simultaneously encourage health consumerism?
- Does health promotion contribute to 'healthism' in which responsibility for health is shifted towards the state rather than the individual?
- Can health promotion be effective without any wider social and political change?

Why is this important for understanding health?

Chapter 1 ends by arguing that there are several reasons why it is important to look at different perspectives about health. Sociology as a discipline plays a crucial role in this area because as this chapter demonstrates sociologists bring to the table a range of interpretations about health, health-related behaviour and health care when theorizing about the subject. Sociology is therefore an important tool in conceptualizing health, health behaviours and the societal relationships that are important to health, as it has developed many useful models for interpreting health and illness. The key concepts of central importance within the discipline are relevant to exploring health for example, social divisions such as class, gender and ethnicity. The exploration of how social divisions relate to health within the discipline has led to a wealth of evidence to demonstrate how health is overwhelmingly socially influenced and determined, prompting much debate and discussion in explaining the existence of health inequalities and the specific mechanisms by which society influences our health. Indeed, sociology has also researched and analysed lay perspectives of health, an area of knowledge and evidence important for adding to professional perspectives, and influencing social policy (see chapter 1 and chapter 5).

Sociology ultimately demonstrates through the lenses of different theoretical perspectives that health is contested, as there is no shared single understanding of health and illness within the discipline. Health is also a very difficult concept to define (see chapter 1). What is shared, however, is the notion that health is social in many ways, that health has to be understood using theoretical and conceptual frameworks and that health and illness need to be researched and explored analytically and critically. Thus, sociology has developed many critical interpretations associated with health, for example, heavily criticizing the medical model of health and the ever increasing medicalization of society.,

Case study

The gendering of mental health.

Sociologists have examined many gender differences in terms of health. One such area of interest is that of mental health because the most common mental health problems, such as depression, are far more prevalent among women (see Foster, 1995 and Bebbington, 1996). Despite this, men are more likely successfully to commit suicide (Biddle et al., 2008), as they often choose a more effective mechanism by which to achieve this. It is still important to consider what social factors play a part in the diagnosis of men with mental illness; for example, are women more health seeking than men and, if so, then why is this the case?

Research has shown that men are less likely to use health services than women (Courtenay, 2000) so in the first instance, less contact with health services means less chance of diagnosis. However, this in itself is not an adequate explanation. So when men actually attend a consultation, do they behave in a way that means they are less likely to be given a diagnosis of mental illness? Sociologists have analysed medical consultations between men and GPs and argue that men relate their emotional experiences to expectations of being male, so they keep a 'stiff upper lip', do not cry, and control their emotions (Moynihan, 1998).

Sociologists have also explored how important the notion of masculinity is in determining diagnoses of male mental illness. Being male and masculine is culturally represented as being both independent and powerful (Newman, 1997), so it has been argued that men are more reluctant to seek help for mental illnesses as they often do not wish to be viewed as less masculine.

So sociology offers some explanation of gender differences in mental illness rates by examining the complex interweaving of the influential role of culture and social influences, which combine to affect health-seeking behaviour, the attitudes of patients and diagnoses.

Summary

- Thinking sociologically about health and illness has led to many interesting analyses of health and health-related behaviour.

- Sociology is a strongly theoretical discipline with many different perspectives that can be used to analyse health and illness from a variety of angles.

- Sociology when critically analysing health has strongly demonstrated that health is overwhelmingly social, showing the importance of social positioning in determining morbidity and mortality. Those who are better positioned within society ultimately have better health outcomes.

Questions

1. Think about the theoretical perspectives discussed within this chapter; which one do you feel is the most realistic in interpreting health and illness?

2. Consider the arguments for medicalization suggested here and think about how these fit with conditions that are often disputed by the medical profession such as Gulf War Syndrome. Why are some conditions disputed when medicalization is seen to be increasing?

3. How much of your own health is socially constructed? Consider the ways in which your experiences of health and illness can be explained within a social constructionist framework.

Further reading

Barry, A.M. & Yuill, C. (2008) Understanding the Sociology of Health: An Introduction. 2nd edn. London, LA, New Delhi, Singapore, Sage Publications.
This is an excellent book that covers the key theories, themes and contexts relevant to understanding the Sociology of health and illness for a reader who is new to the topic and discipline. The book is very reader friendly and a good starting point for those who want to understand how sociology is key in understanding and exploring health and illness.

Giddens, A. (2009) Sociology. 6th edn. Cambridge & Malden, Polity.
This is a huge text that is an excellent introductory textbook to the discipline, covering discussions of education, crime and health by a well-known and well-respected sociologist. The book is well written, colourful and highly interactive. See chapter 10, which concentrates upon health, illness and disability specifically and the section at the end of the chapter that recommends a variety of other resources.

White, K. (2009) An Introduction to the Sociology of Health and Illness. 2nd edn. London, LA, New Delhi, Singapore, Sage Publications.
This is an excellent resource, once again covering all key aspects relevant to introducing students to the discipline of sociology in relation

to exploring health and illness. The book is easy to navigate, taking the reader on a journey through the theories and key areas explored via a sociological lens. The book contains detailed case studies and suggestions for further reading. The book is a great starting point for reading about the theoretical perspectives that underpin sociological understandings of health and illness.

5 Social Anthropology and Health

Overview

This chapter will introduce you to the discipline of social anthropology and demonstrate its relevance to studying and understanding health. The chapter offers an introduction to anthropology as a distinct discipline, concentrating upon culture as a lens though which to begin to explore health, showing that culture is socially located and based and this once again has large implications for health and health-related behaviour. So what are the implications of different cultures in terms of health? The chapter discusses interesting examples of different cultural practices that affect health from across the world. The culture of treatment approaches will also be explored. The chapter will provide analysis of how culture can be both positive and detrimental for health. A case study of anti-social behaviour and attention deficit hyperactivity disorder (ADHD) will be used to demonstrate the influence of cultural context upon health.

What is social anthropology?

Social anthropology is the study of all aspects of society from a cross-cultural perspective. Historically anthropology emerged as the study of the different and 'exotic other', with anthropologists researching non-Western societies, cultures and social worlds perceived as different to the Western developed world. Early anthropologists such as Evans-Pritchard (1937) wrote about life among the Azande people of the Nile/Congo basin, who explained their social world through witchcraft beliefs. Contemporary anthropology, however, is as much concerned with Western culture as it is with exotic others. Within the broad discipline of anthropology there is a large sub-discipline, the anthropology of health and illness, which explores the social and cultural dimensions of health, ill-health, and medicine. Often called medical anthropology, this sub-discipline is concerned with studying patterns of human health, sickness and death by considering both biological and cultural factors. Medical anthropology is therefore concerned with the experiences and practices of health, illness, and healing in different social and cultural contexts. For example, medical anthropologists have researched indigenous African and Asian medicines, local critiques of professional healing systems, differing cultural variations in conceptions of health and illness, cultural universals in health and illness, differing disease patterns, experiences and diagnoses as well as the political and social forces that affect illness and health. Ethnographic studies have demonstrated that illness and medical care are socially constructed (see chapter 3 for discussion of research methods such as **ethnography** and chapter 4 for further discussion on social constructionism) according to the cultural context in which we live. For example, ethnographic studies have shown how therapeutic interventions can be influenced by cultural practices (Prout, 1996), and they have been used to explore the attitudes of professions in relation to health care and health promotion (see Kingfisher & Millard, 1998).

Of special interest to medical anthropologists is the study of enthomedicine, an area examining health-related beliefs, knowledge and practices of cultural groups. Medical anthropology also explores both traditional healing and modern medical technologies. In summary, medical anthropology explores health and illness within its cultural context because culture is important in relation to health in many ways.

Culture and health

The social model of health (see chapters 1 and 4 for more discussion of this) suggests that our individual health is affected by the context in which we live and how we make sense of the world. Defining culture is difficult as it is a contested and debated concept. It has been defined in a variety of ways and is used differently across different disciplines. As a result, for the purposes of this chapter culture is understood as the collective beliefs, assumptions and values that are communicated between people within a society (Boyden, 2004).

> ### Learning task 5.1
>
> **Positive cultural influences.**
> Think about the culture in which you live. Cultural practices are often so deeply embedded in our daily lives that we do not think about them, other than in common sense terms. For example, our attitudes to eating food and meal-time routines, such as eating food together as a family, are part of cultural patterns of behaviour. Similarly, our attitudes to transport are cultural with the UK described in the media as a car dominant society. Health too is culturally influenced with western societies dominated by the biomedical model of health (see chapter 1 for a fuller explanation).
>
> Many of our normal daily activities rooted in culture have a bearing upon our health. How do normal cultural practices affect your health? Reflecting upon your own experiences, make a list of all of the cultural influences that you can think about that may have had a positive effect upon your health beliefs, attitudes and behaviours. For example, do your family and peers encourage you to eat healthily? What are UK attitudes generally like towards smoking and smokers?

Put simply, culture is how we make sense of and understand the social world in which we live. Helman (2000: 2) defines culture as '. . . an inherited "lens", through which the individual perceives and understands the world . . .'. We all live in a specific cultural context that functions as either a positive or negative determinant of health. The learning task above will enable you to explore how culture affects health.

This learning task should have helped you to understand that ultimately health is cultural because the process of giving meaning to behaviours and events such as illness occurrences is a cultural one, shaped by the context in which we live (Timimi, 2005). This is evident when we consider that both our perceptions and experiences of health and illness are influenced by culture and cultural norms. Therefore, not only does culture determine health and illness in many ways, it also shapes our perceptions of illness and views of how we are expected to behave when we are ill. Culture is about meaning too, it is a system of meanings and symbols that influence and shape the way in which people view and define the social world (Corin, 1995). Culture is ultimately related to societal rules. Hence different societies have varying rules and cultural understandings, leading to an array of illness interpretations and experiences. Social norms indicate and prescribe attributes and traits in relation to health and illness. Furedi (2008) argues that people's perceptions of health and illness are largely shaped by the culture in which they are located.

Box 5.1   Example of cultural norms affecting health behaviour.

Krumeich's (1994) study of a 'breast is best' health promotion programme in Dominica shows how women's social position and cultural constructions of gender relate to health behavior (using formula instead of breastfeeding).

- Men's status depends on their virility, the number of sexual partners they have and the number of children they produce, whilst remaining unmarried. Men show to the community that they are fathers of children born out of marriage by providing infant formula. Giving formula is seen to symbolize fatherhood.
- Women, often unmarried, accept the formula as proof of their relationship, which is also an important aspect of female status.
- There are also widely held beliefs about the spoiling of women's milk as a result of negative emotions from relationships, which serve to further limit breastfeeding.
- Beliefs about sexual desires and intercourse also encourage the use of formula because the quality of breast milk is seen to be affected.

Furthermore, '. . . culture does considerably more than shape illness as an experience; it shapes the very way we conceive of illness. A true comparative cross-cultural science of illness must begin with this powerful anthropological insight' (Kleinman, 1977: 4). Here Kleinman is explaining that health is not just embedded within individuals or the social context, rather it is related to a complex interaction between both.

People make sense of their illness experiences within a framework of expectations conveyed via cultural norms. Lupton (1994) argues that individuals construct their understandings of the world, including their beliefs about medicine and disease, from interacting with culture and its products. Thus, Western medicine is a product of culture too; health care, illness and even the doctor–patient relationship are all cultural activities and experiences. Disease and illness are a form of communication reflecting cultural conventions and norms on both an individual and societal level.

Comparisons of different societies provide further insights into how health and illness experiences are framed by cultural practices. For example, comparing experiences of childbirth in the UK with the Netherlands demonstrates different cultural attitudes and practices in relation to the experience. Van Teijlingen (2000) illustrates that childbirth in the Netherlands is viewed as a natural and healthy condition, where medical intervention is not necessary and therefore is limited. Women are supported by a midwife and give birth at home. Comparatively the experience in the UK is much more medicalized, viewed in terms of the risk to mother and unborn child and therefore supervised by medical practitioners at regular intervals, with birth taking place in the hospital setting. It is interesting to note that the Netherlands has a better record than the UK in relation to birth outcomes. So fewer women experience complications and fewer babies die at birth in the Netherlands, despite the use of a much less interventionist approach to caring for women during their pregnancies.

So at a societal level, coherent and organized patterns of interpretations of health and illness exist, which influence the perceptions and behaviour of whole populations. This is a positivist understanding (see chapter 3 for more detailed explanation of positivism) in the sense that anthropologists studying health and illness explore the facts about how and why people behave in the way that they do, and then connect these to begin to explain behaviour. The response to physical symptoms is therefore not just about the disease or illness, because people make sense of their symptoms in different ways and consequently act according to their shared cultural beliefs. Anthropologists have demonstrated this by paying attention to illness narratives and the accounts given by patients. These accounts have been minimized in the West where biomedicine dominates because medical diagnoses are based upon objective observations, with the views of patients therefore losing both relevance and power (Lupton, 1994). However, anthropologists argue that cultural interpretations of illness are still relevant to the medical model and there is a wealth of evidence to support this point.

Box 5.2

Example of cultural interpretations of pain.

Research has shown that pain responses vary culturally. During the early 1950s, Zborowski found that pain was viewed differently amongst ethnic groups when he conducted a study in a New York hospital looking at patients, doctors, nurses and parents of children.

- Old-Americans (by birth) responded with stoicism
- Irish patients denied their pain
- Italian patients were concerned about getting pain relief
- Jewish patients focused upon what the pain meant in terms of their future health

For Zborowski (1952), these differences could be explained by the way in which children are socialised with attitudes to pain being influenced by child-rearing practices. However the study was subjective and so is open to criticism (see chapter 3 for discussion of research bias).

This example demonstrates that the way in which we respond to illness is influenced by cultural context because pain responses relate to the meanings that we have learnt in our own families. Here and in many other studies, anthropological research clearly demonstrates that cultural groups respond to pain in different ways, influenced by social and cultural background. Furthermore, how and whether people communicate pain to health care professionals is also heavily influenced by social and cultural factors (Helman, 2007).

Box 5.3   **Example – Illness behaviour and functionality: Myalgic Encephalopathy or 'ME'**

- ME is an illness with uncertain cause.
- There are different diagnostic criteria used to determine the illness in a variety of countries (UK, USA and Australia).
- Symptoms include muscle spasms, cognitive dysfunction such as memory loss, general symptoms such as sore throats, enlarged glands, joint pains, headaches and flu-like feelings. Symptoms tend to fluctuate in severity.
- ME has attracted much debate about whether it exists and how it can be treated.
- Many sufferers find that their lives are massively disrupted and present with their symptoms when their normal functionality is compromised.

Illness behaviour is also influenced by divisions within societies as well as between them. For example, there are clear differences between social classes. Classic studies found that middle-class people were more likely to exhibit illness and health-seeking behaviour when compared with working-class people experiencing the same symptoms (Koos, 1954). It was suggested that this is because deciding to seek medical attention is often weighed against competing demands from family and work as well as the financial implications of becoming ill. Contemporary research debates whether this is the case in all contexts because those who are lower down the class scale experience higher rates of morbidity and therefore in some instances seek more medical care. Blaxter and Paterson (1982) argued that working-class children's symptoms were only recognized as illness when they were no longer able to play or walk. Other symptoms were dismissed if they did not interfere with functionality, suggesting that minor symptoms were more likely to be ignored within the lower social classes.

How illness affects individual functionality (health as function is discussed in chapter 1) is an interesting explanation for some social class differences in the use of health services. Indeed, there is a wealth of evidence about social variations in health and illness according to social class, gender, and ethnicity all documented since the 1950s and many accompanying attempts to explain them. However, the mechanisms by which social differences work are not yet fully understood. Anthropologists reject the idea of biological determinism in health behaviours, recognizing that social and cultural factors are important but the extent to which behaviour is freely chosen is still highly debated. Examinations of lay accounts of health and illness demonstrate that there exists a complex relationship between the physical, social and cultural factors influencing health.

Experiencing illness

There has been considerable investigation by anthropologists into lay experiences of health and illness. Kleinman's (1998) work, *The Illness Narratives* is influential here, arguing that the state of illness is different to that of disease. Illness can be understood as the social, lived experience of symptoms and suffering as well as the associated behaviour that seeks to rectify the situation, such as seeking treatment and cures. Indeed, studying illness accounts has led to useful insights into the meanings attached to specific illnesses, which Kleinman (1998) usefully categorizes:

- Illness problems – practical difficulties caused by the illness related to socio-cultural expectations. These often include shame associated with disfigurement and loss of 'normal' functioning and frustration associated with not being able to perform usual roles such as work.
- Illness complaints – the descriptions that the patient brings to the practitioner (these do not necessarily include descriptions of the illness problems).

These social experiences of illness and treatment are bound up with cultural interpretations and meanings. People understand illness and disease in a variety of dynamic ways. Health beliefs emerge from dominant discourses such as biomedicine, alternative schools of thought, the media and personal experiences (Lupton, 1994). Despite the dominance of the medical model in the West, the literature about lay beliefs demonstrates that these may differ from biomedical theories (Gillick, 1985; Helman, 1991). More importantly, lay beliefs significantly determine health and illness behaviour and risk perceptions, which has implications for treatment and management of conditions (Breakwell, 2000). Unsurprisingly, lay beliefs of health often stress the holistic aspects and dynamics characteristics of health (Helman, 1991). These views also differ across the lifespan, with older people evaluating their health based upon the presence of chronic conditions and younger people viewing health in terms of functionality in relation to the capability to play sports and psychosocial categories (Backett & Davidson, 1992; Piko, 2000).

> **Box 5.4**　　　　**Example lay accounts of illness – Hypertension.**
>
> Blumhagen (1980) demonstrates a range of lay beliefs about illness causation in relation to hypertension (high blood pressure) amongst men. For example, one patient cited 'family arguments' as the cause leading to symptoms such as 'ballooning veins', 'dizzy spells and flashing lights'.
>
> In analysing his findings he argues that
>
> - 'Folk' beliefs can not be entirely separated from 'formal' medical ones.
> - Individual illness beliefs can be inconsistent and change rapidly.

Lay accounts of illness also demonstrate how patients describe their illnesses using interesting language and impersonal terms. Those experiencing illness may therefore understand their conditions in a broader way than the medical profession do and so the existence of lay beliefs and approaches goes some way to explaining non-compliance and non-adherence to medical treatments.

People believe in a wide range of causal factors leading to illnesses. Lay explanations of illness help people to make sense of their illness experiences. They are based in folklore, influenced by the media, the internet and the medical model to demonstrate illness causation as located within the individual, the environment, the social world or the supernatural world (Helman, 2007). Many lay explanations of the causes of illness are imbued with notions of individual responsibility. The importance of food and mental attitude in relation to staying healthy are central to lay beliefs (Pill & Stott, 1982). For example, staying positive in the face of illness and believing that you will recover, while attempting to maintain control and involvement in everyday life are practices encouraged in some societies. There are also beliefs around illness causation based upon food consumption, so illness can be caused by 'poor diet', you need to maintain healthy eating practices to avoid becoming ill in the first place or eat specific foods that will help you to recover, if you are already ill. The stage of the life-course where people are at is also important in shaping lay beliefs about health and illness, for example, giving up sport for fear of injury and not having the time to be ill are often cited by parents who feel responsible for staying healthy (Backett, 1982; Pill & Stott, 1982). The next learning task asks you to explore lay beliefs in more depth.

The lay beliefs we hold about illness causation in turn influence our attitudes to treatment, our health-seeking behaviour and who we approach for treatment. These are all culturally determined.

Learning task 5.2

Lay beliefs.
Think about the last time that you experienced a common cold.

1. How did you explain the way in which the cold had been caused? For example, by experiencing a change of temperature or by not wearing the correct clothes?
2. Reflect too upon the way in which you have heard other people explain why they had experienced common colds.
3. Make a list of all of the explanations that you have given and heard, then group together the themes that appear in your list.

These explanations reflect commonly held lay beliefs about illness causation in relation to colds. There are also lay beliefs about how to treat colds successfully. Think about what some of these are and if you have ever used any. These reflect cultural practices that are often unrecognized as such because the behaviour is seen as normal.

Culture and treatment

Alternative treatments such as acupuncture are increasingly more accepted by the medical profession in the West.

© F1 Online/Rex Features

Culture affects our descriptions of health and illness, our attitudes and so too our health-seeking behaviour and the treatments that we use. How people understand their health in cultural context also affects the choices they make and how they behave as a result. Medical anthropology has investigated the use of both medical and alternative treatments and why these are used in a number of different contexts. Germond and Cochrane (2010) argue that a striking development in the medical landscape in the West is the extent to which modern medicine is increasingly being used alongside alternative treatments and approaches such as homeopathy, acupuncture and Chinese herbalism. These non-traditional healing approaches have been aggressively marketed as part of the broader trend of the commercialization of treatment. In many societies this mingling of different treatment approaches has always occurred, with pluralistic health-seeking strategies frequently found in multi-cultural environments, although these do vary according to social characteristics such as class (Scrambler & Higgs, 1999), gender, age and religious beliefs. Some complementary approaches such as acupuncture have become part of dominant medical systems in the West, and are used alongside biomedical treatments (Giddens, 2009). Furthermore, Benson and Thistlethwaite (2009) argue that many health professionals are increasingly becoming more open to at least acknowledging, if not working with traditional healers. These changing practices of both health-seeking behaviour and treatment fit with evolving cultural understandings of health and illness. Traditional approaches are also very appropriate in some instances. For example, indigenous people of countries like Canada and Australia can have mental health problems associated with colonialism and rapid cultural change. Therefore, healing rituals and traditional ceremonies are likely to work as a powerful force enabling indigenous people to either gain or reinforce their identity, while reuniting them with the environment; all essential for communal healing (Kirmayer, 2004). In evaluating the success of traditional approaches to healing and treatment, it is not possible to quantify the effects of such approaches as they are influenced by psychological attitudes and expectations. There is also the possibility of the placebo effect with all approaches, both traditional and biomedical (Benson & Thistlethwaite, 2009). Irrespective of the levels of efficacy associated with alternative approaches, there are a growing number of people in the West using them. In some cultures too biomedical approaches are not dominant; they remain unavailable to the masses for their use and are not widely accepted. For example, in Nepal there are approximately forty psychiatrists in a country of twenty-five million people (Benson & Thistlethwaite, 2009). Hence, cultural context remains crucial in determining our attitudes to treatment and health-seeking behaviour.

In their study of health-seeking behaviour in Lesotho, Germond and Cochrane (2010) suggest that 'healthworlds' exist in which health is understood in terms of its social and religious context. So individual healthworlds reflect and demonstrate the common cultural understandings and constructions of health and illness of the society in which they are located. Now complete the next learning task and explore your own healthworld.

The way in which illness is treated ultimately depends upon how it is culturally understood, with many different explanations articulated for the cause of illnesses across cultures. Illness in some cultures is believed to be caused by external forces, evil spirits and possessions rather than biological causes. Therefore, treatment is ritual-based, can

Learning task 5.3

Healthworld as culture.
Think about how the cultural context in which you live determines your healthworld. What is your cultural healthworld and how does this affect your attitude and health seeking behaviour?

Reflect upon the dominance of biomedicine in the West. Is this how you understand health and illness, in biomedical terms? When you are ill do you seek help from the medical profession first? Do you have any other beliefs that explain ill-health too, for example, lay or religious beliefs? Have you ever used alternative approaches and treatments such as homeopathy or acupuncture, and if you have, why did you?

What do these reflections tell you about how your culture affects your attitudes and behaviour in relation to your health? Do you hold multiple beliefs that inform your healthworld?

involve ceremonies to drive away spirits, witchcraft, voodoo and the use of Shamans and traditional healers. Such externalizing systems of treatment tend to locate both solutions and causes as external to the person and instead see them within the interpersonal, social or spiritual realm. Consequently, treatment involves rituals based within families and the whole community (Kirmayer, 2004). Comparatively, Western medicine works within the biomedical model, and is often criticized for being too limited and not considering personal, psychological, spiritual and social factors in illness causation because it tends to be very individualistic in its treatment approach. This tends to lead to a curative approach based upon the diagnosis of diseases. Seeking treatment from 'professionals' is however not the first step in many cultures, as individuals often self-medicate prior to this. Self-medication also varies according to culture and is therefore more culturally dominant in certain locations. Lee (1996) demonstrates that lay beliefs in Korea increase self-medication among middle-class men, who wish to remain independent from medical intervention in controlling their health problems. This trend towards self-medication is part of an approach to maintain and promote health, but it is also based on a long tradition of using plant-based home remedies found within traditional Korean practices and self-reliance. The key point that Lee (1996) makes is that self-medication involves socio-cultural, political and economic dimensions.

Illnesses are described differently across cultures because there are cultural aspects in our descriptions and expressions of our experiences of health and illness. These descriptions are reflected in how health and illness are culturally represented. Lay beliefs exist alongside medical and scientific beliefs, often merging with these too. For

In some cultures, medical treatment is conducted through rituals and ceremonies. Witch doctors for example can play an important role in many local communities.

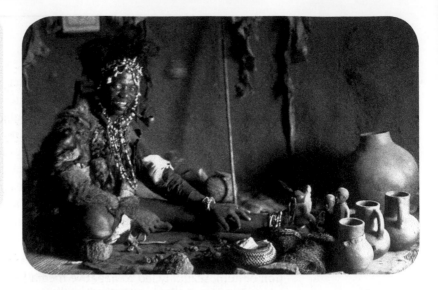

example, Ayurvedic approaches to health are seen as complementary to Western medical practices but there are many overlaps between the systems, with similar diagnostic approaches being applied and the use of medicines as part of treatment. Lay beliefs exist about pharmacological treatments being effective even when there is a lack of evidence to support this, such as in the case of colds and 'flu (Johnson & Helman, 2004). There may also be a relationship between lay beliefs and the placebo effect, which is an improvement in health not attributable to any medication or procedures.

Cultural representations

How illnesses are described and understood varies significantly across cultures. For example, many languages do not contain a word to describe cancer (Dein, 2006) yet this does not indicate that it does not exist. The Western media also convey dominant cultural messages about health and illness via newspapers, reports and broader television programmes. The Internet is also increasingly important in influencing our cultural understandings. These channels all influence our lay beliefs and understandings in a number of ways. Hence, lay beliefs are also strongly tied into cultural representations of health and illness, where perceptions of morality become related to some conditions. Helman (2007) argues that some diseases, especially those that are difficult to treat, explain and control, become symbols for more general anxieties that people have. Hence, some conditions become more than just diseases, they become metaphors (Sontag, 1989). Focusing specifically upon cancer, Sontag argued that metaphorical discourse can be stigmatizing. In the West, cancer is perceived as an uncontrollable, invasive and shameful disease and these views affect both health-seeking

Box 5.5   HIV/AIDs and stigma.

- Societal social norms and myths have been attached to HIV and have lead to some groups being stigmatized more than others.
- Some HIV patients are seen as not blameworthy in relation to their diagnosis, and more worthy victims, for example individuals who became infected after receiving infected blood.
- Other patients have been much more stigmatized because their behavioural practices are less culturally acceptable. So HIV patients who acquire the disease as a result of having sex with multiple partners, being sex workers or injecting drug users have been stigmatized much more.
- When HIV/AIDS was first identified, the prevailing cultural rejection of homosexuality led to negative media headlines and labels such as 'the gay cancer' and the 'gay plague'. The medical journal the *Lancet*, labelled it as the 'gay compromise syndrome'. This negative labelling resulted in cultural stigmatization for those diagnosed as HIV positive.

behaviour, with patients fearful of a cancer diagnosis and how patients are treated too. Attitudes are slowly changing in that cancer victims do now receive much sympathy and positive media attention in relation to various charitable fundraising efforts. Nonetheless, cancer is still often used as an adjective in the media to describe an array of problems such as drug abuse, immigration and crime. AIDs is often negatively described metaphorically too, associated with pollution and ultimately stigmatized (see chapter 4 for a fuller discussion of stigma), with patients facing discrimination because of these views.

Commonly held views of stigmatized conditions are reflected in patients' descriptions of these diseases; often patients do not view disease as part of their body but as a separate entity, an invading force that needs to be removed via appropriate treatment (Lupton, 1994).

Illness metaphors reflect broad cultural trends about attitudes to certain conditions. These illness metaphors are not static and hence may change over time. In some instances illness metaphors are linked to explanations of causation, which are value-laden. For example, explanations of illnesses associated with lifestyle choice are also culturally bounded and heavily value-laden. Self-indulgence and a lack of self-discipline or control are explanatory tools for understanding some conditions. Some behaviour is therefore represented as being socially deviant and illness causing; smoking tobacco, unsafe sex, poor diet and lack of exercise are cited as causal factors in conditions such as cancers, diabetes and coronary heart disease. Indeed, this is true of course, but what needs more recognition is that victims may not be in full control of their choices as these are heavily shaped by their social and cultural environment. There is a sense in which some patients are seen to have caused their own ill-health as a result of participating in risky activities (see chapter 2 for a discussion of risk in further detail). A range of conditions is therefore negatively represented in cultural terms, for example mental illnesses are also associated with negative images in some cultures.

Culture and mental illness

Scheff (1966) argues that in some cultures there are no labels to describe unusual behaviours that make up rule breaking and are seen as deviant. As a result, these behaviours become labelled as mental illnesses. For Scheff, it is labelling that is the primary cause of mental illness. Whatever the suggested explanation, medical anthropologists have written extensively about mental illness, demonstrating that there are no universal categories of mental illness across all cultures. This is indeed borne out in lay descriptions of illness experiences. Fenton and Sadiq-Sangster (1996) describe how Asian women discuss mental distress in a culturally specific set of language terms and how their accounts differ from those of English speakers in important ways. At the same time they describe a syndrome of mental distress that corresponds in a number of features to the category 'depression'. Similarly, in aboriginal culture notions of longing for, crying for and being sick for their country has exactly the same symptom base as depression (Vicary & Westerman, 2004). Anthropological research has also shown differences in understandings in relation to schizophrenia; in some cultures hallucinatory behaviour and suspiciousness are not necessarily seen as signs of mental illness (Pote & Orrell, 2002).

Every culture has established boundaries of normal thought processes and behaviour, accompanied by meanings and labels for those who behave outside those parameters. However, those in one culture who are labelled as mentally ill, may simply be seen in another culture as different: as sages, witches, prophets or simply eccentric. Anthropology also demonstrates that mental health problems in some cultures manifest themselves spiritually and culturally and so have to be solved in the same way. Mental health problems can be linked to breaches of forbidden and scared relationships (Benson & Thistlethwaite, 2008). Consequently, in some cultures there are strong beliefs about the curative power of non-medical interventions with traditional folk medicines and healers the preferred treatment option (Whitley et al., 2006). Healing rituals and traditional ceremonies in places where colonialism and ensuing cultural change have caused mental health problems are likely to be both appropriate and central to community healing (Kirmayer, 2004). There is no single definition of community healing but generally such approaches are about collective action related to the community, in order to bring about positive change. This demonstrates that Western psychiatric diagnoses and treatment approaches may not be accurate or even appropriate in all cultures and circumstances (Benson & Thistlethwaite, 2008). Helman (2007) argues that psychiatric knowledge is to some extent a cultural construction. So culture is a social construction (see chapters 1 and 4 for further discussion of this).

Indeed, not only is mental illness understood differently and treated differently across cultures, cultural context can influence the incidence of mental ill-health. Those who exist in a culture that promotes **resilience**-producing characteristics are much more likely to be able to cope with stress and therefore less likely to experience mental ill-health. Different cultures encourage certain personality types such as hardiness, ego strength, optimism and humour. Hence, mental health problems are heavily socially influenced; feelings such as despair and hopelessness are located in individual brains, but are also related to patterns of interaction with families, communities and indeed wider society (Marsella, 2007) with understandings afforded to individuals through their social interactions with others and society at large. This is related to resilience, with much research evidence showing that more resilient individuals tend to have better health and better mental health (see Friedli, 2009). Chapter 10 offers a more detailed discussion of this.

The cultural context in which mental health is experienced also differs with some societies much more likely to stigmatize those who are diagnosed or perceived to be suffering. This stigma varies according to different conditions too. Now complete learning task 5.4 to reflect upon the stigma associated with the experience of mental illness.

Learning task 5.4

Cultural representations of mental illness.
Think about how the society where you live treats people with mental health problems. What words are used to describe mental health problems and their experience? List all of the words that you can think of and group them into positive and negative descriptions. Which of your lists are the longest? Also consider descriptions of mental illness that are featured in the media. What does this tell you about dominant cultural attitudes? Finally, reflect further about the implications of these dominant cultural beliefs?

This task will help you to understand how our attitudes are shaped by the culture in which we live and experience illness.

Cultural influences upon health

In general, we are often not consciously aware of the culturally patterned nature of our health behaviour since this is taken for granted and feels normal. There are many cultural influences upon health that may not be perceived as such (see chapter 1 for a fuller discussion of notions of what constitutes health) and these can be detrimental and damaging. Cultural influences are negative when, for example, they are supportive of health-damaging behaviours such as drinking excessive amounts of alcohol. However, there may be caveats to this as discussed in the case study at the end of chapter 1. A number of studies demonstrate that the incidence of alcoholism and the regular consumption of alcohol vary significantly between social and cultural groups within and between societies (Helman, 2007). One of the explanations cited for these differences is that alcohol intake is embedded in a matrix of cultural values and influenced by the expectations of different social groups. Alcohol use is inherently cultural; it is related to cultural meanings and specific norms of behaviour. It is also related to the social networks that people have and participate in. Cultural and societal rules underpin what is seen as normal; who is able to drink, who they can drink with and the context in which this drinking can occur. Examining all of these aspects of drinking norms in any culture demonstrates the social roles that alcohol plays. Alcohol use can be used to create identity, and can be important in social relationships too (Helman, 2007). Thus, in many senses alcohol consumption may be socially important in some societies but detrimental to health. Health damaging behaviours can therefore be both culturally supported and acceptable. Further examples include the use of sunbeds and sunbathing to tan skin, despite the associated risk of skin cancer. The concept of an obesogenic environment as a largely negative Western cultural influence on health is also well documented in the literature, suggesting that inactivity, changes in dietary habits and environmental factors all combine to support increased rates of obesity. There are a number of changing trends that have made the environment more obesogenic. For example, increased traffic hazards for walkers and cyclists, reduced opportunities for recreational physical activity, increased sedentary recreation, multiple TV channels around the clock and changes in food production and the availability of food (Hanlon et al., 2010) are all seen as contributing factors within the Western obesogenic environment.

Some commentators have argued that modern Western culture is generally damaging to health. Eckersley (2005) specifically suggests that the cultural aspects of materialism and individualism are detrimental to health and well-being because of their impacts on psychosocial factors such as personal control and social support. Other aspects of contemporary Western culture have also been highlighted as detrimental to health. For example, it has been argued that the 24-hour, round-the-clock culture in which we now live contributes to disturbed

Box 5.6	Different cultural attitudes to obesity as a 'health problem'.

- Obesity is not seen as a health problem in all societies as there are different cultural views about obesity.
- Obesity in some cultures is linked to social status with being fat linked to being wealthy.
- Obesity is also perceived as sexually attractive in some cultures. For example, historically in Mauritania obesity was revered to such an extent that force feeding young women became a common cultural practice. However, changing cultural attitudes are now resulting in force feeding declining, with thinness now culturally equated with beauty (Giddens 2009).

sleep patterns and therefore negative ill-health. Shift work, the advent of new technology and the leisure industry boom have all been blamed for contributing to sleep deprivation, which is ultimately bad for health (Stanley, 2009). It has been suggested that the growing rates of depression, anxiety and the loss of well-being provide the most direct evidence of the degree to which modern populations are feeling over-whelmed as a result of changing social conditions known as modernity (Hanlon et al., 2010). These discussions are located within a specific cultural context in which emphasis is increasingly placed upon lifestyle choices and responsibility for health, discussed within a biomedically dominant culture.

The dominance of biomedicine in the West is culturally pervasive. Medical views on health and illness dominate both public and private discourse, with individuals placing much trust in medical practition-ers and increasingly depending upon medicine to provide answers to both medical and social problems (Lupton, 1994). Medicalization has become culturally dominant and for some commentators this too is a negative cultural influence (see chapter 4 for definitions and discus-sions of the concept of medicalization). Furedi (2008) argues that powerful cultural signals allow individuals to interpret their problems in a medicalized framework, leading to an increase in self-perceptions of illness. This is an interesting analysis in light of the fact that despite huge improvements in medicine and public health, large numbers of society report experiences of long-term illness and disability. Indeed, medical diagnoses offer a definition and interpretation of behaviour and as a consequence allow individuals to make sense of their prob-lems and experiences, while gaining or altering their sense of identity (Furedi, 2008). This contrasts somewhat with the increasing number of subjective reports by people feeling healthier, as reported in survey data. Interestingly, there has been a huge increase in the emergence of new syndromes, whereby social problems are turned into medical complaints. This has also contributed to a prevailing culture of fear and risk found within Western culture (for a broader discussion of risk, see chapter 2). Medicine and the medicalization associated with it are culturally specific to the West. For Lupton (1994) Western medicine itself is culture because it dominates the social arena but yet is not recognized as being socially produced and constructed. The role that medicine plays within society is a product of social relations; medicine can and does support **social inequalities**, depicts both villains and victims and reflects power differentials too. Medicine has contributed to the marginalized position of some groups within society; feminists have long argued that medicine has been a tool to oppress and control women. For example, many feminists have argued that female reproductive functions have become medicalized and male dominated, as well as being used as a way in which to create female dependency (Finkelstein, 1990). Ultimately then medicine is inextricably linked to social processes and is culturally bounded.

The cultural context of behaviour and belief then are clearly important for health. The same behaviours in different cultures may affect health outcomes in different ways. In some non-Western cultures, hallucinogenic drugs are used to obtain states of transcendence and to experience trance states. These rituals may be part of cultural rites of passage and may be experienced over long periods of time. These drugs may be used by shamans or ritual healers. Hallucinogenic drugs have powerful effects upon those who take them; however, the cultural context of their use has an impact upon the experience. For example, the expectations and behaviour of participants, the shaman's visions and the timing of rituals can all be influenced by the use of such drugs. However, many hallucinogenic drugs, highly controlled within non-Western ritual contexts, are used as recreational drugs in industrialized society. These drugs have many known side effects such as psychosis when they are over-used (Helman, 2007). Clearly, culture can be a negative influence in relation to health but so too a positive influence.

Why is this important to health studies?

As this chapter has demonstrated, medical anthropology has been important in highlighting the importance of cultural beliefs, attitudes and practices in relation to health. We are all influenced by the very cultural context in which we are located; therefore our health beliefs, attitudes and practices are also culturally influenced. Culture is an important mechanism from which we draw meanings and understandings in relation to health and illness. Cultural beliefs are often part of a holistic interpretation of the health and illness, allowing individuals to give meaning to their experiences. Anthropology has given voice to many insider accounts demonstrating the importance of holistic interpretations and understandings of health among lay groups.

Case study

Anti-social behaviour, ADHD and the role of culture.

Within Western cultures such as the USA and the UK, diagnosis of attention hyperactivity deficit disorder (ADHD) are increasing, especially among young boys (see Gottlieb, 2002 and Wright, 2003). The condition is understood to be a psychological disorder in which sufferers experience problems concentrating, are unable to focus their attention and find it difficult to learn in the school environment too (Giddens, 2009). Those diagnosed tend to be treated with Ritalin, a drug that is actually a stimulant (Timimi, 2005).

There is no real evidence to support the effectiveness of Ritalin in treating ADHD and no medical tests available to help clinicians diagnose the condition either. It has been suggested that the increasing medicalization of Western society has made it impossible to disentangle the condition from the process of medicalization itself. In America some large-scale epidemiological studies have found that almost half of the children studied satisfied ADHD symptom criteria (Sharma, 2000). Consequently some commentators argue that it is a cultural problem, only diagnosed in the West because of the increasing pressure and stress placed upon children. ADHD is simply a cultural construct that is being presented as a biological fact (Timimi, 2005). ADHD is actually the result of children being exposed to fast-paced living, being overwhelmed by technology, not exercising enough and eating the wrong sorts of food high in fat and sugar content (Giddens, 2009).

So this medical condition is in fact a problem caused by cultural changes which have in turn become medicalized. This is supported by cross-cultural evidence in which medical practitioners view the same childhood behaviours in very different ways. Indeed, ADHD is not a recognized medical problem in many non-Western cultures. ADHD is therefore a specific cultural mechanism that allows people to deal with their growing anxieties about childhood within modern western societies, largely influenced by the macroeconomics of drug companies (Timimi, 2005).

Furthermore, anthropology has debated and discussed how these lay beliefs and approaches to health and illness are rooted within a complex web of knowledge and power. Biomedicine has dominated in the West. Lupton's (1994) book, *Medicine as Culture*, demonstrates this dominance and argues that both medicine and health care are culturally determined. Ultimately our health and health behaviours are socially determined by the culture in which we are located. Anthropological studies have shown that understanding cultural beliefs and interpretations about health and illness are crucial in beginning to explain non-adherence and non-compliance to certain treatments and indeed the choices that patients make when considering treatments. Finally, anthropological understandings show that health behaviours and practices are ultimately culturally embedded and so can be very difficult to modify, which has implications for health practitioners. For example, British lay beliefs about the MMR vaccination (the combined triple immunization of measles, mumps and rubella) being linked to autism (despite much scientific evidence refuting this) have led to a decline in the uptake of the vaccination, which has clear implications for population health. Anthropology can help us to understand such cultural beliefs and therefore may be of use in both managing and changing lay beliefs that oppose medical practice.

Summary

- Medical anthropology is a sub-discipline of social anthropology that demonstrates the importance of culture as a determinant of individuals' understandings and experiences of both illness and treatment.

- Medical anthropology, when critically analysing health, has strongly demonstrated that health is overwhelmingly social, with culture as a key determinant of health beliefs, behaviour and treatment.

- Anthropology shows that health and illness are culturally located and that key social and cultural meanings are associated with health.

Questions

1. Consider the ways in which you describe your experiences of health and illness: how does culture influence these? Are there any conditions that you have experienced that would not be diagnosed within another context?

2. Think about your attitudes to treatment. How much belief do you invest in the medical approach to treatment? Have you ever considered or tried alternative treatments?

3. Pay attention to the media, read newspapers and watch the news. When there are stories that touch upon health, how are these discussed? How are aspects of health culturally determined and discussed?

Further reading

Hahn, R. A. (1995) Sickness and Healing: An Anthropological Perspective. New Haven, Yale University Press.
How does culture influence the definition, experience and treatment of sickness in different societies? This book draws upon both anthropology and epidemiology to demonstrate cultural differences in experiences of sickness and to suggest that understanding these is key to resolving some of the problems of contemporary Western medicine.

Helman, C.G. (2007) Culture, Health and Illness. 5th edn. London, Hodder Arnold.

This is a comprehensive textbook detailing the importance of culture in determining health and illness experiences and behaviour. The book covers the main developments in the field of medical anthropology over recent years and so serves as a useful introduction to a student new to the field.

Lupton, D. (1994) Medicine as Culture. Illness, Disease and the Body in Western Societies. London, Sage.

This book gives a critical analysis of how Western medicine is both experienced and socially constructed. The book provides an overview of the major theoretical critiques of medicine, discusses power relationships and attitudes to medicine. Medicine as culture demonstrates an increasing Western dependence upon the biomedical model, changing expectations around medicine and people's lived experiences of medical interactions and treatment.

6 Health Psychology

> **Key learning outcomes**
>
> **By the end of this chapter you should be able to:**
>
> - understand and describe what health psychology is and how it is relevant to health
>
> - describe, apply and critique some of the key models in health psychology specifically relevant to health behaviour
>
> - appreciate a more critical perspective within health psychology

Overview

This chapter will introduce you to the discipline of health psychology and demonstrate the relevance of this to studying and understanding health and, more specifically, health behaviour. The chapter gives an introductory overview, outlining the specific focus of health psychology within the wider discipline of psychology and drawing on a range of relevant theory. The chapter concentrates on what health psychology has to offer in terms of understanding how people behave, the choices that they make with regard to their health and how this understanding can contribute to designing effective health promotion interventions (see chapter 7 on health promotion). An important theme running through the chapter is the complexity of health behaviour. At the end of the chapter there is an overview of critical health psychology that briefly outlines alternative perspectives and understandings on health behaviour.

Learning task 6.1

Reflective exercise.
Think about a time you tried to change your behaviour (this might be in relation to health or it might not). For example, you may have made a New Year's resolution to eat more healthily.

Reflect on the following:
(a) What made you decide to try to change your behaviour?
(b) What factors influenced this decision?
(c) What factors helped or hindered you in changing your behaviour?
(d) Have you managed to maintain the behaviour change?
(e) If not, what would you do differently next time?

What is health psychology?

As you may have appreciated from learning task 6.1, behaviour change is a complex process that is not simply about the knowledge someone has. There are many different factors involved. Psychology, specifically health psychology, can help us to understand what is involved in behaviour and behaviour change and therefore to design appropriate interventions in order to enable people to take control of their health with a view to maximizing health gain.

This chapter explores contemporary understandings in health psychology and the relevance/application of these to health studies. For some time now there has existed a plethora of evidence linking different types of behaviour to health and illness experience. The emergence of a range of chronic diseases in the most affluent global societies over the last century or so has, among other things, led to a clear link between certain types of behaviour and ill-health. For example, a smoking habit is now strongly linked to lung cancer and being obese is believed to be a risk factor in a range of different diseases. (Note that obesity is not a 'behaviour' itself but is influenced by a range of different behaviours that include patterns of eating and of physical activity.) You can probably think of other examples of this – take a moment to do so.

The focus on behaviours and health originates in the assumptions that behaviour is closely linked to health and that behaviour can be changed or modified in some way (in order to improve health). However, clearly it is not as simple as this, otherwise we wouldn't be facing the public health challenges we currently face (a range of contemporary threats to health are discussed in chapter 2). Health psychology can offer us insight into the way that people think and behave through the development of theory and through research. Health psychology is a branch of psychology specifically concerned with the study of mental processes and behaviour in relation to health and illness. The focus of this chapter will be on health rather than illness, concentrating on explanations and understandings of health behaviour and making healthy choices. As stated, health psychology can be described as a sub-discipline within psychology as a whole and it draws on knowledge from a range of other sub-disciplines within psychology as well as non-psychological disciplines such as medicine and sociology for example (Sarafino, 2002). It is a relatively new area within psychology, having emerged as a discrete branch of psychology only within the last few decades. While maintaining a specific and separate identity, health psychology draws on aspects of other disciplines, including types of research methods (chapter 3 discusses research methods and their importance in relation to health).

Health behaviour

So, if, among other things, health psychology is necessarily concerned with health behaviour, we need to explore what we mean by this. Some would argue that health behaviour is any behaviour that impacts on health in some way. Some also use this term specifically to refer to behaviours that are undertaken to *improve or maintain* health (Straub, 2007). Sometimes the term 'health-related' behaviour is used in the literature so there is some diversity in the use of terms. For this reason this chapter will use the generic term 'health behaviour' to acknowledge the fact that there are very few behaviours that don't impact on health in some way, if we think about health more holistically (see discussion in chapter 1). Straub makes this point very well in the following quote: 'it is difficult to imagine an activity or behaviour that does not influence health in some way – for better or worse, directly or indirectly, immediately or over the long-term' (p. 155). Take a moment to try to think of a behaviour that does not impact on health in some way – there are very few, if any, when health is viewed in a holistic way.

Health behaviour can be distinguished in different ways. Sarafino (2002) specifically identifies *health-protective* behaviour, which refers to any behaviour that protects health status. Examples of this might be wearing seatbelts – can you think of any others? Health behaviours may have a negative or positive impact on health and the judgement of this often depends on the perspective of the person engaged in the behaviour, or of the person observing it, as well as subjective ideas about health and levels of health-related knowledge or understanding.

At the time of writing there is increasing focus in UK health policy on behaviour at an individual level and the role that this plays in addressing short-term and long-term public health issues. Contemporary lifestyles are characterized by certain ways of living and we have seen significant changes in lifestyle patterns associated with developments over time in technology and innovation. For example,

Learning task 6.2

Lifestyle factors.
(a) Make a list of the types of behaviour that might be considered 'lifestyle' factors. To do this you can reflect on your own lifestyle and you may also want to reflect on the lifestyles of the people you come into contact with on a day-to-day basis.
(b) Divide the list into two types of behaviour as follows:
   1. Behaviour that you think might enhance health
   2. Behaviour that you think might be risky to health (or compromise health)
(Bear in mind that some behaviour may legitimately be health-enhancing and risky/compromising to health given the holistic nature of it.)
(c) For each behaviour try to justify why you have decided whether it is health-enhancing or puts health at risk/compromises health (or both). What is the evidence for this?

there has been a general increase in sedentary habits (Marks et al., 2005), which includes less energy expenditure in the workplace and in leisure activities, and this has implications for health. Take a few minutes now to do learning task 6.2.

You have probably come up with a significant list of different types of behaviour attributed to lifestyle that impact on health in some way. It is likely to include things such as dietary choices, levels and type of physical activity, cigarette and alcohol use, etc. The focus on individual behaviour is borne out through the fact that 'ways' of living impact on health and there are a number of chronic diseases for which the largest risk factors are identified as being behavioural in nature (such as certain cancers, heart disease and stroke (Husbands, 2007)). Behaviour has therefore been identified as a key determinant of health (Marks et al., 2005). Other determinants of health are explored in more detail elsewhere in this book (for example in chapters 8 and 10).

Behaviours that promote or enhance health might be defined as those that have a positive impact on health in some way. In learning task 6.2 part (a) you will have produced a list of this type of behaviour. Some examples of health-enhancing behaviours are wearing a seatbelt, regular physical activity, eating healthily and taking up **screening** opportunities. There is empirical evidence to show that a certain set of behaviours *increase* health and longevity. One of the challenges in health promotion is encouraging people to take on or increase health-enhancing behaviours.

'Health-risk behaviours' (Straub, 2007) may be defined as any behaviour that has a negative impact on health, either directly or indirectly, or that may compromise health in some way. In learning task

6.2 part (b) you have produced a list of this type of behaviour. Some examples of health-risk behaviours are smoking, drinking excessive amounts of alcohol, unsafe sexual practices, lack of hand hygiene and eating a lot of foods with a high trans-fat content. These kinds of behaviours have been linked to both short-term and long-term health problems. There is empirical evidence to show that a certain set of behaviours *decrease* health and longevity.

An important point to make here is that a person can engage in both types of behaviour (even at the same time in some cases!). For example, a person might exercise regularly but also eat a high fat diet. In addition, there is clearly some overlap or crossover between health-enhancing and health-compromising behaviours that may depend on a person's beliefs or perspectives. For example, alcohol use may be perceived as beneficial to social and psychological health (raising confidence and self-esteem in social encounters) but has also been shown to be detrimental to physical and mental health if consumed in excess. Another example is smoking. Smoking is now known to be bad for a person's health; however, research has shown that smoking is sometimes used to deal with the stress and strain of everyday life, which could be argued to be a benefit to health, particularly mental health.

In addition, some 'high-risk' health behaviours carry with them a benefit to the person engaging in them. For example people who do adrenaline sports frequently report the fact that taking part in them gives them a buzz and makes them feel good. Consider the case study presented at the end of chapter 1 and at the end of this chapter for more examples of how certain types of behaviour may be seen as health-enhancing and health-compromising.

Different kinds of behaviour

There are several ways in which we might differentiate between different kinds of health behaviour. Hubley and Copeman (2008) provide a framework for differentiating types of behaviour, which is detailed in table 6.1.

We might also distinguish between health behaviour and illness behaviour (actions we take when we are already ill). However, as previously stated, the focus of this chapter is on health behaviour rather than illness behaviour.[1]

There are several different ways of explaining or accounting for why people behave in the way that they behave and why they make the choices that they make with regard to health. Theoretical frameworks and models can help us to further understanding about the processes and factors involved. Firstly let us consider 'determinants' of health behaviour – those things that influence how we behave.

---

[1] For more information on illness behaviour please see, for example, Hubley and Copeman (2008).

Table 6.1. Different types of behaviour (adapted from Hubley & Copeman, 2008).

Decision-based	A behaviour that results from a conscious decision-making process, such as deciding to stop smoking.
One-time	A behaviour which is likely only to be carried out once (or a few times), e.g. sterilization, vaccination.
Routine (Habit)	Something that people do on a regular basis such as teeth-cleaning (often without any conscious thought).
Addictive	Behaviour that is reinforced through biological or psychological dependency, such as smoking.
Custom (behavioural norm)	Behaviour shared by a group of people that reflects a cultural identity, such as specific dietary patterns.
Tradition	Behaviour passed down through generations over time, such as not eating certain foods.
Lifestyle	A set of behaviours that makes up a person's way of life, such as patterns of physical activity and diet.

(Note that the categories are not necessarily discreet and that certain types of behaviour may fall into more than one category).

Determinants of behaviour

This section will focus specifically on psychological determinants of health behaviour. Please see chapters 8 and 9 for more detailed consideration of other types of determinants of health and health behaviour.

Learning task 6.3

Determinants of health behaviour.

(a) Draw a spider diagram of all the things that you think influence health behaviour including as many different things as you can.

(b) When you have run out of ideas, try to spot any patterns or links between your ideas and see if you can group them in any way. For example, you might have listed several things that could be grouped together as being 'social' influences (peer pressure, parents, etc).

(c) When you have grouped the influences on health in some way highlight those that you have identified as being 'psychological' in nature.

One of the ways of understanding influences or determinants of health behaviour is to group them in the following way – those that are psychological in nature, those that are biological, those that are sociological and those that are cultural for example. For the purposes of this chapter we are only focusing on determinants that are identified as being 'psychological'. Sarafino (2002) offers a useful framework for understanding what health psychology is concerned with. He identifies three psychological factors impacting on mental processes and behaviour that are also important for health. In short, these factors are to do with what we *think* about things and why (*cognition*), what we *feel* about things and why (*emotion*) and why we *do* the things we do (*motivation*). All of these factors are important in understanding health behaviour.

Some of the central features of theoretical frameworks designed to provide an explanation of why people behave the way that they do in relation to health are reflected in these three factors. One of the key components of several different models is related to the first factor – *cognition* – and concerns *beliefs*. This part of the chapter will explore some of the theories having beliefs as a key component (also referred to as a 'variable') within them. These include the Health Belief Model, the Theory of Planned Behaviour and Protection Motivation Theory. Before each of these models are considered in turn two types of beliefs central to some behavioural theories will be discussed: self efficacy and beliefs about control.

Self efficacy

Bandura (1977, 1986) defines self efficacy as the belief that we can succeed at something we want to do (cited in Sarafino, 2002) – essentially it is to do with personal judgements about how successful we might be at doing something and is therefore linked with self-confidence. Self efficacy may be an important factor in health behaviour and determining levels of self efficacy may help to predict or understand it. For example it stands to reason that, if you believe you can do something you are more likely to (a) have a go at doing it, (b) follow it through and (c) succeed. People with a high level of self efficacy (strong beliefs in their ability to do something) tend to carry out behaviours that enhance their health, as compared with people with lower levels of self efficacy who tend to engage in behaviour more detrimental to health (Marks et al., 2005; Straub, 2007).

Beliefs about control

Beliefs (or perceptions) about control appear to be very important for health behaviour. Tones and Green (2004) distinguish between several different types of beliefs about control, including *behavourial control*, which they define as 'the possession of skills necessary for translating decisions into action' (p. 93) and which they see as being linked to *cognitive control*, which is to do with gaining knowledge and developing thinking strategies in order to manage different events.

General beliefs about control have been investigated using a construct called Locus of Control proposed by Rotter (1966, cited in Tones & Green, 2004: 93), which determines whether someone believes they are in control of their lives (termed 'internal' locus of control) or that someone (powerful other/s) or something (chance or fate) is in control of their lives. Wallston and Wallston (1982) have taken this idea further in relation to health and developed a health-related measure of personal control called the *Multi-Dimensional Health Locus of Control* scale that basically assesses people's feelings about personal control about their health. People with a high degree of *internal* control tend to believe that they, themselves, are in control of their health, people with a high degree of *external* control tend to believe that they have little control over their health and that their health is determined by factors lying outside their control such as fate or chance. People who score highly on the *powerful other's* dimension of the scale tend to believe that their health is in the hands of other people – usually health care professionals. Clearly where people attribute control in terms of health this will have implications for their health behaviour. For example, people with higher internal control tend to be more likely to adopt health-protecting behaviours than people who believe that their health is subject to the whims of fate or chance.

The Health Belief Model

The Health Belief Model (HBM) is a theoretical framework widely used to try to explain and predict a range of health-related behaviours. It was first developed in the 1960s by Rosenstock, was subsequently developed further by Becker and Rosenstock in the 1970s and 1980s and was originally designed to predict the likelihood that people would take up screening opportunities. It has since been widely applied to a range of other types of health behaviour (Hubley & Copeman, 2008), including smoking, drinking and sexual behaviour (Roberts, Towell & Golding, 2001).

Beliefs are central to the HBM, as indicated by its name. The model accounts for a range of beliefs related to health behaviour, including beliefs about susceptibility to illness and severity of illness (labelled *perceived threat*), beliefs about the benefits and barriers of carrying out a specific behaviour, beliefs about the ability to be able to do something (also called 'selfefficacy' – see later discussion in this chapter) and beliefs about the potential outcomes of a particular behaviour. The relationship of these different types of beliefs to the other variables in the HBM is illustrated in figure 6.1. The HBM seeks to predict the likelihood that someone will take a certain action depending on their assessment of different things according to their beliefs. Key to the HBM is the assumption that people engage in a logical, thoughtful decision-making process where they weigh up the advantages and disadvantages of taking action (i.e. changing their behaviour). For change to take place the positives must outweigh the negatives. This has been called the *cost-benefit analysis*. Models that propose this 'weighing up' process are also sometimes referred to as Value Expectancy Theories. (This underlying assumption has been criticized, however as it implies

Figure 6.1. The
Health Belief
Model.

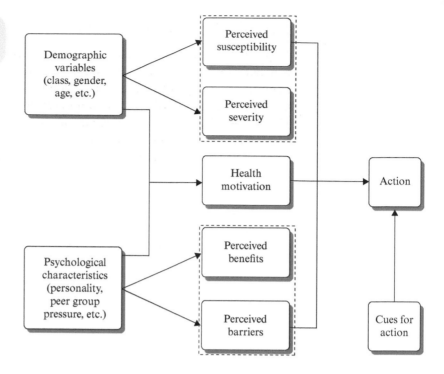

a conscious thought process that is not always present.) Finally the HBM suggests that 'cues to action' are needed to provoke action and that these might be 'internal' to the person concerned (such as experiencing symptoms of ill-health) or 'external', such as health education messages (Berry, 2007).

The HBM may help in predicting or explaining why someone's behaviour may change or not, but the research findings have not been consistent with regard to showing which components (or variables) of the model are the strongest predictors, and there have even been some conflicting findings.

Box 6.1

Application of the HBM to testicular self-examination (might also be applied in a similar way to breast self-examination).

According to the HBM, for a man to carry out Testicular Self-Examination (TSE) he must believe he is at risk of developing testicular cancer, believe that having testicular cancer is serious, believe that carrying out TSE is advantageous (for example, in terms of earlier detection and treatment) and not see carrying out TSE as too costly (for example, as being too inconvenient or embarrassing).

In addition, the HBM proposes that a 'cue to action' is required and this may be in the form of a health promotion message or a diagnosis of testicular cancer for a male relative or friend.

Research and the Health Belief Model

As previously stated, the HBM has been used in relation to a variety of health behaviours and the various variables within it have been examined in many different studies that aim to determine the degree to which the HBM predicts or accounts for health behaviour change. The degree of success has, unfortunately, been limited (Roberts et al., 2001) with evidence suggesting that the HBM accounts for some of the differences in health behaviour but by no means all (Tones & Green, 2004). One of the key difficulties has been that different studies have used different measures and so the predictive value of the HBM is less than it might otherwise be. Nevertheless there is a body of research that has used the HBM to determine the extent to which certain types of behaviour can be predicted and the specific factors involved.

Intentions are also central to different models seeking to provide explanatory accounts of health behaviour. In fact, the notion of intentions is so central that often the focus is on predicting or finding out about intentions to behave in a certain way rather than on the behavioural outcome itself. The Theory of Planned Behaviour and Protection Motivation Theory are examples of models in health psychology that include an 'intention' component as well as variables related to beliefs. Both models are concerned with what factors influence intentions to behave in a certain way. Let's start with the Theory of Planned Behaviour (TPB).

The Theory of Planned Behaviour

The Theory of Planned Behaviour (TPB) is an extension of the Theory of Reasoned Action (TRA) developed in the 1980s by Ajzen and Fishbein. The Theory of Reasoned Action proposes that behavioural intention originates from a combination of two variables – firstly, the 'attitude' that someone holds towards a particular behaviour and secondly, what that person thinks other people think about the behaviour and this includes their motivation to comply with what other people think. This second variable is called the 'subjective norm'.

The Theory of Planned Behaviour (TPB) is also a Value Expectancy Theory and, developed by Ajzen, it adds a third variable to the TRA proposing that behavioural intention results from a combination of attitude, subjective norm and 'perceived behavioural control'. As shown in figure 6.2 the underlying assumption of the TPB (and TRA) is that behavioural intention is then linked to an outcome of behaviour. Perceived behavioural control is seen by some (not everyone) as being the same as self-efficacy, as discussed earlier (see Roberts et al., 2001) and is essentially to do with the degree to which a person believes they are able to make a change to their behaviour. Beliefs about control are important factors in explaining and accounting for health behaviour.

Figure 6.2.
The Theory
of Planned
Behaviour.

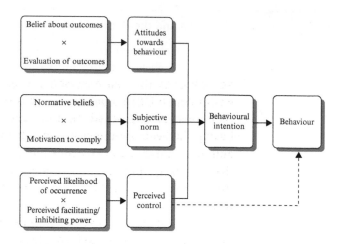

Research and the Theory of Planned Behaviour

Returning to the Theory of Planned Behaviour, there appears to be quite a lot of empirical support for the TPB and it has been used many times to try to predict a range of different health behaviours including physical activity, taking vitamins and using contraception (Berry, 2007). However, although some of the variations in health behaviour can be explained using this model, at best it seems only to be able to predict half of the variance in behavioural intentions and approximately one-quarter of the variance in actual behaviour, which leaves a lot of intention and behaviour unaccounted for. This has led to more recent criticism of it (see Albery & Munafó, 2008). Nevertheless the model is still widely used to investigate a variety of health behaviours, more so than many of the other models that have been developed, and it has been useful in establishing further understanding of a number of variables that influence health behaviour.[1]

Protection Motivation Theory (PMT)

As you will now see, the components (or variables) of Protection Motivation Theory (Rogers, 1975, 1983) reflect similarities with some components of both the Health Belief Model and the Theory of Planned Behaviour. PMT proposes that behavioural intention (intention to carry out a specific health behaviour) results from carrying out two types of appraisal – *threat appraisal*, which includes perceptions about severity and vulnerability and *coping appraisal*, including self-efficacy and beliefs about the effectiveness of a likely response. The motivation to take (protective) action results from carrying out the two different appraisals. A central feature of PMT not accounted

---

[1] For further detail about the application of the Theory of Planned Behaviour in research please see Conner and Norman (2005).

Box 6.2   Application of the Theory of Planned Behaviour to taking up yoga.

According to the TPB a person's intention to start doing yoga would depend on them having a positive attitude towards yoga (believing that it would be beneficial to them in some way), having the belief that they will be able to do yoga or learn to do it and believing that people who are important to them would think that this is appropriate and support them in some way. If all of these factors are in place then the intention to take up yoga will be strong.

The TPB proposes that the stronger the person's intention to take up yoga, the more likely that the person will actually do it (i.e. go to a yoga class, start working to a yoga video).

Theory of Planned Behaviour.

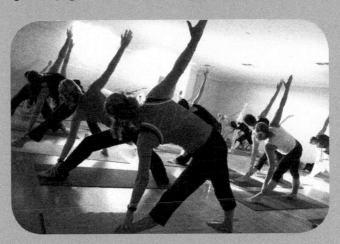

Box 6.3   Application of Protection Motivation Theory to condom use.

When applied to the issue of condom use, PMT proposes that the intention to use a condom results from a combination of a perception of threat to health (from, in this example, vulnerability to sexually transmitted infection) and the confidence the person has (for example, in being able to use a condom, which may be in relation to whether they know how to use one correctly, or whether they have the confidence that they can negotiate condom use during the sexual encounter and how successful this would be in protecting their health).

In this case an *adaptive response* would be using a condom while a *maladaptive response* would be not using a condom.

for in the previous models we have looked at is the role that *fear* plays in determining health behaviour. Therefore, PMT is relevant to situations where a person may be fearful for their health (Roberts et al., 2001). According to PMT an appraisal may result in two different types of responses – an *adaptive* response or a *maladaptive* response. Maladaptive responses may include avoidance, denial, wishful thinking (Norman et al., 2005) or fatalism and hopelessness (Milne et al., 2000). Similarly to TPB the PMT does not really provide a clear or satisfactory explanation of the link between behavioural intention (what we intend to do) and behavioural outcome (whether we actually do it!).[1]

The Stages of Change Model

The Stages of Change Model is also sometimes referred to as the Trans Theoretical Model because it includes factors developed in other theories (Sarafino, 2002). However, for the purposes of this chapter it will be referred to as the Stages of Change model (SCM). The SCM provides a descriptive account of the process of behaviour change and suggests that people move through five stages starting in pre-contemplation, moving to contemplation, then to preparation, action and, finally, maintenance.

The nature of each stage is perhaps self-evident from the label; nevertheless box 6.4 describes the model with reference to reducing the intake of high fat foods.

The key assumption underpinning the SCM is that a person will present in different ways depending on where they are in the process of change. Application of the SCM in practice means that the framework can be used as a mechanism for determining someone's 'readiness to change' and interventions may be designed accordingly. For example, someone in the contemplation stage may need support to move into action. Despite originally being developed with specific reference to addiction, the SCM has been influential in a range of health behaviours. The SCM is distinguishable from the other models we have looked at so far because it provides more of a *description* than an *explanation* of behaviour change processes. Some people have therefore criticized it and maintain that it is neither a model nor a theory since it lacks theoretical constructs (see Roberts et al., 2001). However, it is a useful, and frequently used, framework, which can be used to determine where a person is at with regard to changing their behaviour.[2]

---

[1] For a detailed overview of Protection Motivation Theory using meta-analysis please see Milne et al. (2000).

[2] For a more in-depth account of the Stages of Change Model please see Bunton et al. (2000).

Box 6.4

Application of the Stages of Change Model to changing eating behaviour (reducing intake of high fat foods).

Pre-Contemplation
The person would not be interested in changing behaviour, would not consider their consumption of high fat foods to be problematic and would not want to change their diet.

Contemplation
The person may be interested in changing their diet and eating fewer high-fat foods or thinking about doing so.

Preparation
The person is ready to change behaviour and to have a go at trying to change their diet. They might engage in preparatory action such as getting rid of high fat foods from their store cupboards and fridge or telling their family that they are going to change their diet or learning about how to cook foods that are lower in fat.

Action
The person puts their plans into action and starts to eat a diet which is lower in fat. They have a go at changing their behaviour.

Maintenance
The new way of eating is becomes a part of the person's everyday life.

The SCM also accounts for relapse, which is where a person may return to their previous patterns of behaviour – in this case it'd be eating a lot of high fat foods on a regular basis. This may be temporary and the person may start to move through the cycle again at some point, or it may be permanent.

Critiques of theory

While the models we have considered have provided some useful insights into why people behave in certain ways and developed understandings/driven research, they are not without their limitations. Before you read any further take some time out to do learning task 6.4 as detailed above.

As you will now be aware, none of the models we have considered are able to account for all of the complexity of health behaviour. Each of the models could usefully be criticized individually; however, for the purposes of this chapter, a general critique of the theories is offered in table 6.2. Each criticism is relevant to all of the models discussed in this chapter.

Clearly so far there is not one model that can provide a full

Learning task 6.4

Limitations of models of behaviour change.
So far this chapter has examined a range of specific models of behaviour change in some detail. While the models can contribute to understanding health behaviour they have all been criticized for different reasons.

(a) Take some time out to think about the limitations and short-comings of each model in terms of how they explain, or account for, health behaviour. You may find it useful to refer back to your ideas in the previous learning tasks.
(b) To what extent do the models provide a good explanation for your own experience of trying to change your behaviour detailed in learning task 6.1?
(c) To what extent do they account for all the influences on health behaviour that you identified in learning task 6.3?

explanation for the complexity of health behaviour. The Health Action Model (Tones & Tilford, 2001) offers perhaps a more comprehensive theoretical framework drawing, as it does, on several aspects of the models we have already considered in this chapter.

Health Action Model

The HAM was developed by Tones in the early 1970s (Tones & Green, 2004) to try to include all the major factors that influence health behaviour. You will recognize some of the key variables and components from the other models we have considered reflected in the HAM. It consists of two key sections – one that considers factors influencing 'behavioural intention' and one that considers factors influencing whether an intention will translate into action. (You will recall that this is where some of the models we considered previously have failed to provide an adequate explanation.) The model is rather complex – perhaps necessarily so since it is trying to accomplish many things.

We'll start by looking at the first section in some detail – the one that considers factors that influence behavioural intention. The model proposes that behavioural intention is influenced by a range of interacting factors and suggest that three different systems interact with each other to produce behavioural intention. These are (1) the *belief* system that concerns *cognition* (what we think and believe), (2) the *motivation* system that concerns *affect* (how we feel) and (3) the *normative* system that takes into account social influences on behavioural intention – for example, what other people may think about what we do (note the link with 'subjective norm' in the TPB).

Table 6.2. General critiques of behaviour change models in health psychology.

The models tend to . . .

- Focus at the individual level and not on the wider determinants of health (social, political, environmental, etc.) and so they tend not to account for factors outside the individual that influence behaviour
- Put the emphasis on the individual (called a 'reductionist' approach) (Bunton et al., 2000) and 'objectify' human experience, which goes against a holistic approach (Tones & Green, 2004)
- Promote individualism and individual responsibility for health (Airhihenbuwa & Obregon, 2000)
- View individual actions or behaviour in isolation from the actions or behaviour of others (Hubley & Copeman, 2008) neglecting to consider social influences.

They tend to neglect the role of . . .

- Past behaviour and habit (Sarafino, 2002; Albery & Munafò, 2008; Thirlaway & Upton, 2009)
- Affect ('emotion') (Roberts et al., 2001; Lawton et al., 2009)
- Culture and cultural context (Lin et al., 2005).

They tend to neglect the fact that . . .

- Processes of behaviour change take time and significant change cannot take place over a short period of time (Ramos & Perkins, 2006) and they also over-simplify processes of behaviour change (Abraham & Sheeran, 2005; Berry, 2007).

In terms of research a number of difficulties have been highlighted including . . .

- Problems defining individual constructs (Bunton et al., 2002)
- Limited predictive utility (Abraham & Sheeran, 2005)
- A weak relationship between intention and behaviour – Stephens (2008) argues that other factors should be explored i.e. environmental factors
- A lack of standardization across constructs in experimental design (Conner & Norman, 2005). It is difficult to compare the results of studies that 'test' out the theories because they often use different methods and inconsistent ways of measuring the different components of the models
- They tend to have been developed in specific contexts, which can lead to a 'Western', patriarchal bias
- Much of the research using the models relies on self-report measures that have limitations.
- Whilst many of the models draw upon aspects of sociological, psychological and anthropological theory they tend to neglect political and economic theory (Hubley & Copeman, 2008).

The second section of the HAM attempts to provide a framework for considering how behavioural intention may be translated into actual action (or not!) and what factors influence this process. It identifies a range of 'facilitating' factors that may help

Figure 6.3. The
Health Action
Model.

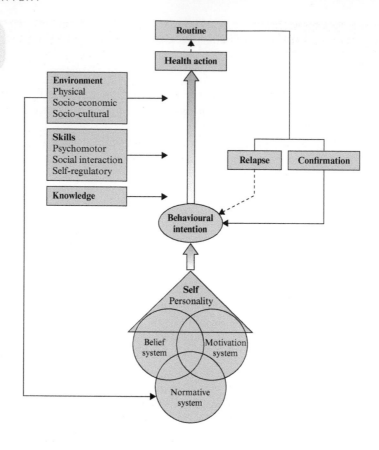

to enable behaviour change. These include a supportive environment, skills and knowledge. However, it should be noted that these
same facilitating factors might also inhibit or discourage behaviour change. For example, a lack of skills and/or knowledge or an
unsupportive environment may hinder behaviour change rather than
helping it to happen. A useful feature of the HAM is that it might be
used to account for (explain) different types of health behaviour such
as single time behaviours and routine behaviours (Tones & Green,
2004).

How is health psychology important?

Among others, Hubley and Copeman (2008) argue that understanding human behaviour is critical to promoting health. We need to at
least attempt to understand why people do the things they do in order
to facilitate change for better health. While this necessarily includes
taking into account the panopoly of wider factors that impact on health
behaviour there is an argument for focusing at an individual level given
the influence that behaviour can have on health outcomes (see chapter
8). There is also significant evidence to suggest that lifestyle interventions can be successful in promoting behaviour change at an individual
level (for example, see Kitzmann et al., 2010). Understanding the

Case study

The practice of sunbathing and using sunbeds.

Concern for appearance (looking tanned) has been shown to be directly linked to increased sunbathing behaviour even when the threat of developing skin cancer is perceived to be a real one (McMath & Prentice-Dunn, 2005). 'Risky' behaviour is maintained, despite the threat because, firstly, the threat is considered to be controllable (read treatable) and, secondly, because some get a lot of pleasure from sunbathing and from having a tan.

Research carried out in America by Geller et al. (2002) examining sunscreen use, sun burning and tanning bed use and the psychosocial variables associated with tan seeking behaviours found that girls are more likely than boys to use sunbeds and that older girls were more likely to than younger girls. The study also found that a preference for tanned skin, having friends who were tanned and the belief in the value of having a tan had an impact on behaviour (infrequent sunscreen use, more frequent burning and increased use of sunbeds).

Sunbathing and sunbed use is a good example of a behaviour which impacts on health in both enhancing and compromising ways. Using sunbeds has been shown to increase the risk of developing skin cancer (Cox et al., 2009). However, people who use sunbeds have reported benefits that can be viewed as enhancing health from a psychological or emotional perspective (increasing feelings of well-being and 'feeling' more healthy).

Sunbed use is a complex behaviour which contributes to a feeling of well-being while damaging health in other ways.

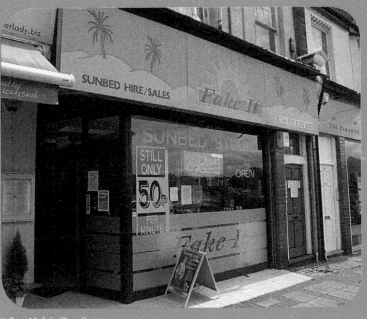

© Ben Melvin/Rex Features

components and processes involved in health behaviour can assist in designing health promotion interventions that have a greater chance of success (Trifiletti et al., 2005; Parker et al., 2004 and NICE, 2006). Tones and Green (2004: 3) argue that 'there is nothing so practical as good theory' and so theory can influence and inform how we implement and evaluate strategies to maximize health, giving us something to work with.

Critical perspectives

Critical health psychology is a specific domain in health psychology in which, among other things, the very notion of 'health behaviour' is challenged. Behaviour is therefore sometimes referred to as 'practices' or 'actions' although these terms (similarly to the way that the term 'health behaviour' has been used in this chapter) also provide a description of specific things that people *do* (Hubley & Copeman, 2008). Critical health psychology is a critical approach to health psychology. It challenges and, as its name suggests, critiques mainstream assumptions and understandings. Marks (2002) argues that the context of social, political and economic forces must also be taken into account and that action to change society must be political. 'It is about influence, power, economics and wealth – its distribution and use' (Marks, 2002: 7).

Summary

- Health psychology is a sub-discipline within psychology that can help us to understand how and why people behave in the ways that they do and make the choices they make in relation to health.

- Health behaviour is complex and influenced by many different factors.

- Models of behaviour change can help in designing interventions to enable people to change their health behaviour.

- Critical health psychology offers an alternative perspective.

Questions

1. Think about the different types of 'health' behaviour discussed in this chapter. Which of these do you think is most influential in terms of long-term health experience and why?

2. How much of your own health is affected by your behaviour? What are the limits of focusing on behaviour as the primary influence on your health experience?

3. Drawing on the contents of this chapter and the explanations for health behaviour what strategies do you think would be most effective in encouraging people to take up healthier practices and why?

Further reading

Abraham, C., Conner, M., Jones, F. and O'Connor, D. (2008) Health Psychology. London, Hodder Education.
This is a useful text that focuses on the application of health psychology to different topics including stress, coping, motivation and behaviour. Part of a series of textbooks on Applied Psychology, this

book provides an overview of the key debates and issues in health psychology research and practice. It is an ideal text to read for further understanding in this area.

Marks, D.F., Murray, M., Evans, B., Willig, C., Woodall C. and Sykes, C. (2005) Health Psychology: Theory, Research and Practice. 2nd edn. London, Sage.

This is a comprehensive, weighty textbook that provides a detailed introduction to health psychology. It covers a range of issues in health psychology and usefully explores the contribution of qualitative and quantitative research to the discipline. In addition it focuses on the application of theory to practice within an inter and multi-disciplinary context.

Murray, M., ed. (2004) Critical Health Psychology. Basingstoke, Palgrave Macmillan.

This is a very useful and interesting edited volume that outlines critical approaches to health psychology and challenges key ideas within mainstream health psychology. It provides a very good overview of contemporary debates that highlight the potential limitations of more traditional approaches within the discipline of health psychology and psychology more generally.

7 Health Promotion

Key learning outcomes

By the end of this chapter you should be able to:

- understand the contested scope and nature of health promotion
- appreciate the value base for health promotion and why values are important for practice
- understand how health promotion practice shapes strategies for health improvement

Overview

This chapter outlines the contested nature of what health promotion is and the scope of approaches that health promotion practitioners can use in their practice. Distinctions and similarities about the origins of both public health and health promotion are described early in the chapter to help readers untangle these frequently interchanged terms. Five frameworks outlining the nature of health promotion are described and examples are used to illustrate the conceptual ideas encompassed within the process of health promotion. Seven principles that underpin health promotion theory and practice have been selected for discussion in order for practitioners to review strategies for health improvement and enhancement. Within the chapter four learning tasks are used to help the reader develop and consolidate understanding of the health promotion approaches and values. Finally, some common criticisms levelled at health promotion are highlighted and countered. A case study at the end of the chapter synthesizes a strategy for addressing domestic violence using Caplan and Holland's model of health promotion as a framework.

What is health promotion?

Health promotion, for many, conjures up notions of media campaigns, handing out leaflets and generally informing people about the do's and don'ts of health-related lifestyle behaviour. However, the scope and diversity of health promotion is much more complex than these simplistic ideas that dominate the public consciousness about a much maligned discipline and practice. Before we consider the academic scope of health promotion it is important to understand what your own perspectives of health promotion may be. Undertake the following learning task.

Learning task 7.1

What do you think health promotion is?

Examine the following activities

- Regulation by local council to reduce the number of fast food outlets
- Traffic-light labels on food
- Practice nurses giving information about how to manage weight
- Food produced in local allotments used in a café staffed by community members
- Soap opera storylines about domestic violence
- Community safety schemes e.g. neighbourhood watch
- Local people protesting about the closure of a specialist centre for cancer
- Setting a minimum wage
- Local authority maintaining local parks and recreation services
- Youth workers setting up dance and boxing clubs in a community centre
- Campaign about drinking and driving
- Higher taxation for individuals earning over £100 000

1. Which would you classify as health promotion?
2. Why did you think this?
3. If you had limited resources, which 3 would you invest in?
4. What shaped your decisions?

After your exploration of this task you will have seen how many activities can be classified as health promotion. Answering 'what is a health promotion?' is more complex that you may recognize. In the next sections we debate where health promotion has come from, together with its scope and nature, by making reference to models of health promotion.

Origins of health promotion

It is important to examine the origins of health promotion in a UK context, so that the contemporary use of this term can be understood. Health promotion is a term often associated, and sometimes interchanged with the term public health. While there is perceived conflict in values and practice between the two, the origins of the two are often in parallel and intertwined. Notions of what Webster and French (2002: 5) refer to as 'co-ordinated community action to ensure a better life' have existed for millennia and represent the ideals of both public health and health promotion. The first public health manifesto developed in Manchester in 1796 as a result of the negative effects of the industrial revolution upon the workforce, acknowledged the root causes of ill-health were determined by social and economic factors rather than biological factors (Maltby, 1918 cited in Webster & French 2002). This is a key feature of the social model of health already discussed in chapters 1 and 4 and one that is especially important when considering what public health and health promotion are. Over time, public health has been categorized in distinct phases that have shaped our perceptions of health promotion and public health today (Hanlon et al., nd). The sanitary phase of 1840 onwards concentrated on environmental engineering to provide clean water and sewerage, improve housing and working conditions. The personal hygiene phase of 1910 onwards (in which health education emerged) emphasized the education of populations about their cleanliness, personal behaviour and therefore responsibility for their own ill-health and health. This provided a springboard for the development of the health education movement and its legacy that we still see today. The Central Council for Health Education was founded in 1927. In parallel, public health departments were located within local authorities where, arguably, they could tackle the environmental and social determinants of health. However, there were also signs of social movements that underpinned the development of health promotion such as the National Unemployed Workers Movement and the Committee against Malnutrition (Lewis, 1991 cited in Webster & French, 2002).

The therapeutic phase (1930 onwards) was characterized by the medicalization of public health and strongly associated with the prevention of ill-health through bio-medical interventions such as vaccination and treatment of ill-health through use of antibiotics. The foundation of the NHS in 1948 reduced the importance of public health and attached even greater value on treatment and care rather than primary prevention, which still resonates in the public consciousness today. The 'new public health' phase (1970s onwards) was an attempt to revitalize the stagnated public health and health promotion professions and respond to the key issues of the day such as widening health inequalities and increasing costs of health care provision in an ageing

> **Box 7.1**   **Common features of new public health and health promotion (Kickbusch, 2003).**
>
> - Commitment to tackling the wider socio-economic and environmental determinants of ill-health (and health).
> - Health has the potential to be created in many sectors, for example education, local government, housing, industry, agriculture, transport as well as health.
> - Focus on individual (although this is contested in public health circles) and population health.
> - **Healthy Public Policy** – all areas of government should be committed to developing policies that create good health (see chapter 11).
> - Inequalities in the health experience are reduced (see chapter 3).

society. This phase saw a return to some of the principles (see box 7.1) of earlier phases and re-emphasizing the importance of drawing on these principles when developing strategies for health improvement and enhancement.

The implications of the complex origins of health promotion and public health are important for several reasons. Firstly, dominance of public health practice by public health medics permeates the UK strategy. Webster and French (2002: 11) argue this is related to the 'assault by the medical profession' to regain the power that was relinquished to health care. Secondly, this affects the type of work that is done for health improvement. Public health is located alongside biomedical approaches to health rather than being structurally aligned to addressing the socio-economic and environmental determinants of health. However, when the historical roots of health promotion are examined it is of no surprise that health promotion is often characterized as only about health education rather than a much broader set of approaches. Thirdly, the health promotion workforce has largely been rebranded as public health within primary care trusts, although the pockets of specialized health promotion service still exist (White, 2009). Consider for example the name of the white paper that makes no reference to health promotion but only to public health; *Healthy Lives, Healthy People: Our Strategy for Public Health in England* (Department of Health, 2010). Lastly, the incoming coalition government continues to threaten both public health and health promotion and plans to return to a model of lifestyle regulation we saw in the personal hygiene phase of 1910 onwards rather than a focus on tackling the social and economic determinants of health (Lansley, 2010). The term health promotion has a more global acceptance and is widely enshrined in the focus of World Health Organization, the global authority coordinating the provision of leadership on global health matters within the United Nations system.

These origins shape our understanding of what health promotion is, where it should be located, i.e. the NHS or local authority, and the nature of how health issues are addressed. In the next section we continue to discuss what health promotion is by drawing on different models of health promotion, outlining the different approaches that can be used.

Tools for understanding health promotion

Models can be a practical way to help us understand phenomena, and analyse what we know, how things fits together and can provide a catalyst to shape approaches about new ideas and ways of working.

A model can be defined as: 'a schematic description of a system, theory, or phenomenon that accounts for its known or inferred properties and may be used for further study of its characteristics' (Free Dictionary, 2009). A good model will provide descriptions of how elements are related and will attempt to provide theoretical understanding. Rawson (2002) defines different types of models in table 7.1.

There are many different types of models and approaches that have been developed to underpin health promotion philosophy and practice. Five different frameworks are discussed below. Each is described and then applied to practice using examples to aid understanding.

Table 7.1. Different types of models.

Iconic model – simple representations of what something looks like in reality and often translates well to practical situations	e.g. Naidoo and Wills (2000) typology of health promotion contains five approaches.
Analogic models – tend to be underpinned by theoretical ideas and are not always based on what currently exists.	e.g. Beattie's (1991) Caplan & Holland (1990)

Tannahill's (1985) model

Tannahill developed his model to act 'as a unifying construct' in order to counter what he saw at the time as **semantic** debates that placed health promotion and prevention of ill-health as separate entities. (Tannahill, 2009: 396). He intended it to be useful for 'planning and doing health promotion'.

The model has three overlapping spheres of activity (Downie, Tannahill & Tannahill, 1996) (see figure 7.1). Prevention – preventive activities are designed to reduce or avoid risks of diseases and ill-health. We can consider preventive services such as vaccination for measles, mumps and rubella. In addition, the overlapping spheres produce preventive health education; examples of this include smoking cessation advice and skills and preventive health protection; examples include legislation to limit tobacco smoking in public places.

Figure 7.1.
Tannahill's
model of health
promotion
(adapted from
Tannahill,1985).

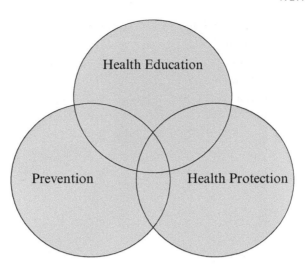

Figure 7.1. Tannahill's model of health promotion (adapted from Tannahill,1985).

Health Education involves communication to enhance health and well-being and prevent ill-health influencing beliefs, knowledge and attitudes. Enshrined in this is the notion of positive health (see chapter 1). An example of health education is developing life skills such as assertiveness, so that young women can negotiate safer sex with their partner. In addition to preventive health education outlined above, health education also overlaps with health protection to produce 'education for positive protection' such as developing skills in lobbying for legislative action e.g. lobbying and demonstration against cuts to child benefits or increasing university fees.

Protection – involves safeguarding populations through legislative, fiscal or social measures. This is rather different now that the term health protection has been appropriated in some circles to mean control of infections and environmental health (Health Protection Agency, 2010). An example of such protection is health and safety legislation at work. The overlapping segments for health protection have already been discussed above.

There are criticisms of this model in that it is not explicitly theoretically derived and is no more than 'simplistic linguistic juggling' (Rawson, 1992: 207). However, Tannahill intended it to be practical for different elements of the workforce to see that they were doing health promotion and contends that this model has facilitated health practitioners, of all types, to consider broadening the scope of their activities rather than simply giving people health-related information.

Beattie's (1991) model

Beattie's 1991 model of health promotion (cited in Naidoo & Wills, 2009) is one of the most widely cited models underpinning health promotion practice. It uses a quadrant structure (see figure 7.2) but considers the mode of action on a continuum. At one end initia-

The passing of legislation to limit smoking in public places is a good example of preventive health protection.

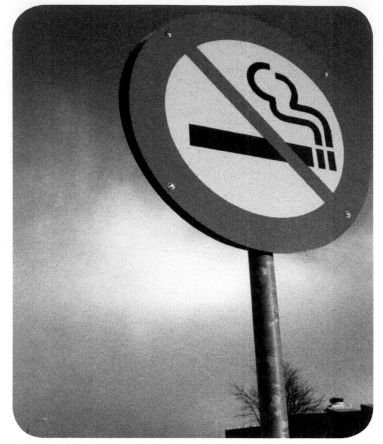

© Kent Rosengaard

tives being imposed (top down) in an authoritarian manner and compared to more autonomous, client-led, bottom-up and negotiated at the other. This continuum refers to a central paradox within health promotion about whether health-related behaviour should be regulated and enforced by authority structures and legislation or whether health-related behaviour should be owned and negotiated by individuals with good information to support decisions about behaviour (see chapter 6 for further discussion about health-related behaviour change). The other continuum refers to the mode of intervention and whether activities are collective (shared between groups or populations of people) or focused on individuals and small groups.

Each quadrant of the model equates to four different approaches within health promotion and these have been applied to alcohol use in order to promote understanding of the model. 'Health persuasion' utilizes action that is aimed at individuals and is led by practitioners. An example is a clinician giving advice about the problems of drinking to excess to a young person who has attended Accident and Emergency after a night out with friends.

Figure
7.2. Beattie's
model of health
promotion
(adapted from
Naidoo & Wills,
2009).

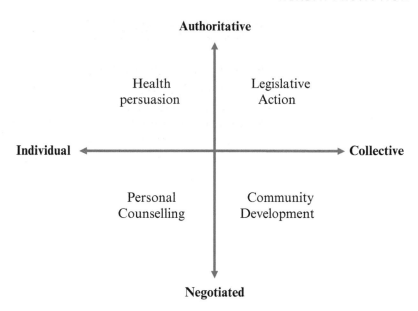

'Personal counselling' is also aimed at individuals but issues are client-defined, client-led, and focus on personal development. An example may be a young person working with a practitioner who feels that they are drinking too much as it relieves the boredom of not being able to get a job. The practitioner may facilitate the young person in developing skills and opportunities for work, or volunteering opportunities that can contribute to work experience.

'Legislative action' includes activities such as social and other policies and is imposed on populations. Examples related to alcohol can include changes in the licensing laws such as bars and supermarkets being able to apply to sell alcohol for longer periods up to 24 hours. This is an attempt to prevent violence and anti-social behaviour when crowds leave venues at the same time under stricter licenses.

'Community development' approaches are linked to empowerment and communities that take action for themselves in addressing health and the wider determinants of health. Community development has been defined as 'action that helps people to recognize and develop their ability and potential and organize themselves to respond to problems and needs that they share' (Scottish Community Development Centre, 2010). An example of community development related to alcohol, is that of the residents of Mill Road in Cambridge, who successfully lobbied the local council not to grant a licence to Tesco to sell alcohol in their area (The No to Mill Road Tesco Campaign, 2010). Community development has also led to successful community initiatives to tackle anti-social behaviour in young people by encouraging other forms of activities to relieve boredom, such as community clubs owned and governed by young people themselves. There are many links here to social capital, as discussed in chapter 9.

Learning task 7.2

Applying Beattie's model of health promotion.

1. Examine all the activities listed in learning task 7.1, for example setting a minimum wage.
2. Using Beattie's model of health promotion, match the differing activities with strategies listed. Where would setting a minimum wage be located within the Beattie model?

- Community development
- Legislative action and policy
- Health persuasion
- Personal counselling

Beattie's model suggests that in addressing a health issue all the four approaches should be used to form a coherent strategy (Stewart & Thomas, 2004). It is evident that not all determinants of alcohol use can be tackled by using a single approach; but if the model is applied, it is more likely that a greater range of social, environmental and economic determinants will be addressed. By completing learning task 7.2 you should be able to understand what health promotion activities fit within each approach stated with Beattie's model

Naidoo and Wills's (2000) typology

This model outlines five different types of health promotion activity.

(a)   Medical preventive approaches are characterized by differing levels of prevention (box 7.2). Primary prevention focuses on population and individual screening and vaccination activities.

(b)   Behaviour change approaches encourage individuals to analyse and change their attitudes so that they can adopt healthier behaviour. These healthy behaviours are generally defined by practitioners. The main examples of this approach are media campaigns to, for instance, encourage no drinking when driving and a social desirability that people should not drink when driving.

(c)   Educational approaches are somewhat similar to behavioural approaches but differ in that they seek only to provide information and skills in order for people to have accurate information and the capacity to change should they want to. It places choice at the heart of the approach. In theory, if people have accurate appropriate information that they understand and also have a set of skills in order to act, then they can decide autonomously whether to continue to smoke or eat fatty food. This means that they have control over their life. This assumes that individuals have free choice and that the social, economic and environmental determinants do not limit choice and action (see chapters 4 and 6 for further discussion about the determinants of health).

(d)   Empowerment approaches. Empowerment is a complex idea but is generally regarded as an approach that facilitates people working together to increase the control that they have over events that influence their lives and health (Woodall et al., 2010) Empowerment can also exist on an individual level when people feel they have control of their own lives and health (again there are links to chapter 9, social support and social capital). Activities where individuals develop capacity and skills such as better coping mechanisms, skills in getting on with other people, or how to manage a budget in tight financial situations could be related to the generation of empowerment.

The second type of empowerment is at a community level. Community empowerment is 'social-action process that promotes the participation of people, organizations and communities towards the goals of increased individual and community control, political efficacy, improved quality of life and social justice. (Wallerstein, 1992: 198). This is more akin to ideas related to social capital (see chapter 9) and to methods such as community development outlined previously in the Beattie model sub-section. In this approach communities work together to identify their own needs and work collectively to address them with the support of practitioners.

(e)   Social change approaches. The goal of social change approaches are to influence positively the physical, social, economic environment in which people live, work and play. These approaches are generally at a policy level and methods of practice relate to lobbying for policy change, policy development and implementation. Redistributive taxation of the wealthy at a higher rate to support the more vulnerable members of society is an example of a social change approach.

Box 7.2   **Levels of prevention (Green & Tones, 2010: 72).**

1.   Primary prevention involves preventing disease by reduction in exposure to risk factors e.g. the use of statins to reduce blood cholesterol levels.

2.   Secondary prevention focuses on early diagnosis to reduce progression of disease e.g. breast cancer screening.

3.   Tertiary prevention seeking to reduce consequences of illness such as rehabilitation programmes or pain relief for people who have experienced heart attacks.

4.   Primordial prevention emergence of social economic and cultural patterns of disease in already healthy cultures.

Learning task 7.3

Behaviour change campaigns.

Examine these short films at the National Archive for public information films as examples of behavioural approaches.

Gimme Five -5 a day

http://www.nationalarchives.gov.uk/films/1979to2006/film page_gimme.htm

Stupid Git John Altman – drink driving campaign

http://www.nationalarchives.gov.uk/films/1979to2006/film page_stupid.htm

Mental health interview

http://www.nationalarchives.gov.uk/films/1979to2006/film page_interview.htm

1.   What is the central message of the clip?
2.   What was your emotional response?
3.   How effective do you think it would be in changing yours or others' behaviour?
4.   Why?

By completing learning task 7.3 this will help you think about how successful behavioural approaches are within the full range of health promotion approaches. This also relates to chapter 6 on health psychology.

Tones and Tilford's (1994) empowerment model

This model brings attempts to synthesize several concepts and is at its heart concerned with empowerment and the goal of enabling people to have control of their own health (Tones & Tilford, 1994). The model contends that there are two major approaches that can be used to underpin health promotion practice and influence health (see figure 7.3). Firstly, health education can raise the critical consciousness of issues within the public's psyche leading to public pressure to influence healthy public policy. A good example of this was the Jamie's School Dinners campaign. Its continued presence in the media and associated pressure on the government ensured that spending per meal on school dinners was increased from 40p to 70p (Morgan, 2006). However, it could be argued that the media focus on food neglected necessary attention on physical activity. Education can influence the agenda setting for healthy public policy. The media and activists can educate politicians and councillors in positions of power to set health agendas.

Health education can lead to individuals having greater control over

The Jamie's School Dinners campaign is a good example of the empowerment model of health promotion.

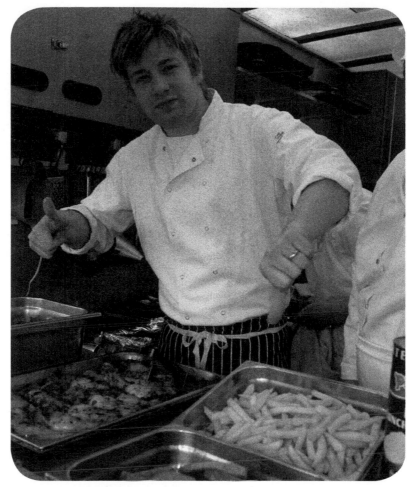

© Julian Makey/Rex Features

their own health (empowerment) by having accurate information and skills in order to make judgements and the capacity to govern their life, health and health-related behaviour. A further mechanism of educative action can change practice within health services to more health promoting activities, for example primary prevention work rather than treatment and cure.

Secondly, the model asserts that healthy public policy is a major approach that can address the wider socio-economic and environmental determinants that shape our health. Healthy public policy is defined as 'an explicit concern for health and **equity** in all areas of policy and an accountability for health impact' (Nutbeam, 1998: 13). A number of healthy public policies cuts across all government departments including the Home Office, which influences public safety and crime, the Treasury, which regulates taxation and has the potential to produce wealth redistribution policies to reduce income inequalities to improve health to the Department for Environment, Food and Rural Affairs, which co-ordinates policy concerning climate change and production

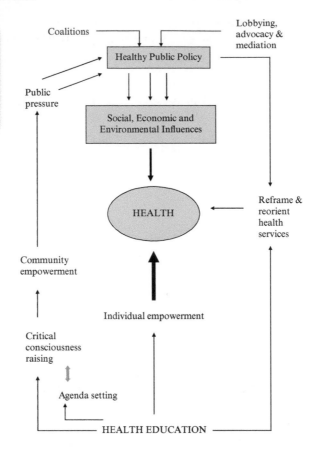

of sustainable food. Healthy public policy is considered in more depth in chapters 11 and 12.

Tones and Tilford (1994) also suggest a mathematical formula for defining health promotion to emphasize the interconnectness and synergy between health education and healthy public policy. This formula encourages us to consider that ONLY by using both approaches will the promotion of health be realized.

Health promotion = health education x healthy public policy.

Caplan and Holland's (1990) four perspectives

Caplan and Holland attempt to use a stronger conceptual framework in the development of what they refer to as a typology rather than a model. The framework is conceptualized around two axes detailed in figure 7.4. One axis refers to a theory of knowledge and how knowledge is generated (see chapter 3 for more discussion of epistemological considerations). Knowledge about health and illness can be perceived as objective and measurable and is related to the biomedical model at one end of the continuum and at the other, knowledge is subjective and relates the individual experiences of health and illness, which may not be quantified. The other axis refers to how society is viewed and ulti-

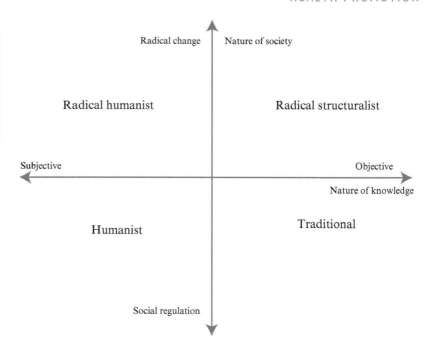

Figure 7.4.
Caplan and
Holland's
model of health
promotion
(adapted from
Caplan &
Holland,1990).

mately will impact on health. At one end of the axis radical change, or what MacDonald & Smith (2001) refers to as social change, states that society is a product of conflict and that those who lack power and consequently have poorer health, struggle against those who have power (see chapter 4 for related discussion about Marxist theory). Therefore, in order to improve health, the structure of society must change. At the other end of the axis social regulation implies that society has an agreed natural order and that deviations from social norms go against this agreed order. Consequently health-related behaviour should be regulated and individuals should comply with received social norms.

Each quadrant or perspective outlines the essential features about the nature of health and health promotion practice. The radical humanist paradigm suggests that a health practitioner develops a mutual partnership with a client and that the clients' viewpoint is valued as they experience health subjectively. The health promotion approach here facilitates personal growth based on the wishes of the client. Power is vested within the clients but supportive methods are used by practitioners

The radical structuralist paradigm proposes that health is measured objectively and is determined by socio-economic and environmental factors. Health and ill-health are created by the unequal distribution of wealth and power. The health promotion approach associated with this paradigm is to change the nature of society by community development or social policy, in order to ensure that power is shared more equally across society.

The humanist paradigm implies that health is defined by the practitioner although the subjective experience of the client is explored.

The aim of this approach is to maximize a 'healthy lifestyle' as defined by the practitioner, by developing clients' own resources and skills. Health education is often utilized by practitioners to facilitate this goal.

The traditional paradigm is related to biomedical ideas about the nature of health (see chapter 1). If health is the absence of disease then health can be brought about by behaviour change to comply with the healthy lifestyle defined by the social norms of society. Power is held by practitioners over their clients. A case study about how this model can be applied to domestic violence is outlined at the end of this chapter.

As we have seen from the above models and typologies, there are many different ways of considering health promotion. Prior to reading this chapter you may have considered that health promotion was only about giving people information. By analysing the models you should now see that health promotion is much more than health education. It ranges from political action for health gain or lobbying for changes in the power and income structures within society to facilitating communities working together to improve their own health. We hope that you can also see overlaps between the different models and that while some models place emphasis on particular elements all the models address the wider socio-economic and environmental determinants of health. An understanding of the models should enable you to have a more fully rounded appreciation of the differing ideas about the scope and nature of health promotion. In addition, analyses of the models should also lead to a more critical set of judgements about what approaches dominate practice and perhaps stronger consideration of which models should be used to more effective ends. Generally, health education tends to dominate health promotion practice, often in a clinical or health care setting. We argue that this is quite a limited approach and is unlikely to lead to sustained changes in health status or will change the circumstances in which people live and experience their health.

In summary, the term 'health promotion' can be defined as 'the process of enabling people to increase control over their health and its determinants, and thereby improve their health' (World Health Organization, 2005d: 1). The differing approaches that are encapsulated within the models forms the basis of how we may go about delivering this process of health promotion. Now we have seen the whole scope of approaches within health promotion it is important to understand the value base that underpins practice. While it is outside the scope of this chapter to discuss all principles and values, we have selected what we feel are the most resonant and transformational in contemporary practice.

Principles and values

The World Health Organization (1986) provides a useful set of values and principles from which to start our discussion. But a more contemporary discourse can be found in Gregg and O'Hara (2007). It is

Box 7.3   **Upstream approaches in health promotion.**

My friend, Irving Zola, relates the story of a physician trying to explain the dilemmas of the modern practice of medicine:

'You know', he said, '. . . sometimes it feels like this. There I am standing by the shore of a swiftly flowing river and I hear the cry of a drowning man. So I jump into the river, put my arms around him, pull him to shore and apply artificial respiration. Just when he begins to breathe, there is another cry for help. So I jump into the river, reach him, pull him to shore, apply artificial respiration, and then just as he begins to breathe, another cry for help. So back in the river again, reaching, pulling, applying, breathing and then another yell. Again and again, without end, goes the sequence. You know, I am so busy jumping in, pulling them to shore, apply-ing artificial respiration, that I have no time to see who the hell is upstream pushing them all in.' (McKinlay, 1979: 249)

not possible to outline a definitive list of values and principles under-pinning health promotion practice but key values have been selected that relate to the ethos of this book.

Focus on upstream approaches

One of the most important considerations in health promotion is the need to address action on the upstream determinants of health (see box 7.3). The term 'upstream' is generally acknowledged to have come from a story told by Irving Zola recounted to his friend McKinlay (1979).

To some degree the whole of part II of this book considers the upstream determinants of health. This notion is inherently linked to the primary and primordial levels of prevention outlined earlier in the chapter. If these determinants are not addressed, then it is likely that health inequalities will worsen and that poorer health status in low-income countries will not improve. This has implications for who we define as a health promotion workforce and how governments fund health promotion work.

Non-victim blaming approaches

Linked to ideas about social constructionism (see chapter 4) and what influences our health, is a non-victim blaming approach to health promotion. Victim blaming is an approach to health education that only focuses on individual action, rather than the external forces that influence an individual person, resulting in blaming people for their health behaviour and related consequences (Hubley & Copeman, 2008). Practitioners should resist victim-blaming, as it does not show understanding of the influences of health behaviour outlined in depth in chapter 6 and in part II of this book. Instead practitioners should consider the social and economic experiences of people's lives and which may explain how and why people behave in the manner that they do.

Evidence base

There have been calls in the last two decades to strengthen the evidence base in health promotion (Green & Tones, 1999; McQueen, 2002; Green & Tones, 2010). Evidence-based practice is defined in chapter 3 on investigating health, but generally is concerned with trying to understand which approaches and methods of working are likely to produce the strongest health improvement. This produces a number of challenges for those in health promotion practice wishing to strengthen evidence base (Waters & Doyle, 2002). The approaches to providing evidence within health promotion differ from those types used, for instance, in clinical interventions where Randomized Control Trials (RCTs) can be applied. This links to the discussion about the nature of evidence outlined towards the end of chapter 3. Notwithstanding the challenges, the principle of generating evidence by providing stronger evaluations of programmes and initiatives as they are developed and implemented and by encouraging the utilization of the existing evidence base by practitioners, are both key principles of practice.

The National Institute of Health and Clinical Evidence produces evidence-based reviews for health promotion practitioners at the following website http://guidance.nice.org.uk/Type/PHG/Published

The Campbell Collaboration, which specializes in producing evidence-based reviews on more socially orientated interventions can be found at the following website http://www.campbellcollaboration.org/library.php

The Cochrane Collaboration, which focuses more on evidence-based biomedical interventions, can be found at the following website: http://www.thecochranelibrary.com/view/0/index.html

Participation and empowerment

These two related methods of working are highly valued within health promotion, as they focus on individuals having control of their lives, a central goal in health promotion. Participation implies 'being present and taking part' in health promotion activities and secondly recognizing that when people participate, what they say should be listened to and acted upon (Lowcock & Cross, 2011). This implies that individuals are perceived as autonomous beings with the inclination, skills and power, to be present, take part and make decisions. In addition practitioners need to value this way of working to be in a position to incorporate participants' ideas. Empowerment discussed previously in this chapter is linked to community development approaches. Arguably, you cannot participate in anything to any degree without being empowered in some way. Participation can therefore be seen as a product of empowerment.

Equity

Equity in health is concerned with fairness and the idea that everyone should have equal right to the fullest health possible. In chapter 2 we outlined different types of health inequality, where the health of populations and communities are different, but the term inequity enshrines an *unfair* distribution of health status. The sociological explanations for health inequalities and inequities are discussed in more depth in chapter 4. One of the fundamental principles of health promotion is that health should be more equally distributed and that health promotion approaches should, as a high priority, address health inequities. Policies and projects are now being evaluated to assess their impact on health equity, to reduce the disproportional impact on those that already experience poorer health, using a technique known as health equity audits (Health Development Agency, 2003)

Ethical practice

Cribb and Duncan (2002: 271) define ethics as 'what is right or good'. We can relate many of the other principles and values of health promotion outlined in the sub-section to notions of ethics, such as equity and non-victim blaming. In the simplistic sense there are two main approaches to ethics. The first is concerned with rules and duties of what is defined as right and good, termed deontology. The second is concerned with the outcomes of actions and what is produced is good and right, termed consequentialism. Both of these ontological positions are important in health promotion ethics, as you will see when you undertake the fourth learning task. An example of a deontological ethical rule is to tell the truth. An example of a consequentialist viewpoint is that the end justifies the means, as when an action such as higher-income earners paying higher taxes to benefit the more vulnerable members of society creates the best health for the whole of society.

There are four major ethical principles outlined in Naidoo and Wills (2009)

- Autonomy – 'Respect for the rights of individuals and their rights to govern their own lives' (Naidoo & Wills, 2000: 91).
- Beneficence – Doing and promoting good but we would need to consider whose good, the individual or wider group.
- Non-maleficence – Doing no harm.
- Justice – People should be treated equally and fairly.

Learning task 7.4

Ethics in health promotion.
Consider the case of the national screening programme for women for cervical cancer.

1. Using the four ethical principles above, consider arguments for and against this screening programme.
2. After you have made your arguments for and against screening for cervical cancer, decide which you think is a stronger argument on ethical grounds.
3. Which ethical principles did you use to make your decisions?

Ethical frameworks underpin codes of conduct in health promotion practice. Learning task 7.4 will help you to think about the moral difficulties that relate to different types of health promotion activities.

Focus on salutogenic models

Salutogenic approaches to health and health promotion are concerned with creating good health, happiness and meaning in life (see chapter 1). This principle of health promotion is greatly neglected in practice although it is now reaching the attention of politicians and policy-makers (Easton, 2010)

Most health promotion activity is centred on the prevention of ill-health and not creating positive health or happiness. Work building social capital via for example volunteering is likely to be a major mechanism to promote meaning in people's lives (see chapter 9) and addressing equity issues has the potential to increase happiness as the unfair health, status and income experienced across societies tends to promote greed and envy.

Critiques of health promotion

Health promotion receives considerable criticism from many quarters. It is important to have a wider understanding of these issues if health promotion activity is be valued and prioritized within health spending. These criticisms can be summarized as follows:

1. As health promotion is so widely scoped and conceptualized, critics suggest that one of the difficulties facing health promoters is that health promotion is everybody's business and nobody's responsibility (Canadian Public Health Association,1996). However, we feel it is important to recognize that different sectors and workforces promoting health are not just those that have a specific health-related job title or work in health care systems but that many

practitioners have the capacity to impact positively on health by addressing wider social, economic and environmental determinants of health.

2. Health promotion regulates lifestyle and choice, by using coercive action enshrined in legislation and leads to a 'nanny state' society. A nanny state is defined as one that over-protects its members by reliance on welfare state and legislation to limit choice in the 'best interests' of the health of populations. An example of this would be the enforcing of the wearing of seatbelts. We can see when using some approaches outlined in the different models of health promotion that practitioners can indeed use policy to improve the health of populations. It is a difficult ethical balancing act to tackle unfair determination of health by factors outside the control of individuals as well as providing the freedom and choice that are so valued within health promotion. It is hoped that by working in empowering ways control and choice will be maintained and that healthy public policy will be made via democratic processes involving collaboration and consultation and a true mandate for action.

3. Health promotion doesn't work. This criticism relates to a weaker evidence base compared to biomedical practice. It is not surprising that health promotion evidence is weaker if is it judged in the same ways as clinical interventions. Health promotion practice is newer and therefore building an evidence base is bound to lag behind biomedical evidence. While there is still a way to go, the evidence that health promotion activity does work is growing.

4. Health education is the main approach used within health promotion practice. Pupavac (2009) argues that the problem with health education in relation to risk and threats to health (see chapter 2) is that there are few incentives to change our behaviour, if we do not expect the changes we make to transform our lives significantly. For this reason a focus on addressing upstream determinants of health is advocated rather than individual behaviour change.

Contribution of health promotion

We hope from an examination of this chapter that you can see that health promotion is the action phase for health improvement. After an analysis of, firstly, patterns of health and the health experience and, secondly, what shapes the patterns and experience of health, health promotion is the process of how to address these issues. The application of the health promotion approaches outlined in this chapter can be found within the case studies outlined in chapter 13.

A number of disciplines outlined in the previous six chapters underpin the theory and practice of health promotion and shape our notions of what and how health promotion should be done. Chapter 1

Case study

Using Caplan and Holland's model to consider different approaches to addressing domestic violence in women.

Domestic violence is an issue about gender power relationships between men and women. It occurs as a global issue, although it is perceived differently by different cultures. There are a number of approaches for dealing with domestic violence. Radical structuralist approaches seek to reduce the power inequality between men and women via legislation and policy work. Radical humanist approaches seek to empower women and provide supportive self-help and other social networks. Humanist approaches aim to work with women so that they can understand and change their and others behaviour and find strategies for change. Traditional approaches would involve education to promote behaviour change in men and also treatment of physical and mental injuries of women. By using these theoretical perspectives, it should be possible to develop a cohesive strategy to address the challenges of changing cultures of violence and values about women.

Radical change | Nature of society

Radical humanist

Provide supportive networks and self help groups and use of safe houses to remove women from violence.

Women to gain more power by developing economic and social power via work and stronger networks.

Radical structuralist

Working to reduce power inequality between men and women through legislation for gender equality.

Issue to be taken seriously by criminal justice system .

Social unacceptability of issue generated through advocacy and lobbying.

Subjective ← → Objective

Nature of knowledge

Humanist

Working with women (and men) directly so they can understand the nature of their experiences and what they can do themselves. Using cognitive-behavioural therapy (CBT) approaches to understand the issues and change behaviour.

Traditional

Treatment of injuries

Educational campaigns about the issue to raise awareness and change attitudes to domestic violence in populations.

Social regulation

outlines what health is so we can define *what* we are promoting. This has implications for what types of methods we use. If health is viewed as absence of disease, then biomedical primary prevention of ill-health via vaccination and screening may be of great importance. If we are trying to use more salutogenic models of health, then we may consider developing resilience and coping strategies when exposed to life stressors.

Feeder disciplines outlined in chapters 2–6 also shape the nature of health promotion. For example, the analysis of risk, risk factors and health behaviour as discussed in chapter 6 links clearly to health education approaches and how we communicate and interpret risk to our health. Structural determinants of health draw more on debates about how societies are structured and organized (see chapter 4). This is linked explicitly to the approach of health public policy (see chapter 11) and the goal of health promotion, where individuals and groups feel they have control over what shapes their health, which may be achieved by employing empowerment and community development approaches.

Health promotion as an interdisciplinary activity offers us the theoretical and practical tools with which to reduce unfair experiences of health, increases life expectancy and offers opportunity for all to meet their health and life potential. There is a large body of evidence that addressing wider socio-economic and environmental determinants in health can lead to improvements in life expectancy and quality of life (Marmot Review Team, 2010)

Summary

- The nature of health promotion is contested and often conceptualized as broad in scope. Health promotion is not simply educating people about the do's and don'ts of a health-related lifestyle.

- There are a number of differing approaches that can be used to address health issues and *all these approaches* should be used to form coherent strategies for health improvement. Approaches that address the wider determinants of health should not be neglected.

- Key values such as equity, ethical principles and non-victim blaming approaches underpin the practice of health promotion.

Questions

1. Do you think that healthy public policy leads to a nanny state culture? How far do you think the state should go in protecting and promoting health?

2. How effective do you think health education strategies are (i.e. giving information and developing skills) in producing gains in health?

3. Is it ever right to use coercion to protect or improve health? For example, seatbelt legislation coerces people to wear seatbelts; if they do not, fines are imposed. There is some evidence that injuries from road traffic accidents have reduced.

Further reading

Naidoo, J. & Wills, J. (2009) Health Promotion: Foundations for Practice. 3rd edn. London, Saunders.

This provides a good all-round text for practitioners and students of health promotion alike. It covers health promotion theory and then has several sections on the different methods that can be used in health promotion practice – for example community development. Other key skills, such as health promotion planning and evaluation, are also developed towards the end of the book. It provides an excellent starting point for people new to the notion of health promotion.

Public Health Action Support Team (2010) The Public Health Knowledge Textbook. [Internet] Available at http://www.health-knowledge.org.uk/public-health-textbook.

The *Public Health Knowledge Textbook* is an online resource that covers all the public health skills and competencies and useful materials for health promotion. There are text-based materials that can be read and interactive materials in the form of videos and learning tasks that supplement the chapters. The e-learning section is arranged more like a module of information and there are quizzes and examinations that can be completed.

Green, J. and Tones, K. (2010) Health Promotion: Planning and Strategies. 2nd edn. London, Sage.

This is a comprehensive text aimed at postgraduates. It takes a strong theoretical perspective and develops many of the ideas that are introduced within this text. While the title implies that it is intended for practitioners planning health promotion initiatives, it debates the central paradoxes facing the discipline and practice of health promotion.

Nutbeam, D. (1998) Health Promotion Glossary. Geneva, WHO.

This comprehensive glossary provides definitions and debates about the most important health promotion terms. It is invaluable for readers faced with an array of new terms who want to understand a new set of vocabulary.

Part III

Influences upon Health

This third and final part of the book considers the wide range of influences upon health by drawing upon Dahlgren and Whitehead's (1991) determinants of health rainbow model in order to give structure and order to understanding different categories of determinants. By understanding this complexity of influences on health at different levels, readers will be able to conceptualize how to address public health issues outlined in the case studies within the final chapter, 13.

Dahlgren and Whitehead's model (below) highlights several of the main factors determining population health. The central feature of the model is several fixed determinants of health such as age, sex and

The Dahlgren and Whitehead determinants of health rainbow.

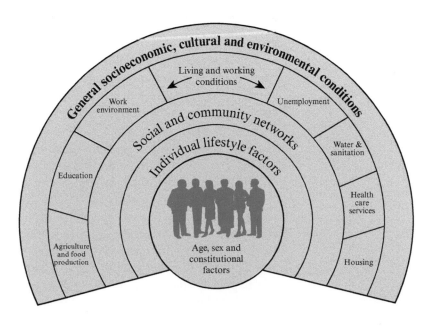

genetics. These are all considered in chapter 8, which critically examines individual characteristics as determinants of health.

The purpose of this chapter is to explore critically individual characteristics in relation to health. As chapter 6 already focuses upon individual behaviour this chapter explores other aspects in relation to individual characteristics including developmental factors such as foetal experiences and age, constitutional factors such as genetic inheritance and social constructs such as gender (how concepts of femininity and masculinity influence health).

Moving outwards, the next layer of Dahlgren and Whitehead's model details the importance of community and broader social influences as determinants of health. So chapter 9 discusses community characteristics and the importance of social and community networks for health protection and promotion. This chapter introduces the reader to concepts such as social support, social capital and social dominance and discusses how these variables mediate health status. This chapter draws upon Marmot's and Wilkinson's (and others') work on autonomy, control and the role of psychosocial pathways in explaining health gradients. The features of healthy communities are also explored, with the chapter debating what a healthy community is and how important this is for individuals living within such environments.

The next layer of the model points to the importance of living and working conditions and food supply (among others) that are needed for the maintenance of health. Therefore chapter 10 pays attention to the physical environment as a health determinant. The chapter explores various aspects of living and working conditions based upon the rainbow model. The chapter analyses several different aspects of our living and working environments such as housing, health care services, water and sanitation, and unemployment and employment. The chapter also considers broader issues such as agriculture and food production.

Finally, Dahlgren and Whitehead (1991) identify the economic, cultural and environmental aspects of society as overall mediators of population health in the outer layer of the model. Hence, chapter 11 discusses policy as a health determinant. The chapter gives a general overview of social policy and then demonstrates that the many facets of policy that exist within our social environment combine to influence and determine our health in a number of ways. This chapter explores how social policy is related to health in a number of ways, looking at how policy is made, discussing the importance of **ideology** within policy and outlining the concept of healthy public policy. Fiscal policy is analysed too. The chapter also demonstrates the importance of the broader policy environment in determining good health, considering how a number of **policy sectors** can all have health impacts.

Chapter 12 then turns to the global context in which health is situated. Although Dahlgren and Whitehead (1991) do not specifically identify the global context of health within their model, there is a case to be made for the importance of the global environment in determining some aspects of health. Chapter 12 therefore explores how health is influenced by globalization in a number of ways. The chapter examines how being part of a global society affects our health in both positive and negative ways, using the concept of globalization as a mechanism to explore global health issues, global patterns of health and disease, global inequality and global health governance.

The final chapter in this book, chapter 13, Synthesizing Perspectives: case studies for action, draws on material from the rest of the book to provide detailed case studies in order to explain how understanding the determinants of health can aid the development of public health strategies and action. Each case study is linked to the Dahlgren and Whitehead (1991) model to demonstrate the range of determinants influencing the health issue. Through the case studies this chapter gives examples of how to address contemporary public health issues using a range of different approaches and methods. The case studies highlight key issues that feature throughout the book and are designed to provide insight and understanding for public health practitioners. Finally, this chapter provides detailed discussion of the Dahlgren and Whitehead model, outlining its strengths and weaknesses and analysing its application to the understanding of public health issues.

8 Individual Characteristics and their Influence upon Health

Overview

The purpose of this chapter is to critically explore individual characteristics in relation to health. It will give an overview of individual characteristics and discuss the influence of these on health experience and their relevance to health studies. Links will be made, where appropriate, with chapter 6, which focused on *behaviour* at an individual level. Rather than individual behaviour, this chapter will explore a range of other factors that influence health and that may be identified as 'individual characteristics'. In doing so the chapter will draw on the individual characteristics specified within Dahlgren and Whitehead's (1991) model, which lie at the middle of the 'rainbow' of determinants of health – the central core of the 'health onion' (Marks, 2002). These include developmental factors such as foetal experiences and age and constitutional factors such as sex and hereditary factors (including genetics) (Barton & Grant, 2006). Social constructs such as gender (how concepts of femininity and masculinity influence health) will also be discussed. In addition, the psychological construct of personality and its links to motivation will be briefly explored as illustrative of how individual psychology can impact on health. A brief consideration of the nature–nurture debate is included. The implication of all of these for health studies will be considered in relation to health promotion across the lifespan using a life course approach. Finally, a case study is presented that considers differential experiences of HIV/AIDS in terms of individual characteristics.

Before we start, take some time to carry out learning task 8.1. This task provides the basis of your reflections for the remainder of this chapter and you will be prompted to refer back to it at various points.

What is this all about?

The individual characteristics listed in the opening paragraph of this chapter undoubtedly influence our health experience through life one way or another. For the purposes of this chapter we are focusing right down to the individual level – on the characteristics we are 'born with' and the biological and social processes that we (generally) have very little control over. In a sense it is a little artificial to consider these things in this way given that, as individuals, we constantly interact with our wider environment on different levels (such as physical and social). The complex relationships between individuals and their environment have been noted by different theorists coming from eco-logical perspectives.[1] For the purposes of this chapter, however, we are going to focus on individual characteristics, in this way making necessary links to other relevant factors as we move through the discussion.

How do individual characteristics influence health?

In learning task 8.1 you will have the opportunity to reflect on the influ-ence of a range of different factors on health. Each of these will now be examined in turn.

Foetal development

The development of the foetus in utero can, and does, have an impact on health for the duration of an individual's life to one extent or another. During the embryonic period, the very first stages of preg-nancy, there is major development of organs and systems occurring. Spina bifida is an example of a condition that can occur when there

---

[1] See for example the 'Behavioural Ecological Model' (Hovell, Wahlgren & Russos, 1997), which assumes a strong two-way interaction between individual behaviour and the environment.

> **Learning task 8.1**
>
> **Individual characteristics and health.**
> (a) Take a few moments to think about how the following indi-
>   vidual characteristics influence, or impact on, health:
> ● Foetal development
> ● Age
> ● Sex (as biologically determined)
> ● Gender (as sociologically constructed or determined – see
>   chapter 4 to remind yourself what this is about if you need to)
> ● Hereditary and genetic factors (you may like to reflect on your
>   own family history here)
> ● Personality
> (b) Make some notes for each area and you will be able to refer back
>   to these throughout the rest of the chapter.

is disruption to these processes. Spina bifida occurs when a specific
region of the neural tube does not develop properly and can cause
paralysis, lack of sensation in the legs and even impaired cognitive
development. This is one example of how disruption in normal development at the foetal stage can impact on individual health experience.
Depending on the severity of the condition, people with spina bifida
may experience health challenges throughout the remainder of their
lives.

Other influences on development at the foetal stage of life come
from our environment. *Teratology* refers to the study of birth defects
and the problems that can arise from environmental influences on
the foetus during pregnancy. Examples of teratogens include alcohol,
cigarettes, drugs (over the counter medication as well as illegal drugs),
exposure to mother's illness and environmental pathogens (i.e. pollution) (Bukatko & Daehler, 2001). Any of these teratogens may impact
on the development of the foetus and the subsequent health experience
of the child/adult. See the later example of Foetal Alcohol Syndrome in
this chapter, which illustrates this.

Foetal programming

The underlying assumptions of 'foetal programming' is that the
origins of some diseases experienced in adulthood are connected
to adverse influences in the early developmental stages of life –
particularly life before birth (as a foetus) (De Boo & Harding, 2006).
This is also sometimes referred to as 'The Barker Hypothesis' after
one of the initial proponents of the idea or 'Foetal Origins Theory'
(Bellingham-Young & Adamson-Macedo 2003). The hypothesis suggests that the foetus makes physiological adjustments in utero in

Box 8.1	The example of Foetal Alcohol Syndrome (FAS).

'FAS is a developmental disorder that can occur after heavy alcohol use by pregnant women' (Strömland et al., 2005: 1121). FAS can cause a range of problems including abnormal growth (pre and post natal), abnormal facial features, mental disability and behavioural problems that undoubtedly impact on health experience through childhood and into adult life. There are a number of complex social factors involved in heavy alcohol use during pregnancy and a range of maternal risk factors associated with FAS including socio-economic status and family/friends with alcohol problems as well as psychological factors (May & Gossage, 2001). The adverse effects of FAS can last into young adulthood and beyond and research has shown that the relationship between the length of time that alcohol is consumed during pregnancy and neuro-cognitive development carries on being significant into early teenage years (Korkman et al., 2003).

response to environmental circumstances that prepare it for life after birth and beyond. Research suggests that foetal experience can influence the development of adult health ranging from, for example, type 2 diabetes (De Boo & Harding, 2006) to depression (Bellingham-Young & Adamson-Macedo 2003). There is also a wealth of evidence that size at birth is related to experience of disease and poorer long-term health outcomes in later life. For example the development of coronary heart disease and cardio-vascular diseases (The Marmot Review, 2010). As Gluckman et al. (2008: 61) state 'many lines of evidence, including epidemiologic data and data from extensive clinical and experimental studies, indicate that early life events play a powerful role in influencing later susceptibility to certain chronic diseases'.

As already stated, a related individual characteristic that appears to be an indicator for future health experience is weight at birth. Birth weight is influenced by a range of complex factors and the interplay between these (Spencer & Logan, 2002). Maternal nutrition is one example of factors that can influence birth weight (Jones, 2002) and this may be particularly important in certain situations such as where access to food with a high nutritional value may be limited. Another example is smoking during pregnancy, which not only influences weight at birth but can also increase the likelihood of miscarriage and the development of childhood asthma (Jaakkola & Gissler, 2004). A study by Nasreen et al. (2010) of 720 women in Bangladesh showed that anxiety and depression during pregnancy is connected to low birth weight. Given the links between low birth weight and infant mortality rates, Nasreen et al. argue that this is as important as poverty or malnutrition.

Smoking and drinking during pregnancy can contribute to health problems via 'foetal programming'.

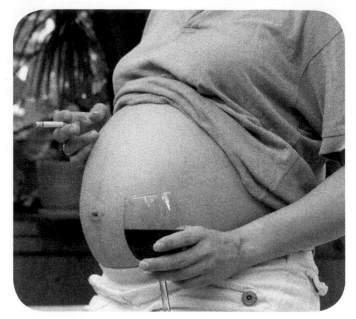

© Julian Makey/Rex Features

Learning task 8.2

The Avon Longitudinal Study of Parents and Children.

(a) Take a few minutes to access the website of the Avon Longitudinal Study of Parents and Children at <http://www.bristol.ac.uk/alspac/>. The Avon Longitudinal Study of Parents and Children in the UK began as the Child of the '90s project. More than 14,000 pregnant women were recruited in the early 1990s to take part in this study, which follows the health and development of the children involved. The study is still on-going. The study has produced a wealth of information and is a unique resource used by researchers the world over.

(b) Focusing on the findings of the study to date, try to identify as many aspects of individual characteristics and health as you can and organize each one according to the headings used in the first learning task in this chapter.

(c) You may also want to look at a similar study taking place in the USA called the National Children's Study, which began more recently. This is specifically examining the effects of environmental influences on children's health and development from birth to age 21 years. Details can be accessed at http://www.nationalchildrensstudy.gov/Pages/default.aspx

Both websites provide a wealth of information and links to follow up that are relevant to the contents of this chapter.

Age

Our age influences our health. We will briefly consider how our health is influenced in different ways at different points during our journey through life. Our health needs and health goals change throughout our lives (Sarafino, 2002) and are inextricably linked to our age. This is also influenced by maturational factors such as development of organic systems, physical structures and our motor capabilities. In terms of age we can categorize our development through life in the following key stages:

- Pre-conception to birth
- Infancy (0–4 years)
- Childhood (including pre-puberty 5–9 years)
- Puberty and adolescence (10–18 years)
- Early adulthood (19 –25 years)
- Middle adulthood (26–50 years)
- Late adulthood (50–70 years and onwards)
- Death and dying

We can take each period of the lifespan in turn and consider the differences in terms of key developmental characteristics – see box 8.2.

Biology and biological sex

There is not enough scope within this chapter to go into a lot of detail about the influence of biology on health. Therefore the focus will be on the influence of biological sex. Whether we are born biologically 'male' or 'female' has an influence on our health experience and health outcomes throughout our lives. This influence begins before birth. For example, male foetuses are more prone to miscarriage than female foetuses. One of the key early findings of the Avon Longitudinal Study of Parents and Children cited earlier is that boys are more prone to almost every minor illness than girls.

Biochemical factors (hormonal factors) are also important in terms of differences between the biological sexes. In women, certain hormones provide a protective factor for some diseases. For example levels of oestrogen are influential in the development of cardiovascular disease and osteoporosis. Reproductive health experience differs according to biological sex. For both sexes the passage through puberty and the development of secondary sexual characteristics are important. For women specifically major events such as pregnancy, childbirth and menopause influence health experience and this links to age as discussed earlier. Biologically determined differences in the origins of certain diseases and illnesses are also physiologically based, for example, to do with the specific male and female reproductive system.

Biological makeup also determines sex-specific illnesses such as those that are linked to male or female reproductive systems (for example, cervical cancer in women and prostate or testicular cancer in

Box 8.2   Key life stages.

Pre-conception to birth – The central features of this period are both the physical development of the embryo in utero and the impact and influence of the process of childbirth. The health and health behaviours of the mother have a big influence on these features. This has already been discussed in some detail in this chapter.

Infancy (0–4 years) – The central features of this period are the acquisition of language as well as physical and cognitive development (learning to walk and to process/make sense of information). Disruption to development at this stage can have a long-term effect on health in many different ways.

Childhood (5–9 years) – During this period physical and cognitive development continues.

Puberty and adolescence (10–18 years) – During this period physical and cognitive development continues with growth spurts and the development of secondary sexual characteristics. There are many features of adolescence that impact on health and health outcomes. For example, 'adolescence is a developmental period characterized by heightened potential for risk-taking behaviours that have important implications for health and well-being' (Smylie et al., 2006: 95). Examples of this type of so-called 'risky' behaviour include binge-drinking and unprotected sex.

Early adulthood (19 – 25 years) – During this period we are fully physically mature adults. Childbirth may be something that occurs here that can impact on health. Major life changes at this, and subsequent stages, can have significant effects on health (such as childbirth, leaving home and developing long-term relationships).

Middle adulthood (26–50 years) – During this period the onset of the ageing process begins, which includes the menopause for women. This process may have an impact on physical functioning and also on emotional well-being. Towards the later end of this time span the ageing process begins, which may impact on physical functioning. The male menopause may also occur later on during this stage.

Late adulthood (50–70 years and onwards) – The ageing process inevitably brings further deterioration in physical functioning and sometime cognitive functioning (in the case of dementia) eventually leading to the final stage of development – death and dying. Retirement can have a major influence on health during this stage.

Adapted from Hubley and Copeman (2008)

men). Biological differences also lead to some biased vulnerabilities to certain diseases. For example, pregnant women are the most vulnerable adult group at risk of malaria and are four times more likely to suffer from it than other adults (Malaria Consortium, 2008). Women's biological vulnerability to HIV is up to four times greater than for men (UNAIDS, 1997), which is believed to be due to anatomy – the area of women's genitals exposed to sexual fluids during intercourse is four times greater than men's and semen carries larger amounts of the virus than vaginal fluids.

Gender

Again, there is not the scope to go into a lot of detail here about the influence of gender on health experience; however, it is important to consider it. One aspect of this is lifestyle factors, which differ according to gendered roles and responsibilities. In addition, socially constructed ideas around feminine and masculine heterogeneity can impact on health throughout life. A dimension of this is to do with who holds power within gender relations. For example, in Zambia men often have the final say about whether a sick child is taken to the clinic or not (because there is usually a cost involved and the men currently hold the power in relation to money within most families in that context). Another example is help-seeking behaviour, which differs according to constructions of masculinity and femininity (see chapter 4). Research shows that women are more likely than men to seek help and advice when experiencing symptoms of ill-health. Although it is a complex phenomenon that requires further investigation, there is a substantial body of evidence that suggests that men are less likely to seek professional help for a range of health issues than women (Galdas et al., 2005). This reluctance has been attributed to a number of different factors but the most significant of these appear to be beliefs about how men should behave according to socially constructed masculine dictates.

Gender differences also exist in a range of mental health experiences throughout life. For example, women are generally more likely than men to experience depressive disorders beginning from puberty and continuing through to adult life (Piccinelli & Wilkinson, 2000). A range of different factors may put women at greater risk for depression than men, including experiences during childhood and adolescence, socio-cultural roles and differences in coping skills. Similarly, gender differences exist in mental health experience in adolescence – deliberate self harm is more common in young women while suicide is more prevalent in young men (Vostanis, 2007).

Hereditary and genetic factors

Illness and disease, particularly in later life, are due largely to the interaction of genetic and environmental factors from very early childhood (Weaver, 2001). Here we will consider genetic and hereditary factors.

'Genetic Endowment' essentially refers to our biological destiny and it can be extremely influential in the development of health throughout life. In learning task 8.1 you had the opportunity to reflect on your own family and the tendencies within it to certain diseases and health experience – characterized by more frequent occurrences. There are many examples of diseases that have a genetic component and that we may have a pre-disposition to developing as we age due to our genetic inheritance. Such examples include degenerative diseases such as dementia, and certain cancers such as breast and bowel cancer. In addition there are also certain hereditary diseases carried on sex chromosomes, such as haemophilia and colour blindness.

Different genes are linked to certain types of characteristics or traits at an individual level. Dominant genes in parents will influence a range of things such as eye colour and height. DNA (Deoxyribonuleic Acid) has become a household term in recent decades and this is the 'genetic command centre' of every human cell. Defects in DNA strands can cause disease and abnormalities. Mutations in DNA may also be genetically inherited. Research has advanced, so that predispositions to certain diseases can now be established in utero by examining foetal DNA (Mameli, 2007). The advantage of this is that an awareness of a pre-disposition to a certain disease may lead someone to change or modify their behaviour to reduce risk factors that lie under their control. For example, cholesterol levels are, in part, determined by genetic factors; however, lifestyle and environmental factors also have a part to play. So someone may have a genetic disposition to developing high cholesterol levels but factors such as smoking, dietary choices and stress will also have influence. The interaction between genes and the environment has been studied in some detail and has a major part to play in the development of disease in later life. For example, Walters et al. (2000) have made a link between genes and chronic obstructive pulmonary disease (COPD) whereby environmental factors such as cigarette smoke might combine with genetic regulation of inflammatory responses that appear to be inherited. So a familial predisposition to developing COPD interacts with environmental factors to increase the risk of disease.

Personality

Personality may influence health in a number of different ways. For example, in terms of what we do and why we do it, as well as how we respond to things. The concept of personality is presented as the construct of 'self' in the Health Action Model (Green & Tones, 2010: 139) discussed in chapter 6. There are some debates in the literature as to whether 'personality' is inherent (something we are born with) or something that is acquired as we develop, particularly in our earliest years. However, there is not the space within this chapter to engage fully with this discussion. For the purposes of considering individual characteristics and their influence on health experience, we are working from the assumption that each of us has a unique 'personality' that may reveal itself through different characteristics and cause us to behave and react in certain ways but that groups of people may share similar personality characteristics. One of the ways in which personality is clearly linked to health is to 'behavioural intention' – a concept we explored in chapter 6.

The construct of personality may be understood in different ways – through identifying and exploring certain traits or types, for example. A popular, but rather simplistic, conceptualization of personality distinguishes between a 'Type A' personality and a 'Type B' personality. Type A personalities are generally seen as being extrovert, competitive and impulsive while Type B personalities are portrayed as being more introvert and easy-going (Bennett & Murphy, 1997). This idea has been criticized on a number of counts; however, there does seem to be some compelling evidence linking certain types of personality to certain diseases, such as research carried out in the 1970s that showed that people with a Type A personality were twice as likely to develop heart disease as those identified as being Type B. The argument for taking into account personality types or traits in terms of health promotion is not about trying to change a fundamental, relatively stable psychological construct but is to do with how behaviours linked to personality types or traits may be changed or adapted to maximize health gain (Green & Tones, 2010). It is important to note here that typologies of personality are subject to criticism (Marks et al., 2005) and are often very culturally and socially bound concepts.

'Risk-taking' is also seen as being strongly linked to personality type (as well as to gender, as discussed earlier in this chapter) and the 'sensation-seeking' personality has also been identified through different measures including a specific scale developed by Zuckerman (1990 cited in Green & Tones, 2010: 141). This is an important idea for health since there seems to be a strong link between taking part in 'riskier' activities and experiencing accident, injury or even death. Examples of 'risky' behaviour are drink-driving, drug taking and engaging in unsafe

Some argue that addictive behaviours such as drug taking are linked to a specific personality type.

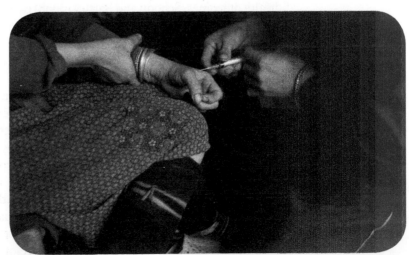

> **Box 8.3**   **Addictive personality.**
>
> Some people argue that there is such a thing as an addictive personality, whereby certain types of personality lend themselves to patterns of behaviour that might be labelled as 'addictive'. The idea behind this is that certain people have pre-dispositions to become addicted to different things (alcohol, drugs, sex, for example). Sometimes this is also linked to hereditary factors. For example, there appears to be a genetic factor in the potential to develop a dependency on alcohol although the bigger picture is usually very complex.
>
> From an individual characteristics point of view addiction can be separated into two types – character type (described as a 'repetitive, stereotyped response to helplessness via compulsive behaviours') and biological disorder resulting in physical addiction (Johnson, 2003). Johnson also differentiates between psychological addictions, such as shopping or gambling, and addictions that can be physical or psychological or both, such as drugs or alcohol. Both can impact on short and long-term health.

sex. There may also be a bio-chemical predisposition to taking risks to do with levels of testosterone that are generally biologically determined, so this is a complicated issue.

Two other concepts linked to notions of personality important for health experience are 'capability' and 'resilience'. These concepts are linked to evidence that we are not all affected by the same things in the same way (Schoon & Bartley, 2008). Facing the same set of adverse circumstances some people may fare better than others and even better than expected. While there are challenges with definition, **operationalization** and measurement of capability and resilience, in the literature and research there is evidence that both of these are important for health and health outcomes. Schoon and Bartley (2008) carried out research exploring the ideas of capability and resilience in relation to growing up in poverty. They found that the family environment played an important role in developing and maintaining capabilities and in fostering resilience. Children from a more supportive family environment were more likely to display this type of characteristic as indicated by engagement with formal educational opportunities. They conclude that 'there is not one major factor that enables individuals to cope with adversity, but rather a combination of influences and measures making a difference' (p. 25).

The BBC *Child of Our Time* series aired two programmes in summer 2010 focusing on personality. This featured a series of tests on the children in the project and the general public determining different personality traits. The programmes reported that by the time we are ten years old psychologists believe that our personalities are fully formed and that they comprise five basic personality traits – extraver-

Learning task 8.3

Personality and motivation.

(a) Consider the quote below in relation to the concepts of personality types and 'motivation'.

'The degree of commitment required to achieve maximal physical fitness might not only militate against social health and, possibly, be inconsistent with cultural norms, it might also be viewed as evidence of obsessional neurosis! Equally, a lifestyle characterized by sloth and self-abuse might lead to considerable happiness and a very successful social life but result in early death'
(Green & Tones, 2010: 13).

(b) To what extent do you agree with the point that is being made?
(c) How is this kind of individual 'difference' important in understanding the influence of individual characteristics on health?

sion, agreeableness, neuroticism, openness and conscientiousness. It is interesting to consider how these traits might impact on health experience and health outcomes. For example, a tendency towards extraversion seems to be associated with higher levels of thrill-seeking or risk-taking. Personality traits also impact on coping ability, which is linked to mental and emotional health experience.

Motivation is a complex psychological construct closely linked to ideas around personality and personality types. The motivation system is one of four systems central to Tones's (1979, 1981 cited in Green and Tones, 2010) Health Action Model[1] that interact together. According to this model the motivation system is 'concerned with feelings (and) refers to goal-directed behaviour' (Green & Tones, 2010: 122). This is essentially to do with what motivates us towards a particular thing (is desirable) and what motivates us to avoid something else (is undesirable). Green and Tones (2010) argue that, in terms of the motivation system in the Health Action Model, motivation operates at four different levels – values, attitudes, drives and emotion. So, in any given situation, we might be motivated by any *one* of these or by a combination of them.

Self-esteem

A related and important individual factor is 'self-esteem'. Self-esteem is a familiar construct in psychology and has become a household word (Baumeister et al., 2003; Tafarodi & Swann, 2001). While there is no agreed definition, self-esteem is often referred to as 'self-worth' and

---

[1] For further, more detailed information about the Health Action Model please see chapter 6 as well as Green & Tones (2010).

> **Box 8.4**
>
> **Levels of motivation (after the Health Action Model in Green & Tones, 2010) applied to the issue of safer sex.**
>
> Values – Strong moral values may motivate people to commit themselves to celibacy or monogamy.
>
> Attitudes – Ambivalent attitudes towards the efficacy of condoms may mean that a person is not motivated to use them during sexual encounters.
>
> Drives – Sex is a drive that is considered, among others such as hunger and thirst, to be a strong motivator for survival. Such a drive may mitigate against safer sexual practice in the 'heat of the moment'.
>
> Emotion – Feelings towards a specific person or about the sexual act may be a strong motivator for or against it.

generally seen as being to do with how much value people place in themselves (Baumeister et al., 2003).

Self-esteem is directly related to health, especially mental health (Naidoo & Wills, 2000). Some even state that it is critical to the improvement of both mental and physical health (Mann et al., 2004). Tones and Tilford (2001) argue that self-esteem is enhanced through processes of empowerment. In terms of health, the higher the self-esteem, the higher the likelihood of making healthier choices. Generally people with higher self-esteem tend to function well in society and people with lower self-esteem tend to struggle (Kohler-Flynn, 2003) which is why it is viewed as an important influence on health at an individual level.

Nature/nurture debate and individual characteristics

One of the key debates around individual development over the lifespan is called the nature/nurture debate. This essentially concerns the extent to which we are programmed by our biology (our genes and biological sex for example), or by our social environment to develop and behave in certain ways. This has implications for health and health experience. Take some time to do learning task 8.4.

As you will appreciate from the preceding learning task the 'nature versus nurture' debate has some relevance to individual characteristics and their influence on health. This was alluded to earlier in the chapter when the point was made that there are differing views about whether personality is something we are born with or something that develops due to our experiences in, and of, life. The 'nature versus nurture' debate is essentially concerned with whether we are a 'product' of our heredity or whether we are a 'product' of our environment.

Learning task 8.4

The nature/nurture debate and individual differences.
(a) What do you know about the so-called 'nature versus nurture' debate? Make notes on what you know already and, if necessary, find out more about this using the internet.

Take some time to answer the following questions:
(b) What are the key features of this debate?
(c) Which of the areas we have examined in this chapter is this debate relevant to?
(d) What can this debate contribute in terms of understanding influences on health at an individual level?

As you will have concluded, health is influenced by a range of different factors including genetic inheritance, personal behaviours and characteristics and the social environment. These factors interact to influence health experience throughout life and individual characteristics play an important and central role.

What does this mean?

The influence of all these factors on health is evident from the discussion that has taken place so far in this chapter. The evidence suggests that health experience varies according to, and is determined by, the result of a variety of individual factors as proposed by Dahlgren and Whitehead's (1991) model of determinants of health. However, it is far from a simple picture. While biological differences may be relatively easily separated out, socially constructed differences (gendered roles of what it means to be labelled 'male' and 'female') present a much more complex picture. There is not the space to consider these kind of issues in great detail here; however, further reading suggestions are offered at the end of this chapter.

There is also the link between individual characteristics and behaviours that needs to be considered in terms of health and health outcomes. Certain behaviours may be expected, or even predicted, of a person based on age, sex and gender. Differences in health behaviour at an individual level may be explained in a number of ways, such as biological, psychological, cultural, social or environmental causes. This was explored in more detail in chapter 6.

A life span perspective

Life course approaches to promoting health are based on the assumption that health experience is influenced by different things at different

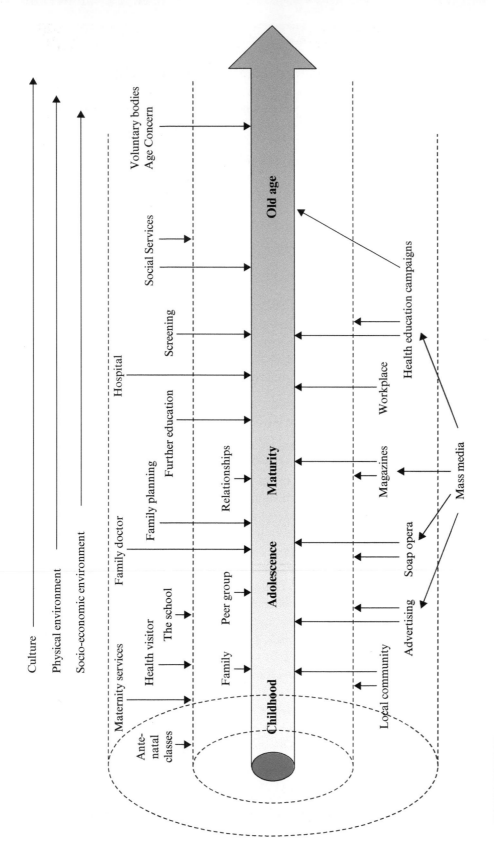

Figure 8.1.
The health career.

Case study

Individual characteristics and the experience of HIV/AIDS.

This case study considers HIV/AIDS and the relationship between this and some of the individual characteristics discussed in this chapter in terms of differential health experience.

Foetal experiences and age

Exposure to the HIV virus in utero or during the birth process can make the foetus vulnerable to infection, although this is not always the case. In recent years the availability of anti-retro viral drugs has significantly reduced the risk of mother to child transmission of HIV. Age has a bearing on the HIV transmission because HIV is most commonly transmitted sexually. Therefore an increase in the incidence of new infections is seen at the point at which young people become sexually active – typically during adolescence.

Biological sex

As has been discussed briefly, women are generally more physiologically vulnerable to HIV infection. In addition to the greater surface area of the female genitalia, referred to earlier, biological vulnerabilities also include a reproductive tract that tears easily, allowing access to HIV, and the fact that vaginal tissue absorbs fluid more easily, including sperm, which has a higher concentration of the HIV virus.

Gender constructs

In many different social and cultural contexts gender has a significant impact on men and women's vulnerability to HIV/AIDS. For example, men are taught to associate prolific sexual activity with constructs of normative masculinity and younger men have the greatest number of sexual partners, yet report feeling at lower risk from infection. Women are often more vulnerable, due to having less power and control and economically or socially being forced into sexually exploitative situations.

Psychological Constructs

Sexual behaviour is clearly linked to HIV infection, and personality traits such as impulsivity and an increased tendency to take risks have been linked to increased and indiscriminate sexual activity, which in turn may lead to increased exposure to HIV infection.

(Adapted from: Gender and HIV/AIDS in the LAC Region available at: www.paho.org/English/hdp/hdw/GenderandHIVPresentation.ppt)

stages in life. This clearly links with the ideas explored under the heading 'The influence of age on health' earlier on in this chapter. Tones and Tilford's (2001) 'Health Promotion' draws on these ideas. The Health Career is a means of conceptualizing how these factors impact on health, as well as opportunities to promote health that will also vary across the lifespan. For example, in early childhood, several things may influence health experience, such as schooling and immediate family. In adulthood, influences will change and different things may come into play, such as significant relationships, the nature of employment and access to health care services. It can be useful to use this type of framework to determine what the key influences are on individuals and to explore the potential to promote health. This is important because we continue to change and develop during the course of our lives and therefore our health needs will also be different at different points in time.

How is this relevant?

Considering individual factors and their impact on health is important in health studies for two key reasons. Firstly, it can help develop and deepen our understanding of health experiences at an individual level. Secondly, an understanding of individual characteristics can help us to design appropriate interventions to promote health. When these factors are taken into account there is an increased likelihood of success. For example, we can design interventions tailored towards specific groups of the population according to different ages, developmental stages, gender and personalities. However, as has been alluded to, it is not a straightforward process because individual factors interact continually with a range of other factors, such as our social, political and physical environment and so these have to be taken into account too. Another way in which this is relevant in the twenty-first century is in relation to the debates around genetic screening and the identification of genes that predispose certain people to certain ill-health. The ethical issues surrounding this debate are enormous.

Summary

- Individual characteristics are many and varied and influence health in a myriad of different ways from before birth and throughout the lifespan.

- Differences at an individual level not only influence health but also a range of other factors such as health behaviour and how we interact with, and respond to, our wider social and physical environment.

- Individual characteristics cannot be viewed in isolation and need to be considered in terms of the complex inter-relations with other systems such as social environment to get a broader view of health and health experience.

Questions

?

1. Think about the different individual characteristics discussed in this chapter. Which of these do you think is most influential in terms of long-term health experience and why?

2. Specifically considering the psychological construct of personality, what other aspects of this might impact on health experience – how and why? Look at the literature – what is the evidence for this?

3. How much of your own health has been influenced by individual characteristics by this stage in your life? Consider the ways in which the contents of this chapter provide an explanation for this.

Further reading

Due to the scope of the contents of this chapter and the many issues that have been discussed, it is not possible to recommend further reading on every aspect. Some selected suggestions are therefore offered here.

Avon Longitudinal Study of Parents and Children http://www.bristol. ac.uk/alspac/
While this is not a textbook, there is a wealth of interesting and accessible information available on the Avon Longitudinal Study of Parents and Children that is highly relevant to the content of this chapter and is worth looking at. You can follow up many of the issues raised in this chapter using this study.

Hernandez, L.M. and Blazer, D.G., eds (2006) Genes, Behavior and the Social Environment: Moving Beyond the Nature/Nurture Debate.
National Academies Press, USA. [Internet] Available at: http://books. nap.edu/catalog.php?record_id=11693#toc
This is an interesting book available on-line at no charge, that picks up a lot of the issues we have touched on in this chapter, specifically the interaction between genetic inheritance and the environment. It reviews these with specific reference to public health and explores key debates in considerable detail.

Kuh, D. and Hardy, R. (2002) A Life Course Approach to Women's Health. Oxford, Oxford University Press.
There are a few textbooks around on life course approaches that focus on different aspects of health. This one, however, particularly looks at women's health and therefore picks up on the biological sex and gender issues raised in this chapter. It specifically links women's life experience to their health in mid-life and beyond.

9 Social and Community Characteristics and their Influence upon Health

Key learning outcomes

By the end of this chapter you should be able to:

- understand and apply the terms social support and social capital in a health context

- understand how processes associated with social support and social capital can influence health

- consider the policy and practice implications of social and community networks for health improvement and reductions in health inequalities

Overview

This chapter considers social and community networks as determinants of health within the sphere of layers in Dahlgren and Whitehead's rainbow model (1991). It bridges the layer between individually constructed determinants of health discussed in the previous chapter and the physical living and working conditions outlined in the next chapter. Wherever possible in this chapter links are made between these layers. Social and community networks are primarily concerned with interactions between groups of people and/or organizations and institutions. Two major concepts, social support and social capital, are defined and debated and evidence presented of the relationship of each to health status. The proposed mechanisms of how social support and social capital influence health are explained. In the final section the implications for policy-makers and practitioners of social and community network influences on health are considered.

As a starting point, it is useful to consider your own social and community networks in the first learning task.

Learning task 9.1

Your social network map.
Consider the past week of your life and the interactions you have had with other people, associations and organizations. Write a list of the types of networks you belong to. It could be a sporting network, a family, a neighbourhood or religious group.

On a blank sheet of paper display your social network map to indicate the nature of your social networks. Below is an example to help you think about your network. However your network will look very different.

The size of the boxes may refer to how important you think each component of your network is and the amount of arrows may indicate the frequency of contact between groups and you; the strength could be indicated e.g. weaker ties could be indicated by a dotted line and direction of the contact (e.g. arrows showing giving and receiving support).

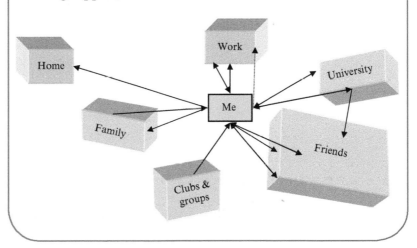

Social and community networks

Before addressing this question directly it is important to unpick some conceptual elements that underpin our understanding of how social and community networks determine our health. This chapter is concerned with how people interact across their networks of communities including family, networks at work, at play and in the whole of life and how these networks can influence our health and well-being. We know that being socially connected to other people is good for our health (Cacioppo & Patrick, 2008) and indeed some commentators would argue social connectedness represents health itself in the form of the specific dimension of social health (see chapter 1).

Social support

Social support is defined as 'information leading the subject to believe [they are] cared for and loved, is esteemed and valued and belongs to a social network of communication and mutual obligation' (Cobb, 1976: 301). Social networks can be analysed in terms of the number of people in the network, frequency of contacts, and the types of support that can be given. You may have considered these issues during the first learning task. House (1981) characterizes four types of social support that also assess not just the structure of the network but the quality of the network.

- emotional (e.g. love, trust, empathy);
- appraisal (e.g. affirmation and feedback);
- informational (e.g. advice)
- instrumental (e.g. tangible help, money and time).

Did you consider not just the structural elements but the quality of your networks in your social network map? In addition Stansfeld (2005) emphasizes an extremely important element of social support for health – that of reciprocity, where you not only receive social support but you are also give social support. Did you consider this issue in the first learning task? What, on an emotional level, made you feel better – giving or receiving social support? This reciprocity has important implications for building connected communities and enhancing the health of communities, which are discussed later in the chapter.

Relationship between social support and health

A large body of evidence now exists showing links between having larger networks and perceived supportive relationships and better health outcomes for physical health (Uchino, 2006) and mental health (Reblin & Uchino, 2008). One of the first rigorous investigations between social connections and mortality came in 1979. Berkman and Syme (1979) found that people who were less socially integrated had higher mortality rates consistently over a nine-year period. However, we must consider the direction of the relationship; i.e. does social support protect against death and poor health outcomes or does poor health mean you will have to develop and maintain less social connections. Berkman and Syme (1979) were able to analyse the direction of this relationship and assess other possible confounding factors such as health-related behaviour and prior poor health that could be linked to mortality rates. They concluded that social support did indeed protect to some extent against premature death. The strongest evidence is between social support and coronary heart disease (Brummett et al., 2001).

Social support appears not only to be linked to mortality but to survival, recovery and prognosis of chronic disease. Survival from heart attacks was predicted by levels of social support (Berkman, Leo-Summers & Horwitz, 1992). Patients with rheumatoid arthritis seem to be offered some protection against depression and further decline in symptoms by experiencing stronger social support (Fitzpatrick et al., 1991).

It is perhaps not surprising that social support appears to be intrinsically linked to mental health status. Durkheim (1951, cited in Stansfeld, 2005) first investigated this by analysing death certificates and found that social isolation was correlated with suicide. Again this is potentially difficult to unpick in terms of causality. Do individuals with mental illness isolate themselves from people, or does mental illness mean that that people cannot develop and maintain or are rejected from their social networks – (termed social erosion)? A small or poor quality social network cannot provide capacity for an individual looking for support for coping with life's challenges and a damaging social network can actually reinforce thoughts of being worthless, hopeless and a failure. Without social support, it is more likely for an individual to develop symptoms of depression (Wade & Kendler, 2000).

The mechanism of action between social support activities, networks and health outcomes is not well understood. However, several interesting interrelated mechanisms are hypothesized and are summarized in figure 9.1.

It is theorized that social support can act along a behavioural pathway where social networks promote healthy behaviours such as physical activity and relaxation and could lead to adherence to treatment programmes and regimes. Consider a mother's or spouse's role in reminders about taking medication. In turn these actions will have a positive impact on physiological process that leads to more positive health outcomes. It is also possible to consider the alternative

Figure 9.1.
Proposed
mechanisms of
action for social
support.
Adapted from Uchino
(2006)

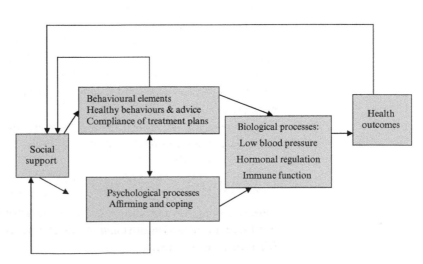

pathway where unhealthy behaviours are promoted through social networks leading to poorer health outcomes. There are links here to chapter 6, health psychology and chapter 8, individual characteristics.

A second and linked psychological pathway attempts to explain the mechanism of action, where social support enhances feelings of self-worth and self-esteem by being valued within the network. The issue of reciprocity may be important here where giving support is as valuable as receiving support. These social outcomes are thought to link to physiological processes such as lowering of blood pressure, and decreases in production of cortisol (a hormone produced in the stress response). An additional mechanism involving the immune system is hypothesized but not well elucidated. Theorell et al. (1995) investigated how higher levels of social support predicted higher counts of CD4 cells in the blood (these are the cells in the immune system that HIV infect and destroy) in men infected with HIV over a five-year period. These links between social support and the immune system have implications in the role social support may play in cancers, which are also mediated by immune system responses.

It should also be noted that not everyone or every network provides positive support. Networks can be damaging as well as supportive.

Social capital

In many ways the concept of social capital builds on ideas that are enshrined in the notion of social support that occurs between individuals within networks but social capital is more concerned with whole community level perspective. The most commonly used definition of social capital is 'features of social organization such as networks, norms, and social trust that facilitate co-ordination and collaboration for mutual benefit' (Putnam, 1995: 67). We can see that this moves the notion of social support from individualized networks to a more ecological or **macro-level** concept. In Putnam's definition, trust in individuals, organizations and communities plays a pivotal role in developing action that enhances life. In his prior work Putnam (1993) also considered civic engagement and identity important in developing social capital. Participation in civic activities can include taking part in political processes such as voting and lobbying about public services, attending public meetings, joining community groups or becoming a school governor.

In order to analyse social capital, different types of social capital have been defined; see box 9.1

Measuring social capital

As we can see from the above, the conceptual framework for social capital is complex and multi-faceted. In order to undertake quantitative work (see chapter 3) investigating social capital and its relationship

Box 9.1 **Different types of social capital.**

Bonding social capital – based on enduring, relationships between similar people with strong mutual commitments such as among friends, family and other close-knit groups.

Bridging social capital – formed from the connections between people who have less in common, but may have overlapping interests, for example, between neighbours, colleagues, or between different groups within a community. 'It acts like a sociological superglue, binding together groups in the community and so can facilitate common action' (McKenzie & Harpham, 2006: 15)

Linking social capital – between people or organizations cutting across status and similarity and enabling people to exert influence and obtain resources outside their usual networks. This type of social capital is important for accessing services such as welfare benefits.

(Office of National Statistics, 2003)

with health, valid and reliable tools need to be developed to measure social capital.

Measurement of social capital has proved difficult for several reasons. Firstly there is no agreed consensus about the definition of social capital, which makes the operationalization of a shared definition problematic (Harper & Kelly, 2003). There are many domains of social capital making development of a short easy to administer tool quite unlikely. Some researchers have overcome this problem by using

Learning task 9.2

Measuring social capital.
1. Examine the definition and types of social capital previously described.
2. List the different domains of social capital e.g. social trust.
3. For each of the domains you have listed try to think about questions you could ask on a questionnaire in an attempt to measure social capital If you were to design a questionnaire to measure social capital what sections would your questionnaire have?
4. Examine the document located on the internet address below, which contains information about the development of a tool to quantify social capital. How does your questionnaire match up? http://www.statistics.gov.uk/socialcapital/downloads/harmonisation_steve_5.pdf
5. What are the strengths and weakness of the questionnaire that Harper and Kelly developed?

more rudimentary indicators of social capital such as how much individuals in a community trust each other. Putnam (2000) developed a comprehensive index to measure social capital and tested it against one question about social trust (presented below) and found as a crude indicator, this question was as useful as the more comprehensive index.

Question – Generally speaking would you say that most people can be trusted or that you can't be too careful in dealing with people ? Choice of answers:

1. most people can be trusted
2. can't be too careful
3. don't know

Some countries including the UK have attempted to measure domains of social capital. Researchers added questions into the **British Household Survey** of 2000 and found the following (Health Development Agency, 2004):

Trust and reciprocity

- Over half of respondents (58%) felt they could trust most or many of the people in their neighbourhood.
- People in more disadvantaged groups were generally more likely to know their neighbours and speak to them daily but less likely to trust their neighbours, or have a reciprocal relationship with them.

Civic engagement

- Nearly 60% of respondents felt well informed about local affairs.
- A quarter felt that they could personally influence decisions in their area.
- Twenty-one per cent were involved in local organization.
- People living in the East of England region were more likely to report feeling civically engaged, compared with the North East region.

Social networks

- Two-thirds (66%) of respondents had a 'satisfactory friendship network'.
- Young people (aged 16–24) were three times more likely to have a satisfactory friendship network than those aged 50+.

Measurements of social capital can be used as performance indicators to consider how well community development or community initiatives are working to build an evidence base (see chapter 3 and chapter 7).

Relationship between social capital and health

The relationship between social capital and health is a complex one precisely because the factors that determine our health, encapsulated in Dahlgren and Whitehead's rainbow model (1991), are also interconnected to social capital. Halpern (2005) provides a comprehensive review of how the social capital is related to economic performance, crime, education and governmental processes and it should now be evident to you that these issues will directly and indirectly influence holistic health status. The more individualistic notions of social capital have already been considered in the section on social support but the upcoming discussion refers to the meso/ecological-level. Good quality empirical work assessing the relationships between **meso-level** social capital and health is more difficult to find. However, there is some evidence about the role that social capital can play in both mortality and income inequality.

Research undertaken between different American States indicates that those that had a greater per capita density of membership in voluntary groups and higher levels of social trust, as gauged by the proportion of residents who believed that people could be trusted, had a more equal income structure and had lower total and disease specific mortality rates (Kawachi et al., 1997). When Russia experienced social disintegration after the collapse of communism, life expectancy decreased. Men reporting high level of mistrust in local government had higher rates of total mortality (Kennedy, Kawachi & Brainerd, 1998).

Hendryx et al. (2002) investigated whether social capital as measured by trust affected access to health services and found that those people who had higher levels of social capital reported better access to health care services.

A sense of belonging (to a group or club) appears to be important in health and is considered an important element of Maslow's hierarchy of need. Campbell, Williams and Gilgen (2002) analysed group membership and its relationship with HIV status. Young men and young women who belonged to sports clubs were less likely to be HIV positive, and young women who belonged to sports clubs were more likely than non-members to use condoms with casual partners. However, unexpected findings came from members of stokvels (voluntary savings clubs accompanied by social festivities). Membership of this group predicted that young men were more likely to be HIV positive. These latter effects could be mediated by social behaviour such as drinking alcohol, which is linked to having sex without a condom. This illustrates the complexity of group membership effects and the difficulties of making simplistic generalizations about relationships between social capital and health.

There is also a smaller body of evidence linking social capital to mental health. McKenzie and Harpham (2006) have produced a good review. As social capital is essentially conceptualized into civic and political activities, an interesting qualitative case study exists from Lusaka, Zambia for women living in informal settlements. Civic involvement and group membership for these women were classified as low and there was perceived disintegration of traditional groups such as credit unions where people both contribute savings and receive loans when needed. Women felt excluded from clubs by men. As a consequence, women felt that they had no influence on decisions that affected their local area (Thomas, 2006). This links to ideas championed by Marmot about the importance of control in influencing health outcomes (Marmot Review Team, 2010)

The mechanisms of action between social capital and health are largely hypothesized. Halpern (2005) provides a useful summary of these ideas. In communities that trust each, other relations between people are likely to be more co-operative and less stressful. Family, neighbours and friends may provide all four types of social support as a consequence, generating an increased climate of trust.

In and between communities where meso-level inequalities exist this is damaging to health. Take this example given by Karl Marx: 'A house may be large or small as long as the surrounding houses are equally small it satisfies all social demands for a dwelling. But if a palace arises beside a little house the little house shrinks to a hovel . . . more dissatisfied and cramped' (Marx, nd, cited in Marmot & Wilkinson, 2001: 1234). This notion of seeing the effects of unfair and unequal economic, educational, occupational and social distributions may impact the behavioural and psychological pathways already outlined in the section on social support.

In communities that participate more in social and civic activities and trust in their networks and organizations, public services may be more efficient and more abundant. In addition there could also be an effect whereby trusting societies are more likely to care about one another and therefore provide a political mandate for policies that redistribute wealth via taxation of the most wealthy or for strong welfare state structures that protect the most vulnerable in society. (See chapter 4 for discussion of health inequality and social divisions and chapter 12 for global health inequalities.)

We have seen how both social support and social capital seem to play important roles in health outcomes. Berkman et al. (2000) have synthesized these relationships in an overarching model that integrates the phenomenon at different levels.

To some degree this builds on the model depicting the mechanisms of social support in figure 9.1. Berkman et al. (2000) argue for a stronger consideration of the macro upstream elements that shape social process in the development of health (also see connections to chapter 7). The conditions that may favour development of social capital and social support are influenced by the socio-political structure of society. The following example illustrates how these processes

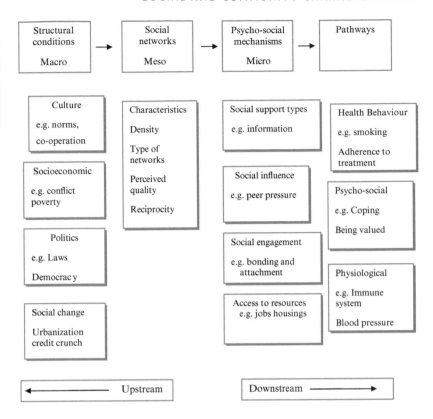

Figure 9.2. How social networks impact upon health (adapted from Berkman et al., 2000).

work synergistically for health gain. At a meso-level we know that democratic societies tend to have fewer health inequalities and better population health (Wilkinson & Pickett, 2010). More **egalitarian** societies tend to engender a spirit of reciprocity fostering closer bonds and bridges, greater spirit of social support leading to direct physiological process that shapes our health.

These upstream influences are also discussed in more depth in chapters 10, 11 and 12.

Learning task 9.3

Example of a connected community?
Examine the Alt Valley Community Trust website @ http://www.communiversity.co.uk/

This trust oversees a range of community-based projects through its Partnerships – we are working together activities.

1. In what ways does the project foster social support?
2. In what ways does the project build social capital? Can you see evidence of bonding bridging and linking social capital?
3. In what ways do you think that these projects could influence health?

Settings for social and community networks

It is possible to contextualize social and community networks using a settings approach (see links with chapter 7). Two settings that have been widely researched are the family and faith-based organizations.

The family

The family structure is considered to be one of the most fundamental foundations and sources of social capital and social support. Fukuyama (1999: 17) asserts that 'families are obviously important sources of social capital everywhere'. However, alternative views exist that relate to the notions of bonding and bridging types of social capital. It is argued that the sometimes strong bonds and trust within families lead to relatively weak bonds and trust outside the family (Winter, 2000). Given that one of the most important aspects of social capital depends on civic engagement, the family unit can sometimes work against the development of social capital.

However, families appear to contribute to social capital in two main ways. Firstly, within the family bonding social support processes influence a range of individual outcomes. For example, strong relationships within the family are linked to children's development and educational outcomes, which will in turn be linked directly and indirectly to health outcomes. This is more akin to social support. As norms and trust can be modelled within a family setting, a transfer of values can take place shaping patterns of social capital-related activities. An example could be parents and children existing in a potentially reciprocal relationship where tolerance and caring for others is fostered. Secondly, bridging social capital, allows links between family and community to be developed. Consider how children may act as a conduit to participation of the family in wider community networks. Attending sporting activities with children can lead parents to meet other parents. This type of social capital is rarely researched.

Debates about the nature of the family as a setting cannot be removed from sociological dilemmas about how families are defined, how the term has become idealized as a prescriptive 'nuclear' family structure and how the increased divorce rates and decline in marriage act upon social capital. However, this example, serves to illustrate how families with disrupted patterns of bonding can still develop supportive links and enhance social capital. Supportive family ties are an important source of support for people in prison. Evidence shows that by maintaining family ties during incarceration, prisoners are less likely to re-offend, more likely to find employment on release and better equipped to reintegrate back into society (Ditchfield, 1994; Woodall et al., 2009). Family ties can also act as a psychological buffer to the detrimental effects of imprisonment and can improve the mental well-being of prisoners (Dixey & Woodall, forthcoming). The Prison

Box 9.2	The importance of family ties for health: The Jigsaw Visitors' Centre at HMP Leeds.

The Jigsaw Visitors' Centre based at HMP Leeds is an innovative prison visitors' centre, which aims, among other things, to improve the health and well-being for prisoners and their families. Working in partnership with the prison and other service providers, the visitors' centre surpasses the provision provided at most prisons in the UK, offering support, advice and information for all those involved in the visit. An evaluation of Jigsaw underscored how the visitors' centre improved the quality of visits and contributed towards the maintenance of family ties through the help and support it provides. Prisoners interviewed as part of the evaluation suggested that the visits organized by Jigsaw enabled them to feel part of the family unit. Imprisoned fathers noted the importance of keeping links with their children and described how visits organized by the Centre were important ways of maintaining their family role. (Woodall et al., 2009)

Further information can be found at Jigsaw Visitors Centre in Leeds website @http://www.jigsawvisitorscentre.org.uk/index.html

Service recognizes the benefits of family contact, as most prisoners are permitted regular communication with their families. This can be through letter writing, telephone conversations and through prison visits. Little research has been done on the prison visit, but recent work shows that from the prisoners' perspective, the visit is a time of great anticipation and excitement, but for families and partners this can be a stressful and unsettling experience (Dixey & Woodall, forthcoming). Prison visitors' centres can provide a source of support for these families and can also help to maintain relationships through making visiting easier and more 'user-friendly'. Some argue that these centres are an essential part of a modern prison service and help to address the government's health inequalities agenda (Woodall et al., 2009).

Faith-based organizations

In some societies faith-based communities can dominate social networks. For example in Durban churches were the main form of group that women belonged to outside their family (Thomas, 2006). Enshrined in many religious doctrines are strong notions of social capital. However, faith can also serve to divide and segregate communities therefore eroding social capital.

Faith-based organizations can develop social capital firstly, by providing places for people to meet and extend their networks, secondly,

Box 9.3   Examples of social capital developed by faith-based organizations.

(cases from Furbey et al., 2006)

(a) Places creating potential for linking and bridging social capital
The new St Peter's Centre in Coventry is used by many groups from all communities: Sikh, Hindu, Muslim, Somalian, Afghan, Iranian and Kurdish.

St Mary's Community Centre in Sheffield is widely used by different groups where bridging social capital is evident between the professionals and other paid workers in the centre '. . . Most of us, we are ignorant really of the backgrounds of many Asian families. I learned a lot from [the Asian People's Project manager] about where Asian families are coming from and how difficult it is for them to live in our society': quote from project worker.

(b) Provision of services
An example of linking social capital comes from Gujarat Hindu Society in Preston. A Lancashire Gujarat Health Users Forum was made up of professionals and members of the community who delivered culturally sensitive services and accessed funding to provide a Learn Direct Centre offering training and advice, which was used by all members of the wider community.

(c) Community forums and advocacy
Faith-based organizations can act as catalysts for community development and setting up 'linking' networks. For example IMPACT in Sheffield, whose mission was to bring together a wide and diverse set of institutions into a civic organization that encourages co-operation on issues and concerns they share.

by providing culturally specific services for the community, thirdly to advocate for social change on behalf of the community via community forums (Schneider, 2004).

Implications for policy and practice

We have argued that the role that social and community networks play in health are important. It should be evident that social capital has the potential to influence a large range of policy sectors such as education, crime, economic development and so on and that the sectors are also intrinsically linked to health status. This has a number of policy and practice implications (Halpern, 2005). A particularly good analysis is provided by the Productivity Commission (2003). A major assumption underlying policy development is that policy can stimulate social capital. This is refuted by some commentators who suggest that social capital is by nature a bottom-up process that arises organically from within communities. However, some evidence exists that social capital can be generated (Pronyk et al., 2008)

Globally, community networks are in decline. At a bare minimum, national and local governance should consider mechanisms that do not further erode community participation in civil and social activities. This may take the form of how communities are organized geographically and physically through planning structures. Spaces and places are needed to foster bridging and linking social capital.

Local governance mechanisms should include strong active and non-tokenism representation from community. Encouraging strong genuine community participation in decision-making with local and regional structures should foster trust and ownership within communities.

Investing in processes of action such as community development that respond to the needs of the community, and cultivating bridging and linking social capital, has the potential to be effective.

Stimulation and pump-priming funding of key sectors and settings may go some way towards developing social capital. Supporting families via schemes such as SureStart has the potential to increase social capital.

Mentoring schemes may provide fruitful access to bridging social capital. Schemes such as adult mentoring of children's reading programmes and business mentoring for individual entrepreneurs are likely to build both economic and social capital.

Creating a culture of volunteering provides one of the most important vehicles for developing reciprocal relationships and is one of the most powerful mechanisms for individuals to feel valued in and by their communities.

The final learning task of this chapter and case study will allow you to consider the different policy and practice implications of generating social capital.

Mentoring schemes such as this are an effective way of developing bonds within communities and building social capital.

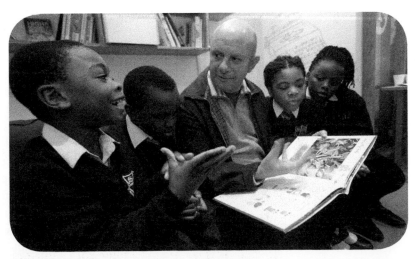

© Heathcliff O'Malley/Rex Features

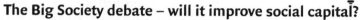

Learning task 9.4

The Big Society debate – will it improve social capital?
Read the following excerpt from the Improvement and Development Agency (IDeA) website outlining David Cameron's community policy initiative 'The Big Society' (2010).

'. . . The government wants to give citizens, communities and local government the power and information they need to come together, solve the problems they face and build the Britain they want. They emphasize that building this Big Society isn't just the responsibility of just one or two government departments but of every department and of every citizen too.

Some broad policies to help take forward the Big Society framework have already been agreed by the coalition government as the first strand of a comprehensive programme for the government. These are the following:

● Giving communities more powers
To radically reform the planning system to give neighbourhoods far more ability to determine the shape of the places in which their inhabitants live
To introduce new powers to help communities save local facilities and services threatened with closure, and give communities the right to bid to take over local state-run services
To train a new generation of community organizers and support the creation of neighbourhood groups across the UK, especially in the most deprived areas

● Encouraging people to take an active role in their communities
To take a range of measures to encourage volunteering and involvement in social action, including launching a national 'Big Society Day' and making regular community involvement a key element of civil service staff appraisals
To take a range of measures to encourage charitable giving and philanthropy
To introduce a National Citizen Service. The initial flagship project will provide a programme for 16-year-olds to give them a chance to develop the skills needed to be active and responsible citizens, mix with people from different backgrounds, and start getting involved in their communities

● Supporting co-ops, mutuals, charities and social enterprise
To support the creation and expansion of mutuals, co-operatives, charities and social enterprises, and support these groups to have much greater involvement in the running of public services
To give public sector workers a new right to form employee-owned co-operatives and bid to take over the services they deliver. This will empower millions of public sector workers to become their own boss and help them to deliver better services

To use funds from dormant bank accounts to establish a Big Society Bank, which will provide new finance for neighbourhood groups, charities, social enterprises and other nongovernmental bodies.' (IDeA, 2010)

1. Do you think these proposals will generate social capital?
2. What do you think some of the barriers could be in implementing this set of proposals?
3. Do you think that these initiatives will address social class or income health inequalities?

Social and community networks

Social health is an important dimension of health in its own right and has been relatively neglected in the discourse about health where physical health and more latterly mental health have tended to dominate (see chapter 1). This chapter has emphasized how social actors and processes are intrinsically and cyclically linked to the other dimensions of health, namely physical and mental health, in order to conceptualize holistic health. Examining the social and community processes that shape our health has implications for how we value our social relationships and how we shape our societies and communities to tap into this under-utilized set of resources. Understanding the concepts of social support and social capital should enable us to unpick the impact of social connectedness on health. This chapter has outlined the significant body of evidence existing that supports the relationship between strong and high-quality social support and increased social capital, enhancing and protecting health and preventing ill-health.

Social capital has been in the political consciousness for the last two decades and has begun to permeate health promotion practice and civic activities. As debated earlier in the implications for policy and practice section, this should allow us to consider what strategies need to take place in order to strengthen social networks and community participation. The next case study represents a strong approach to developing social support and social capital.

Summary

- A significant body of evidence exists that supports causal relationships between social support and health outcomes. Social support can act both positively and negatively either to damage or enhance health.

- The effects of social capital on health are complex because of the multi-factorial nature of health determinants. However, there is relatively good evidence that increased social capital leads to better health outcomes for the whole of society.

Case study

Zambian Open Community Schools, Lusaka.

Zambia Open Community Schools (ZOCS) is a non profit-making and non partisan non-governmental national organization that offers opportunities for orphaned and vulnerable children excluded from education because of fees, expense of uniforms and poor availability of schools to attend community schools. While education is the major goal, the school also attempts to generate bridging and linking social capital by strengthening connections between families and the school and the school and the local community.

At its heart the school aims to generate income for sustainability and has a farm attached including a fish farm and farm shops. The farm is staffed by local community members who receive a wage for their work. Low-cost food is sold to the local community and profits are ploughed back into other projects. A school feeding programme where children receive a free meal has encouraged attendance at school and improved educational outcomes.

The school space also houses workshops where mothers, fathers and older children can develop practical skills woodworking, weaving and enterprise and entrepreneurialism. A training for transformation (TFT) programme develops skills for communities and school staff to lobby for social change and extra resources.

The school utilizes both qualified and unqualified teachers and provides a strong framework of mentorship and in-service training to boost quality of teaching and build capacity.

Direct health issues are addressed in health education programmes, particularly peer education and counselling programmes for HIV.

In addition ZOCS as a collective actively seeks opportunities to influence national policies on children's welfare, advocating for government to support community schools and the right to education for all children.

This provides opportunities for the disadvantaged and attempts to build social capital.

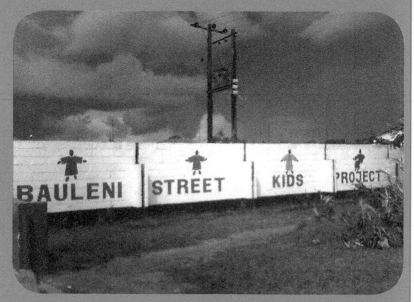

Further information can be found at their website http://www.zocs.org.zm/index.php

- The mechanisms of action for the processes influencing health are not well elucidated but models are highlighted for social capital and social support.

Questions ?

1. Do you want to feel part of your community? What are the reasons behind your answer?

2. What should the balance be between communities having power, decision-making and ownership of services vs strong systems of welfare and public services provided by local or central government?

3. Do you think that the voluntary sector should deliver services that the state has usually provided?

Further reading

Stansfeld, S. (2005) Social Support and Social Cohesion. 2nd edn. In Marmot, M. and Wilkinson, R.G., eds, Social Determinants of Health, 155–78. Oxford, Oxford University Press.

This chapter provides an accessible starting point to understand the relationship between social support, social cohesion and health outcomes. It provides a useful introduction to the central ideas about social and community networks that influence health.

Halpern D. (2005) Social Capital. Cambridge, Polity.

This is a comprehensive text about the nature of social capital in all its forms. However, it also provides a smaller bite sized chapter about the relationship between social capital and health. Useful examples are given from a variety of cultural contexts.

South J., Branney P., White J., Gamsu M. (2010) Engaging the Public in Delivering Health Improvement: Research Briefing. Centre for Health Promotion Research, Leeds Metropolitan University.

This short research report outlines a number of initiatives in which local people have successfully been involved in enhancing health in their communities and is intended for practitioners who may wish to consider involving the public in health improvement activities.

10 The Physical Environment and its Influence on Health

Key learning outcomes

By the end of this chapter you should be able to:

- describe and understand some key physical environmental influences on health

- critique some of the key physical environmental factors influencing health drawing on current research and debate

- further appreciate the extent the physical environment in which we experience our life influences our health

Overview

The purpose of this chapter is to explore critically how our physical environment impacts on our health and health experience. This chapter will give an overview of the physical influences under discussion and how these can, or may, influence health. In doing so, the chapter will draw on the key features of one of the outer 'onion' rings of Dahlgren and Whitehead's (1991) framework for identifying and understanding influences on health. These include agriculture and food production, water and sanitation, housing, the working environment, unemployment, education and health care services. (Note that this is not an exhaustive list of factors within our physical environment that can, and do, impact on our health; however, it is not possible to discuss every aspect of the physical environment within the confines of this chapter.) The chapter goes on to consider the relevance of the discussion to health studies. Finally, a case study is presented that considers the different aspects of living and working conditions discussed in this chapter in relation to a specific context – the Cape Malay families of the winelands of the Western Cape in South Africa.

Learning task 10.1

The physical environment and health.

1. Take a few moments to think about how the following aspects of the physical environment might impact on health and health experience:
(a) Agriculture and food production
(b) Education
(c) Different working environments – for example, manual versus non-manual jobs (also consider the impact on health of being unemployed)
(d) Water and sanitation
(e) Health care services – consider the type of services that might be available in difference contexts as well as access to health care services. For example, consider this in relation to a high-income country such as the USA and a low-income country such as Bangladesh
(f) Housing

2. Make some notes for each area because you will be able to refer back to these throughout the rest of the chapter.

Before we start, take some time out to carry out learning task 10.1. This task will provide the basis of your reflections for the remainder of the chapter and you will be prompted to refer back to it at various points.

What is this all about?

The aspects of the physical environment selected in the opening section of this chapter all impact on, and influence, health and health experience in some way. For the purposes of this chapter, we are concentrating solely on these factors; however, this is not an exclusive list of factors within the physical environment that can affect health. You can probably think of quite a few more. As pointed out in the discussion in chapter 8, it is a little artificial to consider these kinds of things in isolation, given the complex interactions and relationships between the different factors that influence health. For the purposes of this chapter, however, we are going to simplify and focus the discussion in this way. Firstly, two theoretical frameworks for understanding physical influences on health will be discussed – Lalonde's (1974, cited in Earle, 2007b) Health Field Concept and Busfield's (2000) typology of health and illness.

The Lalonde Report, *A New Perspective on the Health of Canadians* published in 1974, signalled a significant shift in the way that health was thought about that has influenced the development of public health and health promotion over the past few decades. Central to this document was a model by Lalonde – the Health Field Concept – which proposed that health could be improved by addressing four different factors – individual lifestyles, health services, human biology/genetics and environmental influences. The discussion in this chapter addresses two of these factors – health services and environmental influences.

Busfield (2000) offers four types of explanation of health and illness[1] as follows:

Type 1 – Explanations to do with individual behaviour (this links to the discussion in Chapter 6).
Type 2 – Explanations to do with individual attributes and circumstances (this links to the discussion in chapter 8).
Type 3 – Explanations to do with the material environment and allocation of resources (this links to discussions in chapter 4, chapter 11 and chapter 12).
Type 4 – Explanations to do with social relationships and human subjectivity (this links to the discussion in chapter 9).

As a starting point for this chapter it is useful to refer to Busfield's 'Type 3' explanation which concerns the physical environment and its influences on health. According to Busfield's typology, our material environment and the way that resources are allocated and distributed have a significant impact on health. In turn, these factors are influenced by the way that society is organized politically and economically (Busfield, 2000). We will explore Busfield's Type 3 explanation in more detail with specific reference to the different factors within this chapter.

Physical environment (living and working conditions)

As Green and Tones (2010) argue, health is influenced by environment in many ways – both directly and indirectly. In learning task 10.1 you have had the opportunity to reflect on the influence of some specific factors of the physical environment on health and health experience. Each of these will now be examined in turn.

Agriculture and food production

Without doubt, food is vital to health and for sustaining human life. For example, as Busfield (2000) argues in her type 3 explanation of health and illness, malnourishment leads to increased susceptibility

---

[1]   For more information about Busfield's (2000) four types of explanation of health and illness please follow up the full reference provided in the reference list at the end of the book.

to illness and disease. Research and experience shows that over- or under-consumption of specific types of food can be detrimental to short-term and long-term health. In addition to the *availability* and *types* of food, the *production* of food is also a vital contributing factor for health. Agriculture and food production are influenced by a number of different things including manufacturing and marketing processes, political systems and economics. Agriculture links with health in several different ways – it is important for good health as it provides food and also, in many countries, materials for shelter and it is also a source of livelihood for many people in lower-income countries (Hawkes & Ruel, 2006). There have been many recent debates about the nature of food production and scares associated with production and manufacturing processes. Take some time out to do learning task 10.2.

Nearly a billion people globally do not have adequate access to clean drinking water, a basic requirement for health.

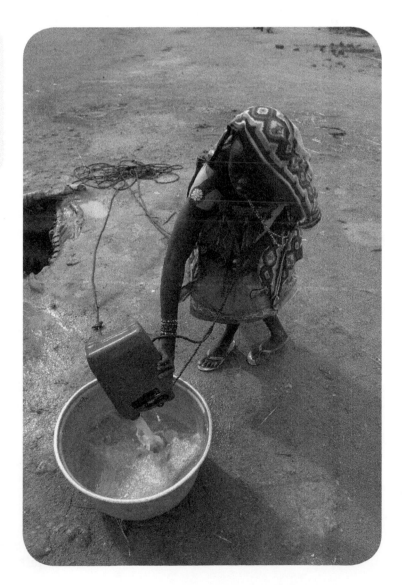

Learning task 10.2

Food scares and health.

1. Using the internet, see if you can find any information about food production and threats to health. As a starting point you might want to use the following examples:
    (a) Eggs and salmonella
    (b) Beef and BSE
    (c) Genetically modified crops

2. Consider the different factors involved in the food production 'chain' in relation to the specific issue you are investigating and how this might impact on health.

3. Who or what regulates food manufacturing and production in relation to the issue/s you have investigated?

Busfield (2000) argues that 'the contamination and adulteration of food . . . is always a major threat' (p. 47). The vulnerability of whole populations to this was recently evident in the so-called 'China Baby Milk Scandal' of 2008. The apparently deliberate contamination of baby milk with an industrial chemical reportedly led to the deaths of at least six infants and caused a further 300,000 babies to be ill (Macartney, 2009).

A related issue is that, in line with wider processes of globalization (discussed in more detail in chapter 12), the majority of food manufacturers are now owned and governed by large multi-national companies that are very powerful and have increasing control over all aspects of the food chain (Lee & Collin, 2005). Regulation of food production processes are increasingly centralized and influenced by bodies such as the European Union (Busfield, 2000).

Lee and Collin (2005) point out that the recent pace of change in the global food trade is 'unprecedented'. This has resulted, they argue, in massively increased food production – 'more than enough to feed everyone on the planet' (p. 43). Given that there are still parts of the world where people do not have enough to eat, there is obviously a problem with the *distribution* of food that links to Busfield's Type 3 explanation about the material environment. At the end of the year 2008, the World Food Programme estimated that there were almost one billion people worldwide without adequate nutrition (World Food Programme, 2009). The term 'food security' has been defined in many different ways (Food and Agriculture Organization, 2003) but it basically refers to *access to* and *availability of* food. While an in-depth discussion cannot take place here, these are two key issues related to food production that are central to health in terms of the physical environment. Another term used in the literature is 'food desert', which 'describes neighbourhoods and communities that have limited access to affordable and nutritious foods' (Tarnapol Whitacre et al., 2009). Again, this is related to access and availability of food. Food deserts can exist in any context including high-income countries.

Excess calorie intake is one of the factors contributing to the rise of the overweight and obese – particularly in the so-called 'Western' context. A number of theories abound as to why we are seeing such an increase in weight among certain populations. Examples are theories that make reference to the 'obesogenic environment'. This term refers to the role environmental factors may play in determining both nutrition and physical activity (Government Office for Science, 2007). Kumanyika (2008), among others, argues that factors such as higher than average availability of fast food outlets and lack of opportunities within the environment for physical activity are relevant and may contribute to above-average levels of food consumption and inadequate levels of physical activity leading to increased likelihood of childhood obesity. This has implications not only for health during childhood but also into adulthood as a substantial amount of research appears to show that an overweight child is likely to remain overweight into adulthood (for example Cole et al., 2000) with all the associated long-term health risks.

Water and sanitation

Before we discuss this aspect of the physical environment and living/working conditions further, take some time out to do learning task 10.3.

In learning task 10.3 you have considered a specific threat to safe water and sanitation – open defecation. CLTS is a successful approach to addressing this issue that has been used in many different countries and contexts across the globe in the last decade or so.

Access to clean water and adequate sanitation facilities are key requirements for good health. In more affluent societies the provision of these is something that we tend to take for granted. However, UNICEF

Learning task 10.3

Community-led total sanitation (CLTS).
Using the internet, see what you can find out about community-led total sanitation.

(a) What is it all about?
(b) With regard to this aspect of the physical environment, how does open defecation impact on health?
(c) What are the key features of CLTS and how do these work together to improve sanitation in rural communities?

Homelessness is a significant risk factor for a range of mental and physical illnesses.

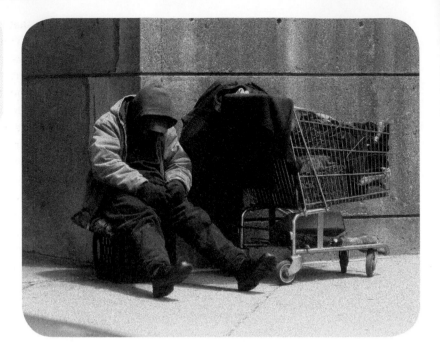

(2010) estimates that, globally, just under one billion people do not have access to clean water and 1.2 billion have no access to sanitation facilities and have to practice open defecation. Improvements in sanitation in Britain in the 1800s, led to massive improvements in public health (Busfield, 2000). However, contamination of water sources, whether through faecal matter, chemicals or industrial waste, remains an issue and a threat to health to a greater or lesser degree around the world.

Estimates are that 'water problems' affect around half of humanity (Shah, 2010). For example, approximately 1.8 million children die each year due to diarrhoea largely through contaminated water sources. Water and sanitation deficits have major repercussions for health, especially in low-income countries. Donaldson and Scally (2009) argue that, from an international perspective, the provision of safe water is an 'aspiration' and it should be increasingly seen as a precious resource.

A recent example is the worst drought in Russia and the Ukraine for decades occurring in summer 2010. This is predicted to have a long-term knock-on effect on global food prices (including meat and poultry) because Russia is the second largest producer of barley, which is also used as animal feed (Wray, 2010). Given the recent effects in the last few years of worldwide economic recession it is likely that the least well-off in society would be most affected by this outcome.

Housing

As Donaldson and Scally (2009) argue, the link between housing conditions and health has been established for some time in Britain.

The period of rapid urbanization in the nineteenth century led to severe overcrowding in towns and cities and resulted in conditions of rampant disease, such as the spread of communicable infections like tuberculosis and cholera. The sanitary reforms of the same period focused, among other things, on improvements in housing with massive effects on public health (Earle, 2007b). Despite the fact that it is difficult to control for confounding factors when researching the link between housing and health, there appears to be some evidence that damp and cold housing may be linked with respiratory illnesses (Evans et al., 2000). In addition, poor quality housing can add to a general burden of stress. Homelessness is another issue of relevance here. Being completely homeless or living in temporary accommodation can put people at increased risk of mental – including drug and alcohol misuse – and physical illness (The Queen's Nursing Institute, 2007). This is a global issue. As of July 2009 the UN Refugee Agency estimated that there were '42 million uprooted people waiting to go home' (Guterres, 2009).

The growth of urban slums, exacerbated by the migration of rural populations into towns and cities, means that nearly half the

Western media attention has traditionally focused on starvation; however malnutrition has a significant and enduring impact on health in lower-income countries.

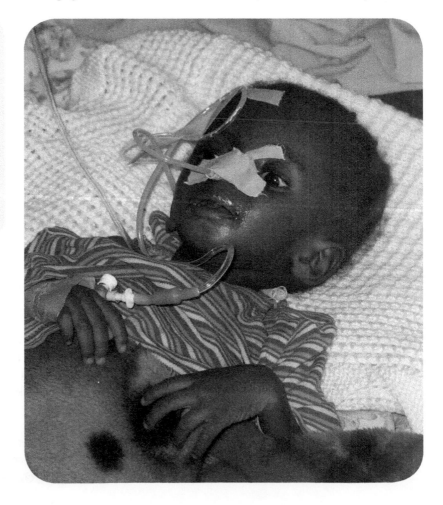

> **Learning task 10.4**
>
> **The influence of the working environment on health.**
> (a) Take some time out to consider the effect of the working environment on health beyond what you did for learning task 10.1.
> (b) Consider whether there might be differences according to type of work, gender roles and age for example.

population of the world now live in urban areas. As of 2005, there were approximately one billion people living in slum conditions (Millennium Development Goals Report, 2007). The impact on health of living in these types of conditions are many and range from threats to personal security to issues directly related to overcrowding, such as rapid spread of air- and water-borne infectious diseases.

A further issue related to housing is clean indoor air. Clean air is essential for good health. However, 2.5 billion people in developing countries have to rely on solid fuels ('biomass' such as wood and charcoal) to meet their energy needs – for cooking and keeping warm. This results in indoor air pollution from, for example carbon monoxide, which kills approximately 1.8 million people every year (World Bank, 2008), contributing to the global disease burden. Another form of potential air pollution within the 'home environment' is cigarette smoke. Secondary or passive smoking appears to have significant detrimental effects on non-smokers (Barnoya and Glantz, 2005; Semple et al., 2007). A recent campaign in the UK, 'Smoke Free Homes', is aimed at reducing the risk to others, especially children, from second-hand smoke. A number of towns and cities across Britain are now working towards becoming smoke free. In the UK all work places are smoke free by law but this does not ensure that the working environment is healthy because it influences our health in complex ways. The final learning task of this chapter encourages you to think about the relationship between the work environment and health.

The working environment

Given the amount of time we spend in the workplace during our working lives it is important to consider the influence of the working environment on health. This can be done in three ways – in terms of working patterns, in terms of the physical working environment and in terms of psycho-social impact.

Working patterns can, and do, influence our health. Most obviously, working irregular shifts has been shown to be detrimental for both physical and mental health and increases risk for a variety of illnesses and disorders including high blood pressure and certain types of cancer, as well as anxiety and depression (Shields, 2002) and compromises pregnancy outcomes (Knutsson, 2003). There appear to be three possible reasons for this – disruption to sleep patterns, patterns of unhealthy behaviour associated with working shifts and stress (Scott, 2000; Knutsson, 2003).

Another feature of the working environment that has received attention in recent decades is 'Sick Building Syndrome' (SBS). According to Burge (2004) Sick Building Syndrome is 'a group of mucosal, skin and general symptoms that are temporally related to working in particular buildings' (p. 185). Workers experience a range of symptoms caused by the condition of the building in which they work, usually in relation to factors such as air temperature, humidity and lighting levels. Illnesses related to 'sick' buildings also include viral infections and toxic reactions. Since the symptoms of SBS are difficult to test objectively and typically clear up within a short time of leaving the building, there are quite a few sceptics about its existence (Burge, 2004). Nevertheless, it appears to be something that impacts subjectively on the health of many people, reducing productivity and increasing absenteeism (Epstein, 2008).

In terms of the influence of the working environment and health, the Whitehall Studies carried out in the UK have been highly influential. These were two longitudinal studies carried out on British civil servants. The first began in 1967 and was carried out over ten years. The second began in 1985. The Whitehall studies have sought to investigate the social determinants of health and have produced a number of significant findings. For example, low levels of work demand, control and support have been associated with higher rates of absence (North et al., 1996). Hierarchical workplace relationships and perceptions of imbalances in power have been linked to workplace bullying, which in turn have been linked to absenteeism (Salin, 2003).

More recently, Aronsson et al. (2002) compared differences in work conditions and health in Swedish workers in temporary and permanent employment. They found clear differences between the two groups and that generally the permanently employed had better health than those in temporary employment. Another Scandinavian study with a sample of 5001 Danish employees found that worsening self reported health over a five-year period was linked to repetitive work, high psychological demands, low social support, high job insecurity and high ergonomic exposures (Borg et al., 2000). This is significant because, as Borg et al. point out, self-reported health is a powerful independent predictor for total mortality.

Unemployment

In 1995 a systematic review on the impact of unemployment was published by Lin et al. The review concluded what, instinctively, we might predict it would – that being unemployed is detrimental to health. Although Lin et al. (1995) demonstrated a strong relationship between unemployment and adverse health outcomes the causal nature of this was less clear from their review. They concluded that this is because there are likely to be many other factors contributing to the picture. The key question, as Lin et al. succinctly put it is – 'does unemployment cause poor health, or it is more likely that poor health causes unemployment?' (p. 531). The review links unemployment to a range of adverse health outcomes including suicide, deaths in road accidents, physical and mental disorders and increased alcohol consumption and seems to suggest that there is more epidemiological evidence that unemployment causes ill-health than the other way around.

More recently Stewart (2001) states that a number of studies indicates that people who are unemployed experience higher death rates than people who are employed. This is still the case when potential confounding characteristics are accounted for (such as social class, age, marriage, sex and occupation). Stewart points out that there are three main reasons why there is a link between unemployment and death rates – firstly, unemployment decreases health status, secondly people with impaired health status are more likely to become unemployed for periods of time and thirdly, people with impaired health status are more likely to remain unemployed. However, as Kessler et al. (2009) argue, the experience of being unemployed is not the same for everyone. Despite the fact that there is a lot of research that shows that being unemployed is detrimental to health and undoubtedly has a negative impact, we still don't know much about why this is the case. In an attempt to understand the specific impact on mental health Kessler et al. analysed the experience of being unemployed by considering a range of different stressors created or made worse by it. They concluded that two main mechanisms cause adverse affects specific to mental health. Firstly, that unemployment results in increased financial pressure that has negative health effects and secondly, that it increases individual vulnerability to other unrelated life events.

With regard to mental health Artazcoz et al. (2004) investigated the impact of unemployment to see if there were any effects associated with gender, family roles or social class. Their findings suggested that being unemployed affected men's mental health more than women's mental health and that these observed gender differences were related to social class and family responsibilities. Interestingly the findings pick up on gendered health issues referred to elsewhere in this book (see chapters 4 and 8). Family responsibilities seem to increase the effects of unemployment on mental health for men – perhaps given societal expectations about their traditional masculine responsibilities as primary providers or 'breadwinners'. For the women in the study, however, their traditional feminine role as caregiver seems to act as a buffer for the adverse mental health effects of unemployment.

Education

While it might not be immediately obvious what the causal mechanisms are, education has an important influence on people's health and their lifestyles later in life (Donaldson & Scally, 2009). Ross and Wu's (1995) findings suggested that there are positive associations between education and health. They offer three categories of explanation for this – firstly, work and economic conditions, secondly, social-psychological resources and thirdly, lifestyle. Let's consider each of these briefly in turn. Ross and Wu's findings seem to suggest that work and economic conditions are important – the more educated you are, the less likely you are to be unemployed. You have considered the impact that being unemployed can have on our health in learning task 10.1. The more educated you are, the more likely you are to work full time in fulfilling, subjectively rewarding work all of which significantly improves health outcomes. Social-psychological resources such as life skills, resilience and social skills receive attention because the more educated you are, the more likely you are to report a sense of control over your life and your health and greater levels of social support, both of which are conducive to better health experience. Finally, the more educated you are the less likely you are to adopt health-damaging practices such as smoking and take up health-enhancing practices such as regular exercise – all of which are associated with good health. Ross and Wu (1995) therefore conclude that high educational attainment improves health directly, and also indirectly.

More recently, in the UK context, Sir Michael Marmot, Chair of The Marmot Review (2010), pointed out that people who have university degrees live longer and have better health than people who don't. At the other end of the educational spectrum there is evidence to show that providing quality primary-level education to young girls in low-income countries greatly benefits later maternal and child health (UNICEF, nd). 'Educated girls also have higher self-esteem, are more likely to avoid HIV infection, violence and exploitation, and to spread good health and sanitation practices to their families and communities' (UNICEF, nd). One of the Millennium Development Goals (see chapter 12) highlights the importance of education for girls, recognizing the massive impact that this has, not only on the health of the girls themselves but on the health of their future children. Hammond (2004) argues that learning can have a range of psycho-social benefits, including increased self-esteem and self-efficacy, increased purpose and identity and better social integration, all of which can help to promote mental health and the ability to cope better with ill-health generally. However, the relationship between education and health is very complex. Research also seems to suggest that children who experience poor health generally don't do as well educationally (Case et al., 2005) and this could be due to a number of different factors. In addition to having lower educational attainment the same children, as adults, also have lower social status and experience poorer health, perpetuating the so-called 'Cycle of Deprivation' (Joseph, 1974) or 'Cycle of Disadvantage' (Rutter & Madge, 1976) both cited in Welshman (2002).

Health care services

While the role of health care services in improving population health is continuously under debate (Nolte et al., 2005; Taylor & Hawley, 2010) the quality and availability of health care makes a huge difference to health outcomes within any given population. Maternal and infant experiences are one example of where this is strikingly the case. These differ considerably according to whether a woman lives in a low-income or high-income country. Let's first consider some of the evidence for this. According to UNICEF (nd) a woman dies from complications of childbirth every minute – about 529,000 per year and the vast majority of these deaths occur in low-income countries. To put this in perspective it means that a woman in sub-Saharan Africa has a one in six chance of dying in pregnancy or childbirth compared to a one in 4000 risk for a woman in a higher-income country. This is a huge disparity. While there are many different reasons why this might be the case there is a lot of evidence to suggest that lack of access to ante-, peri- and post-natal care plays a major part. It is argued that access to skilled care during these important periods is key to saving women and children's lives (UNICEF, nd).

In the UK the so-called 'Post Code Lottery' is a label used to describe relative differences in the provision of health care related to geographic location. There are several areas of health care provision and associated health outcomes that seem to depend on where you live – hence the 'post code' label. For example, Lyon et al. (2004) studied response times, distance travelled to the scene and location and survival of non-hospital cardiac arrests and concluded that survival is heavily influenced by the response time and distance. The closer you live to an ambulance dispatch point the better your chances of surviving a heart attack. Cancer care is another aspect of health services provision in the UK that varies from region to region (Bungay, 2005; Clarke et al., 2008).

In the USA, one of the wealthiest countries in the world, access to health care services is far from equal, although the new administration under President Barack Obama is making efforts to increase access and affordability of health care for the whole population. Research by van Doorslaer et al. (2006) suggests that this type of disparity is not peculiar to the USA. They carried out a study that examined access to health care in terms of use of general practitioner services in 21 high-income member countries of the Organization for Economic Co-operation and Development. They concluded that, even though general practitioner services were relatively evenly distributed, better-off sections of society made more use of services, even more so when private insurance or private care options were offered.

What does this mean?

As Lalonde pointed out in 1974 and Donaldson and Scally (2009), among others, still argue, the physical environment (our living and working conditions) has a large part to play in our experiences of heath. As stated previously, the issues that have been discussed within this chapter are not exhaustive. There are many other factors of our living and working conditions that impact on health. Some additional examples are natural and manmade disasters, climate change (Macdonald, 2006), out-door air pollution (Donaldson & Scally, 2009), solid waste disposal (Leonardi et al, 2005) and transport. Did you come up with any other ones earlier on?

In addition we would also need to consider our socio-political environment and how this can impact on our health and well-being. This has been referred to in more detail elsewhere in this book (see chapters 4 and 11). The discussion in this chapter is indicative of the way in which different living and working conditions might impact on health but necessarily focuses on a few key factors using Dahlgren and Whitehead's (1991) model as a point of reference. Importantly, as argued by Green and Tones (2010), although this is not explored in detail here, different environmental factors may interact with each other to influence health. For example, 'poverty is associated with poor housing, diet, education and health care . . . leading to fewer life chances overall' (Green & Tones, 2010: 87). These issues link to the arguments put forward in chapter 11 (on policy).

How is this relevant ?

It is important to consider factors within the physical environment and how these can influence health and health experience. This is for a number of reasons. Once we can identify environmental factors affecting health we are then in a position to address them and potentially make a real difference to health outcomes. There is also the potential to influence health policy, how fiscal decisions are made and where resources to improve health are aimed. As Donaldson and Scally (2009) argue, decisions carried out at a local, national (and international) governmental level in many different fields – from education to the built environment – may ultimately have an effect on population health.

A central underlying principle of health promotion first mentioned in the Ottawa Charter (WHO, 1986) and later picked up in more detail in the Sundsvall Statement (WHO, 1991) is that in order to promote health we need to be creating supportive environments, among other things. Supportive environments for health is about influencing our living and working conditions in order to maximize health gain. The UK Public Health White Paper of 2004 – Choosing Health: Making Healthier Choices Easier (DH, 2004) signals the importance of creating and maintaining environments where people can make better choices for better health.

The 'settings' approach, another key concept in health promotion, is also relevant here (Hubley & Copeman, 2008). The settings approach takes into account the direct effect of the setting itself on health as well as providing an opportunity for promoting health. The term 'settings' covers a wide range of different contexts, from the physical to the geographical to the virtual, from the home to towns and cities and from schools to workplaces and communities. Hubley and Copeman (2008) define a 'setting' as 'a specific context/location from which to carry out health promotion' (p. 34). Unquestionably the idea of settings has relevance to any discussion on the influence of living and working conditions on health and many different settings offer different opportunities to promote health.

Case study

The physical environment, health and health experience in a South African context.

This case study considers the different aspects of living and working conditions discussed in this chapter in relation to a specific context – the Cape Malay families of the winelands of the Western Cape in South Africa. Note that, for the purposes of the case study broad generalizations are made.

Several factors may influence health outcomes for families in this specific context.

Health care services: Facilities for health care may be lacking and be unaffordable for families on relatively low wages. Families may have to travel from remote areas to access health care other than basic clinical services.

Agriculture and food production: Access to good nutrition may be affected by the amount of money that is available to spend on food, which can be limited by low wages and by local provision of food.

Water and sanitation: This will vary, however; access to clean water may come from stand pipes and toilets in existence may be pit latrines. Houses with piped running water and flush toilets are relatively uncommon.

Working environment: Most of the work is manual labour, which involves the processes connected with the grape-growing and wine-producing seasons. This brings associated risks, such as from accident and injury as well as seasonal work.

Housing: This will tend to be fairly basic with whole families living altogether in relatively few rooms and differing physical standards of housing infrastructure.

Summary

- There are many aspects of the physical environment that impact on health and health experience throughout life through our living and working conditions.

- Research into these factors, and the impact of them, is challenging because, while positive relationships and associations can be demonstrated, the causal mechanisms (how and why) can be harder to determine.

- The relationship between our living and working conditions and the way that we live our lives is very complex and involves the interaction of a large number of different factors that are hard to separate from each other.

Questions

1. Think about the different aspects of our living and working conditions discussed in this chapter (and others mentioned). Which of these do you think is most influential on health and why? What is the evidence for this?

2. With specific reference to the settings approach to promoting health, how might health be improved within a particular setting; for example, you could consider prisons, schools, hospitals or neighbourhood settings.

3. How much of your own health is influenced by your living and working conditions? Consider the ways in which the contents of this chapter provide an explanation for this. What would you add to this 'onion' ring layer of Dahlgren and Whitehead's model?

Further reading

Due to the scope of the contents of this chapter and the many issues that have been discussed, it is not possible to recommend further reading on every aspect. Some selected suggestions are therefore offered here.

Taylor, G. and Hawley, H. (2010) Key Debates in Health Care. Maidenhead, Open University Press.
This is a very good source of central, topical debates in health care. Although it is primarily focused on issues impacting on the UK and USA, there are examples from other international contexts throughout that are useful. The book is structured around addressing key questions relating to health care provision that can be applied to many different contexts.

MacDonald, T.H. (2005) Third World Health: Hostage to First World Health. Oxford, Radcliffe.
This book clearly explains the persistence of inequalities and inequities in health in lower-income countries and the relationship between

global health and wealth. It debates some of the major issues raised in this chapter using case studies to bring these to life in the discussion. It is a very interesting and accessible read and highlights some key issues and debates.

Scriven, A. and Hodgins, M. (2011) Health Promotion Setting: Principles and Practice London, Sage.

This is a comprehensive text offering a wealth of information about settings in health promotion. It is an edited volume which contains a number of chapters by authors with expertise in different areas related to settings. It includes discussion of different settings such as prisons, hospitals, schools, workplaces, cities and universities. It also goes into considerable depth about the settings approach to promoting health.

11 Policy Influences upon Health

Key learning outcomes

By the end of this chapter you should be able to:

- understand what social policy is and how the policy-making process works

- understand how social policy influences individual health in a variety of ways both positively and negatively

- identify and understand the principles of healthy public policy

Overview

Social policy is recognized within the Dahlgren and Whitehead (1991) framework as a determinant of health encompassed under general socio-economic, cultural and environmental conditions. This chapter gives an overview of what social policy is generally. More specifically it demonstrates that many facets of policy exist within our social environment that combine to influence and determine health in a number of ways. This chapter will answer key questions such as what is social policy and how does social policy influence and affect our health? This chapter will explore how social policy is related to health, beginning by exploring the ideological basis of policy to demonstrate that values are crucial in formulating policy and influencing health, not always positively. The chapter answers key questions such as how important are health services as a determinant of good health, and what is healthy public policy? The chapter explores policy clearly and specifically related to health and demonstrates the importance of the broader policy environment in determining good health; for example education, welfare and transport policy can all have health impacts. Finally, the chapter examines how crucial fiscal policy is in terms of health, using a case study to illustrate how recession affects government policy, which in turn affects health.

What is social policy?

Social policy can be described as a field of activity decided upon and implemented by the government, a course of action and indeed a web of decisions rather than a single decision (Hill, 1997). Policy usually is a stance towards a particular topic (see the discussions of ideology later in this chapter), and involves a cluster of related decisions and actions often dealt with in a consistent fashion (Harrison & Macdonald, 2008). Social policy is often concerned with tackling social problems and bringing about change, yet it can work in a number of opposable and generalized ways:

- to keep things as they are (maintaining the status quo) or to try to change things
- to give privilege or advantage to certain groups, or instead to try to treat people equally
- to promote equality or alternatively to extend inequality
- to promote certain, specific values or to accommodate a range of diverse values
- to change individuals (or indeed groups) or to change environments.

Policy therefore can work in a variety of ways and hence affect health in a variety of ways. The policy-making process in which policy paths are determined is also complex and dynamic, itself subject to a range of influences from various groups and stakeholders who have an interest in directing policy. Blakemore and Griggs (2007) argue that the wider social and environmental influences on what happens to us in the doctor's surgery or hospital are reflected in government policy. This is affected by the cost of services and the money available to fund these rising costs for example associated with medications, public expectations and developments in medical technology are key in policy-making. They define health policy in two ways:

1. as the efforts made by the government to improve health through both services and medical treatment
2. as any activity undertaken by the government that affects health and illness.

Policy is thus made on a number of levels. Chapter 12 discusses policy made internationally with the aim of making global improvements but policy is also made on a national and regional level. For example, the UK's National Health Service is governed nationally hence policy related to the service is made by the government, through the Department of Health. However, it is not just the UK government who influence policy-making in relation to the NHS. Policy actors include a range of other people such as civil servants, professional bodies, expert advisory groups, interest groups, user groups and the media. The roles of these different groups vary within the policy process; for example, the media and interest groups often serve to raise issues effectively and to get policy problems on the agenda but they have no role in implementation once policy is created. Certain issues become important in policy terms and make it onto the policy agenda. The media has often played a role in the UK in framing specific health issues as important, for example, the unavailability of life-prolonging drugs for cancer patients has had a wealth of media attention, as has the refusal of treatment for patients based upon certain criteria such as their refusal to stop smoking, change their lifestyle or because of their obesity. It is not just the media who play a part in influencing the policy agenda, powerful corporate interests group can often work with politicians and government officials to negotiate and lobby, as a mechanism to serve their private corporate interests particularly within the USA

Learning task 11.1

The UK Media and MMR

- In 1998, Dr Andrew Wakefield published the findings of a study in the *Lancet* suggesting a link between the MMR (measles, mumps and rubella) vaccination and autism.
- The media reported the findings and continually backed Dr Wakefield, even when his claims were disputed by a number of different experts, demanding parental choice in choosing single vaccinations rather than the combined MMR that is currently available on the NHS.
- The UK Government and Department of Health did not change immunization policy and so the MMR triple vaccination remained free for NHS patients, whilst single vaccinations were only available privately.
- Brendan O'Neill wrote in the *Guardian* (16.6.2006) that the media should 'hang their heads in shame' for creating a climate of fear about the MMR vaccination, which resulted in decreased immunization rates and the resurgence of more measles cases.

1. Use the Internet to find out more about the media reporting about the MMR vaccination and the subsequent decision of the government not to make any policy changes.
2. Take time to think about the ethical debates that emerge as a result of the media reporting of the issue. You may wish to give consideration to 'scaremongering' and its implications.
3. You also might want to think about which societal groups were more likely to be negatively affected by both the reporting and government's refusal to change policy.

(Crinson, 2009). Thus corporate lobbying and the role of the media has raised ethical questions in relation to the policy-making process. The following learning task will help you to think about the role of the media and its influence upon the policy-making process.

This learning task demonstrates that the relationship between the state and individuals affected by its policies is complex. It is also a useful starting point to discussing the presence of power within the policy-making process. Power plays a part in the policy-making process, with the pluralist view being that power is spread throughout society so that no one group holds power over others. Comparatively the elitist view is that policy choices are dominated by the upper social classes, the ruling elite who wish to continue to keep power and play a dominant role in society.

Clearly, the policy-making process is incredibly complex and consequently how policy is made and works in practice is therefore debated. Academics have characterized policy-making using a number of different models, broadly described as follows:

> Rationalist – in this model policy-makers are assumed to have a good understanding of the problems relevant to the policy-making process and are consequently able to choose different options and make clear, rational decisions in relation to policy.

> Incrementalist – in this model policy-makers are assumed not to start with a blank sheet and they also do not have perfect knowledge about the issues encompassed within the policy-making process. Often policy-makers have to respond to changes and as a result these are small and incremental.

> Pluralist – within this model, policy is understood to emerge from the interaction of different parties at all stages of development and implementation.

> Institutionalism – this model suggests that policy is created by government institutions and that there is a very close relationship between policy-making as a process and such institutions because policies are implemented by them.

> Policy communities – this model depicts policy as being made within specific communities via networks such as those that exist between public and private actors. It is essential that these networks are uncovered and explored in order to gain understanding of the policy-making process.

Hogwood and Gunn (1984) describe nine stages of the process, Jenkins (1978) outlines seven and Rose (1973) describes twelve. The three key stages described by Harrison & Macdonald (2008) are

1.   the public policy agenda – how and why do issues come onto the agenda?

2. alternatives and choices – are policy choices rational?
3. implementation – are choices put into action and if so, how so?

The locus of power within policy-making is particularly important when thinking about public health policy because the state intervenes in a number of different ways in relation to population health.

Social policy as a determinant of health

Social policy determines health in a number of ways, with health policy encompassing a variety of activities such as disease prevention, health promotion, welfare, and the support of caring systems. Health policy can be described as efforts by the government to improve health, welfare and medical treatment. Much academic focus upon health policy within the UK is related to the exploration of the National Health Service (NHS). Similarly, in other countries reforming the health care system and implementing effective policies has dominated debates; for example in the USA, Barack Obama has made several controversial and often opposed changes to the provision of health care insurance schemes. Health care policy tends to focus upon the medical services delivered within hospitals and across communities, in hospitals or doctors' surgeries – hence the large amount of attention afforded to the NHS. This is also a complex area, with Harrison & Macdonald (2008) arguing that there are significant contradictions evident within the politics of contemporary health care. The activities of the NHS are certainly crucial in caring for health but there are also broader policy areas relevant to health. The delivery of measures aiming to tackle health-related problems such as alcohol consumption, obesity, inactivity and more specific health promotion programmes, such as recent work to tackle swine flu via a vaccination programme, are all relevant to health. Furthermore, health policy is important in attempting to tackle inequalities by trying to change the circumstances in which people live such as housing conditions, the local environment and the distribution of income in society (Hudson et al., 2008). In recent years in the UK, there were many health-related policy changes introduced by the New Labour government geared towards increasing the health of the nation, with the notable example of the **social marketing** programme, Change4Life, launched in 2009, with the slogan 'Eat Well, Move More and Live Longer'. Health policy can also be controversial and receive negative public responses.

Health policy change is also further complicated because of its inter-relationship with other policy areas. Hudson et al. argue that this interconnectedness of policy areas and policy dilemmas is one of the reasons why policy delivery is such a complicated aspect of government because it is incredibly difficult to deliver a finished policy solution. This is because the interconnectedness of policy areas makes it notably hard to predict how a change in one area may impact upon another

> **Box 11.1**
>
> ## Example of public reaction to potential policy change.
>
> On 26th September 2010 a newspaper article described a public outcry at a proposed rewards system to encourage behaviour change amongst certain groups of people.
>
> A number of schemes were investigated as potential future policy options including
>
> - Dieters to be paid for losing weight
> - Pregnant women to be given shopping vouchers for stopping smoking
> - Children to be rewarded with toys when they have eaten their vegetables
> - Rewards for over-weight parents walking their children to school
>
> The schemes were opposed by a number of commentators who argued that lifestyle changes should not be rewarded and that the evidence base for the effectiveness of interventions is unclear (Donnelly 2010).

Learning task 11.2

Making health policy work.

Verdung (1988) argues that if you look hard enough, policy instruments can be reduced to three simple mechanisms.

1. Carrots – meaning incentives and rewards such as remuneration
2. Sticks – meaning regulation and punishment
3. Sermons – meaning advice, guidance and information provision

Think about all three of these approaches in relation to reducing alcohol consumption in the UK. If you were a policy maker tasked with creating policy to reduce overall drinking rates within the general population, think about the above policy mechanisms and answer the following questions,

1. How might carrots work to reduce drinking levels?
2. How might sticks work to reduce drinking levels?
3. How might sermons work to reduce drinking levels?
4. What would be the limitations of all of these approaches if they were to be implemented?
5. How might the implementation of this health policy affect other policy sectors?

---

policy sector. Delivering the goals of any policy is also complicated, as the policy can be 'remade' during the implementation process by those responsible for delivering it on the ground. Indeed, formulating policy is itself a complex process, as learning task 11.2 will help you to grasp.

Current policy issues

There are many challenges faced by current health and welfare services in the UK and across the world. The issue that often receives most media attention and discussion is that of continued funding challenges. When the NHS was established, it was not possible to envisage the demands that the service would face or indeed the advancement of medical science in developing new treatments, which are often extremely expensive. There have been considerable improvements in medical treatment, such as anaesthesia and keyhole surgery, as well as changing priorities and needs from patients, compared with those existing fifty years ago (Blakemore & Griggs, 2007). Pioneering new treatments, medication regimes and equipment all add to the cost of health care provision, and money for health spending is a finite resource, leading to difficult policy decisions about what can and cannot be funded. Chapter 2 discusses contemporary threats to health in detail and considers the implications of some of these threats in relation to service provision and finance.

Historically the health service predominantly treated acute conditions and life-threatening infectious diseases. Now the health service is faced with dealing with long-term conditions and chronic illnesses such as asthma, mental illness and diabetes (Blakemore & Griggs, 2007). There are also many health issues posed by demographic changes, with an ageing population arguably placing more demands upon health care resources and increasingly costing the service more money. Moore (2008) argues that an ageing population in the UK poses the question of whether some patients have more right to treatment than others. There are some commentators who argue that an ageing population does not necessarily mean there will be a spending crisis, suggesting that, as most acute resources are spent on people in the last year of their lives, then it is irrelevant whether they die at age sixty or eighty. This may be the case in some instances; however this argument is based upon the assumption that people will have a good quality of life until their final year, and given the increase in lifestyle-associated chronic conditions, this is not always going to be the case. It is more likely that the older population will carry a disproportionate burden of age-related conditions such as dementia, heart problems and cancers; therefore the cost of treatment is likely to rise as the population ages. There is, of course, large uncertainty about this because the impact of such changing demographics has yet to be experienced and so remains open to debate.

Furthermore, lifestyle-related health conditions are placing more strain on health services. For example, the cost of obesity, diabetes, sexually transmitted infections and alcohol-related diseases are consistently increasing year on year. These conditions have caused much debate about the responsibility we should take for our own health. This is coupled with rising expectations held by the UK public about what can be achieved by contemporary medicine. The 2002 Wanless Report estimated that NHS spending would need to be more than doubled in the following twenty years. Wanless also described three possible scenarios in relation to how much responsibility individuals would take and how this relates to projected costs, the implication being that if we all become 'fully engaged' then we will cost the health service less than if we make 'solid progress' or even worse 'slow uptake'. Even if the fully engaged scenario was to be achieved by 2022, health spending would still need to be doubled (based upon 2002 prices) to a massive £154 billion. If the worst-case scenario of slow uptake were to be realized, then even more funding will be required, estimated at £184 billion. In 2006, his follow-up report, commissioned by the Kings Fund suggests that despite record levels of investment, the NHS is not on course for the fully engaged scenario. Wanless (2007) was critical about current policy and the way in which the determinants of health were being tackled, arguing that there has been a lack of investment in public health initiatives and citing concerns about lifestyle-related health problems such as those associated with growing rates of obesity.

These issues reflect the complexity of health care challenges and the issues associated with the **rationing** of services. It has been argued that if the NHS is to cope with the full burden of unhealthy lifestyles and the burdens associated with an ageing population, then it can no longer do this as a fully comprehensive service (Moore, 2008). There are questions about how health care provision can be based upon need, how need can be defined, and who ultimately makes such decisions. Furthermore, as the NHS is free at the point of consumption, patients often have no idea of the cost of the services and the treatment that they receive and research also suggests that patient expectations are rising in relation to the treatment received.

All of these challenges to the NHS are related to broader concerns about the limitations and scope of the service. Concerns about the limitations of the NHS are not new and have been expressed in a number of ways since its inception (Klein, 2006). These rationing challenges are also being experienced and debated in many other countries, often resulting in the creation of specific bodies with responsibility for making recommendations in relation to the provision and funding of health care. The UK organization that assumes a central role in rationing is the National Institute for Clinical Excellence.

The British Welfare State

The British Welfare State has a complex history and is just one particular type of welfare model. Esping-Anderson (1990) argues that there are different types of welfare systems around the world, each based upon different ideologies and principles. This is important because the organization of both health and welfare systems fundamentally shape

Box 11.2   Rationing health care – the role of NICE in the UK

- Many of the difficult policy decisions associated with treatment are now made by an independent organization called the National Institute for Clinical Excellence (NICE), established in 1999.
- NICE regulates which treatments are available free of charge on the NHS. It reviews evidence about treatment regimes, the effectiveness of medications and conducts cost-benefit analyses in order to produce recommendations or rejections of proposed drugs and treatment pathways.
- NICE also produces national guidelines in an attempt to bring about equality of treatment across different geographical areas (see chapter 10 for discussion of the postcode lottery).
- NICE has no role to implement the recommendations that it makes.
- NICE has attracted controversy and criticism. For example, the development of NICE has significantly reduced the power of doctors to prescribe medicines that they think are the most clinically effective on the grounds of cost (Crinson 2009).
- NICE has also attracted negative attention for some of the decisions it has made, for example restricting anti-cancer drugs such as Herceptin (Tait 2006).
- Despite these issues, NICE has gained recognition outside the UK and has been considered as a template for use within other healthcare systems.

Box 11.3   Important debates in the provision of welfare

- What constitutes a basic human need? There are many debates about what 'need' actually means.
- How can welfare states ensure that all members of society have access to basic human needs and entitlements?
- How should welfare be funded? Should it be through taxation? Should the private sector be involved in funding? Should there be a mixture of provision (this is often called a 'mixed economy' of care)?
- How should welfare services be delivered and who should deliver them? Should it be the state? Should it be families? What about the role of the market in this process?

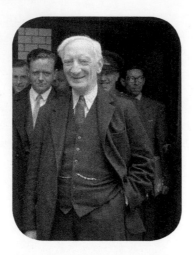

William Beveridge (1879–1963). The Beveridge Report of 1942 provided the impetus for the British Welfare State.

who has access to the services that are provided. Welfare states are a mechanism for meeting the basic needs of the population, and these are a crucial area of social policy research. However, there are many complex debates based around the provision of welfare.

While there are many debates about which model of welfare is the best, once a nation has a model then it is rare for it to have a major shift in any radical way. This is certainly true of the British Welfare State, established during 1945–50 as a comprehensive and universal welfare system, underpinned by the principle that the state should provide a range of services to support the population, funded through general taxation, from cradle to grave. The founder of the British Welfare State is William Beveridge, whose 1942 post-war report identified that there were five giants threatening the UK population.

- Want – people did not have sufficient income
- Idleness – unemployment because there were not enough jobs
- Squalor – poverty and poor housing conditions
- Ignorance – gaps in educational provision
- Disease – poor health made worse by a lack of affordable and accessible medical care.

These five giants underpin the modern welfare system, which is based upon five pillars of social security (related to want), employment, housing, education and health (Hudson et al., 2008). The Beveridge Report (1942) provided the basis of several key policies in post-war Britain enacted through several acts of parliament including

- The Education Act 1944
- The Family Allowances Act 1945
- The National Health Service Act 1946
- The National Insurance Act 1946.

Together these acts established a number of welfare benefits and enabled mass education and health care free at the point of consumption for the UK population. The welfare system has evolved massively since then but its principles and provision have fundamentally remained the same. This tends to occur in most countries with the chosen mechanisms of welfare provision remaining the same and alternatives not often implemented (Hudson et al., 2008). Thus, there is some level of policy inheritance that occurs, despite changes in government. This is called path dependency (Pierson, 2004) and shows that policy mechanisms can shape political interests as well as being influenced by them (Hudson et al., 2008). Thus, the British Welfare State has remained the same, despite a number of flaws. Blakemore and Griggs (2007) highlight a number of problems with the UK welfare system arguing that poverty persisted because benefits for some groups were set too low. National Insurance contributions were also set too low resulting in provision always being topped up with income from tax payers. There are many debates about the future provision of welfare in the UK as its continuation requires higher levels of taxation from a population that will need to work for longer (Glennerster, 2003). The British welfare system is currently facing huge cuts in its funding, after the Coalition Government Spending Review of October 2010 (BBC News, 2010). This has led to many debates about the future of welfare provision of the UK and the basis upon which the current UK coalition government is making cuts. There have been arguments made suggesting that cuts to public services are not simply a response to the UK's financial debt, but are also part of the new government's plans to shrink the welfare state and reduce the role of the public sector in service provision because of their ideological standpoint. Ideology is important in relation to the politics of welfare as the dominant ideological viewpoint of a government will impact upon their approaches to welfare provision and therefore, health.

Ideological and political values

Health and therefore health policy are political because population health is related to the actions of the government and the policy environment in which people live. Politics is important in health care within every country, with governments intervening in health care provision across the globe in a variety of ways. Values are commonly found in health policy and of course in politics too. There are many different clusters of values in policy-making, often associated with different political approaches and parties and we each hold our own ideological viewpoints, which influence our attitudes to health and health care. Table 11.1 outlines several different ideological perspectives and discusses how they relate to health. These descriptions are simplified massively but the key point here is that ideology underpins health care policy as well as beliefs about the provision of and payment for health care. The table gives an overview of the key aspects of various ideological viewpoints and the likely impact that such schools of thought have upon health.

Table 11.1. Ideological positions and their implications for health.

Ideological school of thought	General key points	What does this mean for health?
Conservatism	<ul><li>Seeks to maintain the traditional order of society.</li><li>Recognizes that inequalities exist and that they are inevitable.</li><li>Sees the role of the state as minimal with too much provision creating welfare dependency.</li><li>Values the **private sector** in service provision such as the delivery of health care.</li></ul>	<ul><li>Historical rejection of the UK Black Report (see chapter 4).</li><li>Reductions in public expenditure.</li><li>Expansion of the private sector.</li><li>Business principles applied to the UK NHS, the internal market was used to increase efficiency via competition.</li><li>Increased inequalities.</li></ul>
Liberalism	<ul><li>Essentially focuses upon freedom of choice.</li><li>Sees individuals as important. Individuals should behave responsibly.</li><li>Neo-liberalism is a global economic approach scaling back the state and public spending and encouraging privatization.</li></ul>	<ul><li>Modern liberalism has involved increased state intervention to reduce the effects of the market, so increased state provision of health care.</li><li>In comparison, neo-liberalism advocates reductions in spending on health and increased privatization.</li><li>Neo-liberalism shifts responsibility onto individuals who should adopt healthy behaviours.</li><li>Increased inequalities.</li></ul>
Socialism	<ul><li>This is a broad school of ideology, with differing meanings.</li><li>Originally associated with Marxism, which advocates revolution against the state.</li><li>Contemporary socialism has involved governments attempting to reform the state, and to increase state intervention in the provision of services.</li></ul>	<ul><li>Expansion of services including the provision of health care.</li><li>Concerned with equality in treatment and provision (the UK NHS is socialist in its underpinnings).</li></ul>
Nationalism	<ul><li>This is a belief system rather than an ideology per se, and has been employed by a variety of different governments.</li><li>Sees nations as self-governing, for example, Scotland.</li><li>Sees shared national identity as important in promoting social cohesion.</li></ul>	<ul><li>The effects upon health will depend upon the overall political context in which nationalism is employed.</li><li>Scottish health policy has seen an expansion of the UK NHS, with no prescription charges.</li><li>Some nationalist approaches have been damaging for health because of reductions in public spending.</li></ul>

Table 11.1. (continued)

Ideological school of thought	General key points	What does this mean for health?
Feminism	• There are a number of different feminisms. • Feminism generally raises the importance of gender relationships. • Liberal feminists attempt to overcome discrimination in the legal sphere. • Radical feminists focus upon the oppressive content of domestic relationships between men and women.	• Feminists have drawn attention to inequalities in health care diagnoses and treatment, arguing for service provision change and equality.
Environmentalism	• Term applies to a broad range of ideas • Recognizes the global environmental crisis and the importance of the environment. • Advocates sustainability and policies that do not damage the environment.	• The link between the environment and public health is emphasized here. • Public health needs the ecosystem to support it. • Encourages sustainable development to reduce inequalities. • Encourages reduction in carbon usage and ecological footprints.

The British NHS, established in 1948, is based upon the principle of health care as a right for every citizen, including the provision of care as comprehensive, universal and free to all at the point of consumption. The policy literature refers to this as institutionalism, an ideological position associated with left liberals and Fabians. The NHS has been subjected to a variety of political interventions since its creation in 1948 but despite much modernization and changes in services, structures and treatments, NHS principles have largely remained the same and were confirmed as such in 2000, in the NHS Plan. Navarro and Shi (2001) argue that population health is the best in countries that have social democratic governments, after analysing evidence from a range of countries including Sweden, Denmark and Austria. These countries tend to use high levels of taxation to fund their extensive welfare states, which allows increased health, education and family support services. The principles of equality and redistribution of health are seen as fundamentally good for health. Furthermore, other countries' health care systems operate differently and have a different ideological basis, leading to a variety of health outcomes. For example, health care in the USA is underpinned by neo-liberal ideology, which results in more inequality and poorer health outcomes (Kaiser Family Foundation 2009). Furthermore, all of us as individuals in society have our own beliefs

> ### Learning task 11.3
>
> **Ideological beliefs**
> What is your ideological standpoint in relation to health care? Read through the following statements – do you agree or disagree? Then think about what this tells you about your political values, referring back to the table (11.1) that summarises key ideologies?
>
> - People are responsible for their own health behaviour.
> - People who need to be hospitalized after binge drinking should pay for their treatment.
> - People who can afford to pay for private health care should not have to contribute to the funding of public health care.
> - Health is a commodity and therefore can and should be bought and sold in a competitive free market system.
> - All health care systems should be in public control.
> - The state should intervene, for example by using legislation to influence moral choices such as the termination of pregnancies.
> - Health care should be free for all consumers at the point of consumption, irrespective of whether they have contributed to paying for the care in any way.
> - If you adopt unhealthy lifestyle choices such as smoking and eating fatty foods then you should pay for the health care you require as a result of your behaviour.

and these viewpoints affect our attitudes in relation to the provision of health care. Learning task 11.3 will help you reflect upon your own ideological beliefs.

Health services as a determinant of health

Medical treatment may enhance health and the organization of health care systems fundamentally shapes who has access to the services that are provided. There are inequities of access to most health care systems and there are many debates about this (Hudson et al., 2008) that receive media and public attention. However, there is an array of evidence to demonstrate that health and illness are determined by many factors other than individual treatment. As chapter 4 demonstrates, our health is overwhelmingly social and chapter 5 also shows the importance of culture and cultural beliefs in influencing and determining our health. This 3rd section of the book demonstrates numerous influences upon health. There is also evidence that suggests that only 25% of the health of a developed population is attributable to its health care system (Harrison & Macdonald, 2008).

Moreover, the UK National Health Service currently faces many challenges in providing care. Acute illnesses and infectious diseases are no longer the predominant concern, as these have been replaced by long-term chronic conditions such as diabetes, various forms of mental illness and other illnesses that cause long periods of disability prior to death (see chapter 2 for a full discussion of contemporary threats to health). Consequently, health services are increasingly being used to manage and control the symptoms of such chronic conditions rather than as a curative service (Blakemore & Griggs, 2007). In light of this, many sociologists have argued that modern health care services are better known as 'sickness services' because of their focus upon treatment within a biomedical framework. The UK NHS model of health care favours clinical interventions to treat illness and disease, rather than dealing with environmental and cultural factors that cause ill-health in the first instance. The NHS uses a downstream approach, with health promotion campaigners and workers arguing for more upstream work that will prevent and tackle the actual causes of ill-health before they reach the point where treatment is required (see chapter 7 for a more detailed discussion of health promotion). This upstream work could be developed and delivered within the remit of healthy public policy.

Healthy public policy

Healthy public policy is policy that has a clear and explicit concern for health. For example, the 2006 health bill in the UK ensured that smoking was made impossible in almost all enclosed spaces and workplaces across the country. The primary objective of this healthy public policy was to reduce exposure to second-hand smoke for workers and the general public, with the secondary objective of reducing overall smoking rates. The overall impact of the smoking ban on improving health is unlikely to be clear until twenty or even thirty years on from its implementation. However, it is hoped that smoking-related diseases such as lung cancer and coronary heart disease will significantly reduce in number, and that smoking will gradually become less socially acceptable, further extending health benefits. Early research indicates that there have been some positive results. Shepherd (2008) cites The Smoking Toolkit Study, published 1 July 2008, which predicts a dramatic decline in smokers, estimating that in the ten years following the ban as many as forty thousand deaths will be prevented. Shepherd (2008) also quotes a Daily Mail newspaper article that suggested that in the nine months after the ban there were approximately three per cent fewer heart attacks compared with the same period the previous year, amounting to 1,384 fewer hospital admissions. These figures can be challenged because it is difficult to compare year-on-year statistics for changing smoking rates and heart-attack incidences due to the variety of influences upon both of these. From a policy-making perspective the ideal is of course to reduce smoking rates via such an approach.

Box 11.4 **Healthy Public Policy – tackling UK inequalities.**

- *Saving Lives: Our Healthier Nation* (DoH 1999) – White Paper committed to narrowing the health gap.
- *The NHS Plan 2000* (DoH 2000) – set targets to reduce inequalities in health by 10%, measured by infant mortality rates and life expectancy at birth.
- Programme of Action for Tackling Inequalities (DoH 2003) – setting further targets and outlining delivery mechanisms for inequality reduction at a more local level involving local authorities, primary care trusts and the Sure Start Programme (a dedicated service aimed working with families).
- 2005 (DoH) status report examining progress showed that gaps in inequalities had actually widened, although the numbers of children living in poverty had decreased.
- The Programme of Action remained in place until 2010 but there were very few further statements made and tackling inequalities slipped off the political agenda (Crinson 2009).

There was specific healthy public policy introduced within the UK as a direct attempt to tackle health inequalities under the New Labour Government, 1997–2010. This followed the commissioning of a report by Sir Donald Acheson, the Chief Medical Officer of the time. Acheson (1998) produced an independent report arguing that material disadvantage was the ultimate cause of health inequalities. This led to policy development that demonstrated a political willingness to use government policy to tackle inequalities (described in box 11.4) although no additional funding was made available (Crinson, 2009).

There has also been a move to create healthy public policy on a global scale with several examples already in existence such as the Framework Convention on Tobacco Control and the Kyoto Protocol on Greenhouse Gas Emissions (Labonte, 2010). Although these policies are part of a global recognition that health is a social product, they have received criticism for failing to be radical enough in attempting to tackle health inequalities (Crinson, 2009). Furthermore, as the determinants of health are so broad, healthy public policy needs to have a broader focus than just health.

The broader policy environment

The overall policy environment affects health, even if such policy is not clearly intended to determine health. There are many government activities affecting health and illness; for example, the taxation of certain products, the regulation of air and water pollution, the safety of food and the working environment (Blakemore & Griggs, 2007).

The introduction of compulsory seatbelt wearing exemplifies the way in which the broader policy environment (in this case, transport policy) can have significant impacts on health.

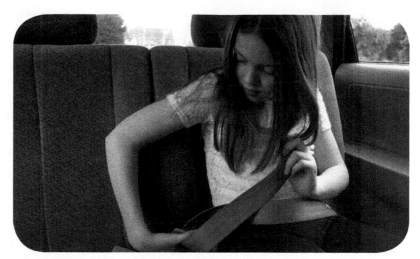

© Karen Town

There are academic arguments that suggest the biggest health outcome gains have resulted from public health measures that do not rely upon medical interventions such as removing impurities from water and improving nutrition (McKeown, 1979). Indeed, an example of transport policy that has had massive health benefits is the introduction of compulsory seatbelt wearing in the UK in 1983, when it became law for those travelling in a car to wear seatbelts. Although this social policy is classed as transport policy, it has had clear health benefits by reducing the number of deaths in car accidents across the UK significantly. Another example of a policy that aims to achieve health improvements is the UK Winter Fuel Payment, an annual tax-free payment for residents born before 1950, which helps them to keep warm in winter. This additional funding is likely to have health benefits such as reducing fuel poverty and cold related illnesses among the older UK population.

The broader policy environment can also be detrimental to health. For example, the policy to generate power via the use of nuclear reactors can have devastating effects. The 1986 Chernobyl disaster led to a radioactive cloud contaminating Europe, and has undoubtedly caused many long-term health effects that are little understood (Crinson 2009). This has led to some arguing that nuclear power is simply not safe. However, the disease and deaths associated with burning fossil fuels are much higher and often less recognized, for example in the media. Changes to the UK licensing laws made in 2005, allowing extensions to the hours in which alcohol can be sold led to what critics called a twenty-four-hour drinking culture (BBC News, 2005). These changes were criticized in relation to potential negative health outcomes associated with additional alcohol consumption in a country where death rates for chronic liver disease and cirrhosis have risen in recent years and are well above the European average (DoH, 2007b). The following learning task will help you to think about how health is influenced by a variety of policy sectors.

Learning task 11.4

Policy Sectors and health implications

1. Outline as many UK government departments as you can. If you are finding this difficult go to the Direct Gov Website and use the directory http://www.direct.gov.uk/en/Dl1/Directories/A–ZOfCentralGovernment/index.htm

2. List the policy focus of these different departments, and some example policies.

3. Think about how these policies may impact upon health. For example, think about anti-social behaviour policy and how this may be helpful in combating the negative mental health implications that might be associated with the experience of anti-social behaviour.

This learning task will help you to understand that holistic health is influenced by policy from many different sectors, rather than just health policy per se. It is in this overall context that the importance of fiscal policy needs to be considered.

The importance of fiscal policy

The NHS receives government funding and is a core part of health care provision; however, it does not attempt to tackle the determinants of health. Policy can be used as a mechanism to try to change people's social and emotional well-being and improve their health by generally tackling the economic circumstances in which they live. There is a large bank of evidence showing how income levels are strongly correlated to the health of people. Those living in the most unequal of societies face more mental illness (including drug and alcohol addiction), lower life expectancy and higher infant mortality, obesity and teenage pregnancy rates (Wilkinson & Pickett, 2009). What is important in tackling these health problems is not money generally but the scale of the inequality that exists; where we are in relation to other members of society is crucial in terms of our own health and welfare. Policy is also important here because it can act as a mechanism to try to redistribute income or it can further extend inequality by widening income gaps between the poorest and the richest sections of society. Fiscal policy, that is, policy concerned with money and general economics can be used then in such circumstances to try to tackle some of these problems. Policy can be designed to try to support those on lower incomes for example to redistribute income by applying progressive taxation rates. By reducing inequality in society then health inequalities should also decrease.

Thus, Wilkinson and Pickett (2009) argue that income distribution provides policy-makers with a way of improving the well-being

| Box 11.5 | UK Fiscal Policy to Tackle Inequality – Some Examples of New Labour's Approach |

- Introduction of Working Tax Credits (2003) to provide additional financial benefit for those on lower incomes who work, through a means tested benefit.
- Introduction of Child Tax Credits (2003), again to provide additional income for those on lower incomes with dependent children. Again this is a means tested benefit.
- The Child Trust Fund was created as a long-term tax-free savings and investment account for children. The government gives every eligible child a voucher to start their fund (the payments are now being significantly reduced from 2011).

(DirectGov 2010)

of whole populations. The UK New Labour government implemented several fiscal policies between 1997 and 2010 in an attempt to begin to tackle societal inequalities.

Despite these attempts to effect social change via both fiscal policy and specific policy aiming to address inequalities, evidence suggests that these policy interventions have had little effect. Thomas et al. (2010) report on the extent of inequality in premature deaths across different geographical areas in Britain, showing that despite government interventions health inequalities have not reduced and that in some cases they may have actually widened. They conclude that social inequalities in mortality rates are influenced by complex and long-term processes and as a result changes in fiscal and social policy are unable to tackle inequalities. Wilkinson and Pickett (2009) similarly argue that such policy has failed, suggesting that this is because rather than reducing inequality, most policies aimed at dealing with health and social problems attempt to break the link between deprivation and associated problems instead of tackling the root of the cause. This demonstrates that policy has limitations in terms of what it can achieve. The current UK government (the Conservative and Liberal Democrat coalition) is developing policy in relation to inequalities but is already encountering criticism for attempting to reform the NHS in line with neo-liberal principles because this is likely to impact negatively upon inequalities.

Social policy and health studies

As this chapter demonstrates, social policy can influence our health in a number of ways both positively and negatively through a number of different policy sectors. The discipline of social policy is a crucial underpinning to the health studies field because it enables us to examine critically how social policy acts as a determinant of

Case study

Challenges to health in times of recession.

All welfare provision is subject to rationing but especially so when countries face recession and increased financial challenges. So how will the UK's 'credit crunch' of 2008 and subsequent recession the following year affect health? In previous recessions, there were massive challenges to funding public services, with cuts made particularly within housing and education (Klein, 2010). Crowther (2008) documented the impacts of previous recessions showing that during the 1970s, the UK government borrowed money from the International Monetary Fund which insisted on a reduction in public spending as a condition of granting the loan. Consequently, public spending was reduced and the plan to build new hospitals was halted. There were also pay disputes resulting in strikes. The recession of the 1980s, again posed challenges to the Thatcher government of the time, reducing levels of investment. In an attempt to increase funding for the health service, there was an attempt to introduce direct user charges in some areas, leading to a public outcry. As a result, Mrs Thatcher did not introduce the charges and reassured the public that the NHS was 'safe in our hands'. The 1990s recession, led to attempts to increase the efficiency of the NHS and insufficient investment, although spending was not cut. These lessons from previous recessions indicate that

- Welfare and the public sector will be negatively affected
- the rationing of certain services and treatments may increase
- priorities will be determined

The NHS has however often remained protected from massive changes and large reductions in investment because of its continuing public popularity. For example, in the 1979 election both political parties committed themselves to giving financial priority to the NHS, despite general economic problems (Klein, 2010). Similarly, in the Comprehensive Spending Review of 2010, the NHS budget remained protected but there are clear plans for improving efficiency which are likely to involve changes being made.

health. Furthermore, by studying social policy it is possible to see how ideological values, beliefs and ideas are used to shape both policy and practice in relation to health. The field of social policy is incredibly complex and the policy environment is constantly changing, so it is important to understand the dynamics involved in the formulation of policy as these clearly impact upon the broader determinants of health and the provision of welfare including health care. The British NHS is based upon specific values about who is entitled to receive state support and at what level. This shows the importance of social policy as a tool to meet basic human needs and links into some of the key debates and concepts related to the provision of welfare. These include defining need, ethical considerations in relation to human rights and the impact of welfare upon equality. Welfare systems are important in addressing these issues and important in relation to health because welfare can be used as a mechanism to address the structural determinants of health. Social policy ultimately shapes the economic and social context in which we experience health and so understanding it is crucial for a health studies student.

Summary

- Social policy as a discipline is crucial in helping us to understand how the social and economic environment in which we live influences our health through the mechanisms of health and welfare systems.

- Health and welfare policy are important determinants of health, underpinned by complex ideological values and beliefs.

- Health policy and healthy public policy are important for our health, but the complexity of the social policy field means that many policy sectors are important in determining health outcomes.

Questions

1. Do you agree with the statement that health is political? Think about the involvement of politicians in shaping health service provision and examine media reports discussing health to help you to form a conclusion.

2. Think about your own ideological values, which learning task 11.3 helped you begin to explore. What would these mean if you were a policy-maker tasked with improving public health? Reflect upon the likely consequences of your ideological approach for specific societal groups such as those who are more vulnerable.

3. Think about the focus of current UK health policy (it is mostly concerned with the provision of health care). Do you think that defined action at a societal level is needed to improve health and focus upon preventative measures, or do you feel that public health policy has clear limitations?

Further reading

Crinson, I. (2009). Health Policy. A Critical Perspective. London, Sage.
This book provides the reader with a critical discussion of the key areas of UK health policy particularly. This is a useful introduction to readers with little knowledge of the area as it covers the policy-making process; the development of the NHS; health care governance; health promotion; and the comparative analysis of health care systems

within the EU and US. The book provides some interesting analysis of history, theory and politics.

Klein, R (2010) The New Politics of the NHS. From Creation to Reinvention. Oxford, Radcliffe.
This book provides a key overview of the NHS, from its inception to current day. It is a chronicle of the NHS since its foundation and discusses all aspects of the Health Service, detailing the many changes that have occurred. It is a really useful introduction to readers without any prior knowledge of the NHS and the policies associated with it.

Buse, K., Mays, N. and Walt, G. (2005) Making Health Policy Work. Maidenhead, Open University Press.
This book is an excellent introduction to the issues of power and process within the social policy field. It is written as an overall guide and has sections on policy analysis, power, the public and the private sectors, policy-makers, implementation and the interaction of research and policy. The book also draws upon examples from the sub-national, national and international level.

12 The Global Context of Health

Key learning outcomes

By the end of this chapter you should be able to:

- understand how the global context influences individual health

- understand how inequality on a global scale affects and determines health

- identify how globalization impacts upon health in a number of contradictory ways

Overview

Although the global environment as a determinant of health is not depicted within Dahlgren and Whitehead's (1991) model, there is still a clear case to be made for the importance of the global environment in influencing and determining individual health. The chapter therefore introduces the notion of global society and discusses the implications of our location within this realm in relation to health. This chapter considers how being part of a global society affects health both positively and negatively; it also considers how global health issues are framed by the processes associated with globalization. Globalization is a process influencing patterns of health and disease, inequality, the environment and the governance of health, which are all discussed in this chapter. A case study of female health problems is used to demonstrate how powerlessness is a key factor in the poor health of large numbers of women in lower-income countries.

Why is global health important?

Health is bound up in global relationships; the global context in which we are located influences our health. The notion that we live in a global society is supported by evidence showing that trends and relationships exist between health and well-being in many societies across the globe. Many commentators argue that our individual health is increasingly conditioned and determined by both global processes and relationships (Yuill et al., 2010). There are a number of health problems and issues that require tackling on a global scale, hence the need for global solutions (see chapter 2 for a discussion of contemporary threats to health, many of which are global). Davies (2010) argues that health is a political issue impacting at the local, national and global level especially as any death and much ill-health is the result of local, international and political decisions. A United Nations Commission set up in 1999, found that the disproportionate disease burden experienced by lower-income countries was a massive threat to global wealth and security (Brundtland, 2003), and that millions of poor people die from preventable and treatable conditions simply because of their societal position (Sachs, 2001).

In addition, the World Health Organization (2008) has identified a number of health challenges that exist on a global level

- One fifth of all global deaths in 2004 were children under five, often as a result of malnutrition.
- Smoking-related lung cancer is the leading cause of cancer-related death for men.
- Ischaemic heart disease and cardiovascular disease are the leading causes of death in the world.
- In Africa, the main cause of death among 15–59 year-olds is the HIV/ AIDS virus. HIV/AIDS is responsible for 40 per cent of female deaths in Africa.
- The global burden of mental illness is also increasing, with depression resulting in many instances of disability.
- Road traffic accidents are also increasing across the globe as a result of increased numbers of cars and urbanization.

How does the global context influence health?

Globalization

Globalization has been defined in a number of different ways within the academic literature and it does have many components. Social, cultural and economic aspects of life are all important in relation to the changing social world, and they are all components of globalization. Global social change is not a new phenomenon but the rapid change that has occurred over the last three decades is said to be unprecedented. Globalization is the increased social, economic and political interconnectedness of the world. Giddens (2009: 126) defines globalization as 'the fact that we all increasingly live in one world, so that individuals,

Box 12.1

Example – areas where globalization impacts upon health (Lee 1998).

- The spread of disease within and across countries (are epidemiological patterns changing and what implications are there for the prevention and treatment of disease?)
- The global financing of health care (how has the globalization of finance influenced health care funding?)
- Global trade and production (are more regulations needed to protect health?)
- Global information (are there inequalities in access to health care information?)
- Global governance (who are the key players and is their role positive in terms of improving health?)
- Global law (what global health issues need to be dealt with via the legal system?)

groups and nations become ever more dependent'. Globalization is defined in a number of ways but it encompasses economics as well as social and cultural aspects and hence is important in relation to health. The idea of an interconnected global society has raised several questions about health especially as many more health issues are now being conceptualized as 'global' and therefore in need of global solutions .

Pro-globalization commentators suggest that liberalization increases trade, which increases growth and wealth and ultimately decreases poverty (Labonte, 2010). There are also broader arguments about the importance of the cognitive dimensions of globalization. For example, Scholte (2000) writes about the continued growth of global consciousness as a positive benefit of globalization. Thus, there are ideas about the importance of our global neighbourhood, the common global social problems faced by the entire world and there has been the development of a global discourse about both health and welfare. However, the relationship between the processes of globalization and health are complex and there is a large amount of literature arguing that globalization has exacerbated inequality, therefore worsening health for some. There has also been a globalization of health trends, as a result of the globalization of unhealthy lifestyles. For example, increasing food consumption combined with inactivity is resulting in a number of health problems across the world. Heart disease, stroke, cancers and other chronic conditions are seen as the result of such lifestyles. The consumption of increased levels of alcohol and risky sexual behaviours are also cited as problematic for global health with increasing rates of liver problems and sexually transmitted infections as a consequence. The following learning task will help you to explore how globalization is affecting health. There is a large amount

> **Learning task 12.1**
>
> ### Globalization debate.
> Look at the following website and read in more depth about globalization; http://www.sociology.emory.edu/globalization/
>   This will help you to complete the following task.
>   Debate whether globalization is good or bad for health.
>
> 1. Make a list of points to support both sides of the argument, reasons for why it is detrimental to health and also reasons for why and how it can benefit health.
> 2. Which of your lists was the longest?
> 3. Finally, reflect upon how your position in the global world may relate to the impact that globalization may have upon your health. If you lived in a different place, perhaps a lower income country, consider how the relationship between health and globalization might differ.

of evidence suggesting that the relationship between globalization and health is contingent upon where you live, as well as your level of income. However, it is not just income that matters; it is standards of living and access to services. Stiglitz (2006) argues that development is often accompanied by urbanization, which has left many cities in developing countries squalid, congested, noisy and with dirty air and poor sanitation (see chapter 10 for more detailed discussion about how these affect health). These conditions are certainly not beneficial for good health. So the relationship between health outcomes and globalization has been and continues to be debated. It is clear that health and health care are affected by globalization in a number of ways.

Migration

One of the most devastating impacts of the increased movement of people around the globe associated with globalization has been the increased spread of deadly epidemics. This global spread of infection has a long history and it still continues today (see chapter 2 for more discussion of contemporary threats to health). Although better knowledge and capabilities exist in relation to dealing with the spread of disease through increased mobility, it is clear that threats from emerging and re-emerging infectious diseases are increased by globalization (Feacham, 2001).

Globalization has also resulted in the increased mobility of health professionals across borders. Migration has resulted in what is called the 'brain drain'; high proportions of doctors and nurses who are trained and educated in their own countries; those often have huge

Box 12.2   Example – Health Tourism.

- Consumers of health care services access treatment in other countries in which they are not residents.
- There are many reasons for health tourism such as long waiting lists, high costs of elective treatments such as cosmetic surgery at home, and easy travel.
- At the international level, health tourism is an industry sustained by 617 million individuals and it is growing year on year (Carrera and Bridges 2006).
- India will potentially receive $2.2 billion from health tourism by 2012 (Macready 2007).

health problems; then they leave to work in the developed world, where pay and conditions are much more favourable. Macdonald (2006) argues that the UK National Health Service simply could not function without the staff it gains from other countries. Increasing demands for health professionals in the Western world are likely to continue this brain drain and exacerbate the problem. In Zimbabwe from 1990 to 2000, 840 out of a total of 1,200 medical graduates emigrated. In the year 2001, over 2,000 nurses from Africa left to work in the UK (Sanders, 2005).

Indeed, it is not just health professionals who travel. Health consumers are patients who are also increasingly travelling to access medical care in what is often termed health tourism.

However, despite countries receiving additional income from health tourism, it is not possible to say whether this extra income is invested into domestic health care systems (Blouin, 2007). This rise in medical tourism emphasizes the privatization of health care, the growing dependence on technology, uneven access to health resources and the accelerated globalization of both health care and tourism (Connell, 2006). Many commentators therefore argue that health tourism only benefits a small number of people and draws resources away from public health care, therefore bringing little benefit to local populations (Davies, 2010). Furthermore, health care systems in affluent countries may also bear additional burdens in the sense that they face associated costs such as the treatment of infections acquired while abroad, and botched procedures.

Trade

A further area where negative health impacts are often discussed is in relation to trade and the globalization of markets. Bettcher and Lee (2002) argue that although global trade offers opportunities for public health improvements, it is not possible to overlook the negative health

Box 12.3   Example – Trade and negative health consequences.

- There is a large amount of evidence to demonstrate the importance of breastfeeding for the health of the mother and the infant. It is also economically advantageous as it costs nothing.
- Despite the existence of the code for marketing of breast-milk substitutes, created by the WHO during the 1980s, there are often violations of the rules such as free samples being provided in hospitals in poorer countries such as Thailand, South Africa and Bangladesh (Macdonald 2006).

impacts of financial liberalization and trade, such as the extended marketing and promotion of harmful products such as tobacco. There are many transnational corporations across the globe, operating within a framework of free trade entering into the economies of lower-income countries. Macdonald (2007) argues that as a result of neo-liberal globalization, such companies have worked unethically to increase their profits and therefore have had a negative impact upon health.

The marketing of formula milk is just one example. The drive for economic growth has also increased the consumption of processed food and cigarettes (Graham, 2010). For example, in Bangladesh 80 per cent of the population live on less than $2 per day but smoking rates among 35–49 year-old men are extremely high at over 70 per cent (World Bank 2003). Poorer countries as a consequence face a double burden of disease as they experience high levels of infectious diseases and also increasing rates of chronic conditions due to lifestyle (Graham, 2010).

The promotion of formula milk in the developing world has provoked serious debates about the impact of globalized trade on public health.

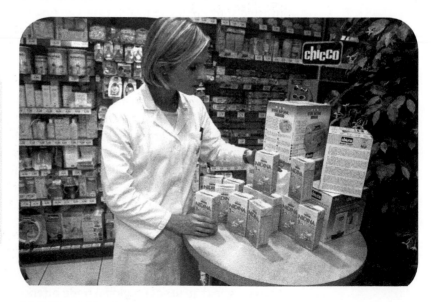

© Luigi Nocenti/Rex Features

Similarly, pharmaceutical companies work globally and have received massive criticism for the way in which they have tended to operate, excluding access to prescription medicines for large numbers of people on the basis of affordability. The existence of TRIPs (trade related aspects of intellectual property rights) is seen as the main problem. The existence of TRIPs means that drugs developed by private companies remain owned by the companies and protected by copyright. This prevents the production of cheaper generic drugs for a number of years. Approximately 80 per cent of the world's population lives without access to essential medication (Leach et al., 2005) so the existence of TRIPs has been heavily criticized. Some commentators have argued that TRIPs is necessary in order to protect the profit of these large companies so that they can invest further money into research and development. However, this is questioned by others who argue that such companies are simply profit driven.

Some of these concerns are now being addressed in initiatives such as the Global Alliance for Vaccines and Immunization (GAVI), which attempts to address such inequalities by encouraging more

| Box 12.4 | Example – Pharmaceuticals industry and global health. |

- Economic considerations are massively influential in the development of new drugs (Kaufmann 2009).
- The common diseases affecting lower income countries do not attract research funding because market forces determine levels of spending (Macdonald 2006).
- Only 5% of the money spent on medical research and development is directed towards diseases which affect lower income countries (Scuklenk 2003).
- In the last quarter of a century there have been 1400 new drugs launched but only four of these were for malaria and just thirteen for tropical diseases (Kaufmann 2007).
- Western research remains focused upon infectious diseases such as HIV/AIDS, multi-drug resistant tuberculosis and pandemic influenzas (Davies 2010).
- The costs charged by large pharmaceutical companies for essential medication means that those who are least able to afford such costs are paying them (WHO-WTO 2002).
- The existence of trade agreements means that prices of drugs particularly those for AIDS have risen to unaffordable levels (Stiglitz 2006).
- There is clear evidence that political and economic power is absolutely fundamental for deciding who is treated, for specific diseases, when and where and indeed for how much (see Aginam 2005).

Learning task 12.2

Transnational corporations, health and ethics.
A large TNC, 'Bigpharma' has established a new laboratory in a medium sized city in India. The company has advocated the positive benefits of its establishment as local job creation and the provision of free health checks for those participating in clinical trials. The local inhabitants are generally poor, they are not educated to high standards and there are very few formal employment opportunities. The country's legislation is weak in relation to health and safety, and there is some evidence of corruption in government.

1. Think about how this company may have an impact upon the health and wealth of the local population.
2. List both the advantages and disadvantages of its presence.
3. Reflect upon power, choice, control and ethics.

research into the common diseases that affect lower-income countries. However, whether significant changes will occur remains to be seen. Attempts to overcome such problems by the WHO's creation of an Essential Drugs List have also been problematic because some drugs do not meet the criteria set for the list. Furthermore, an area seldom discussed is that of pharmaceutical companies conducting off-shore clinical trials. Trials in poorer countries can be conducted relatively cheaply and can increase health service coverage by providing health checks for those who participate in them. However, the positive consequences of such trials are open to debate; the trials may be controversial and exploitative (Angell, 1997). In addition, the power of the pharmaceutical industry may be enhanced in lower-income countries because of less finance and less regulation within government departments. The learning task above explores these issues.

On a global scale, pharmaceutical companies and indeed other large transnationals can exert more influence than entire countries, as many are simply richer than lower-income countries (Stiglitz, 2006). This financial power has led to a number of negative health impacts in addition to the issues already discussed. One example is the explosion at the Union Carbide Plant in Bhopal in India during the 1980s, which killed more than twenty thousand people and damaged many more people's long-term health (Stiglitz, 2006).

The environment

Globalization is also argued to be a massive threat to the environment, causing environmental damage and therefore contributing to health consequences (Feacham, 2001). The increased movement of people

Learning task 12.3

Climate change and health.

What are the likely challenges to public health services that result from global warming?

Make a list of all of the problems that health services may face when trying to deal with the plethora of problems caused by climate change. You might wish to start with basic points about challenges to funding and staffing levels and then develop your list from there.

The WHO has published a wealth of literature about health and climate change, so visit the web-site to expand upon your ideas in addressing this challenge – www.who.int

across the planet not only affects the spread of disease but it also has an impact upon the environment, notably contributing to climate change. Globalization contributes to climate change in several ways, for example, as a result of increased travel and pollution, the increased demand and use of energy sources and the consumption of products and associated waste. Wilkinson (2005) argues that new environmental threats are emerging through complex and extended pathways that are global in their reach. As global environmental change occurs, public health will be challenged. Health is certainly threatened by climate change in a number of ways (see the more detailed discussion of this in chapter 2). However, the likely effects of climate change are still open to debate as it is not known how severe these impacts will be, although it is likely that they will affect the most vulnerable disproportionately. The learning task above will help you to think about how climate change will affect health and therefore health services.

Inequalities

There are massive inequalities globally in relation to health and despite economic growth large variations still exist across the globe in relation to life expectancy. The relationship between income and health is complex, with those living in high-income countries tending to experience much better health and life chances than those in lower-income countries, as demonstrated by differential life expectancies in table 12.1. However, although people may live longer in some countries, this does not mean that they are in good health for the duration of their lives or that they achieve good quality of life. This is demonstrated in table 12.1, which compares how long people live with how long they are healthy for. The difference in the figures demonstrate that on average people experience several years of ill-health, so living for longer does not mean living in good health.

Table 12.1. Comparison of life expectancy and healthy life expectancy.

Approximate Life Expectancy (years)	Healthy Life Expectancy (years)
Afghanistan – 42.6	Afghanistan – 35.5
Iceland – 80.1	Iceland – 72.8
Zimbabwe – 37.9	Zimbabwe – 35.5
UK – 78.2	UK – 70.6

Source: http://www.worldlifeexpectancy.com/

This table also demonstrates the large variations in global life expectancy, showing that lower-income countries tend to have poorer life expectancy. However, wealth is not simply a good predictor of high life expectancy. Wilkinson (1996) has demonstrated the importance of relative income in relation to health within societies. Wilkinson and Pickett (2009) also show that health outcomes fail to rise rapidly in countries when income reaches a certain point, showing that economic growth is not simply beneficial for health per se. The world's richest country, the USA, has lower life expectancy (77.0) than countries with less income (such as Sweden 79.7 and Japan 80.7). There are also middle-income countries that have higher life expectancy than might be expected. Sri Lanka is one such example, with average life expectancy of 73.1 (World Bank, 2002; UNDP, 2003). Sri Lanka and Cuba are both examples of high health achieving countries as a result of national level policies that created access to basic social services (Mehrotra, 2000). This demonstrates the importance of government investment in services such as clean water and sanitation, education and basic health care (Sen, 1999). Achieving good health in a low-income country can be compounded by poor sanitation, polluted water, lack of education, poor health care and a much higher risk of exposure to infectious diseases.

Poverty and the powerlessness that is associated with it negatively affect the health of those experiencing it. The World Health Organization has stated that extreme poverty is the most serious cause of disease, with 70 per cent of deaths in developing countries attributable to five causes that can be easily and cheaply combated; pneumonia, diarrhoea, malaria, measles and malnutrition (WHO, 1995). In 2001, the deaths of two million people could have been prevented simply if they had been given access to uncontaminated food and clean drinking water (Kindhauser, 2003). Those in weak social, economic and political positions, such as women, are much more at risk of certain conditions such as malnutrition, violence, sexually transmitted infections and respiratory conditions. Indeed, women and children bear the brunt of global health inequalities. In 2007, women made up sixty one per cent of HIV infections in sub-Saharan Africa (UNAIDS, 2007).

Access to life-saving drugs in lower-income countries has improved but is still a significant problem, demonstrating continued global inequalities.

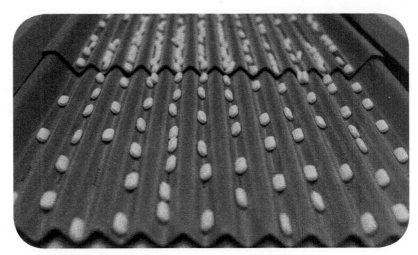

© Edward Webb/Rex Features

In addition there are many deaths from maternal mortality (Hill et al., 2007). Put simply, within all societies death rates are typically highest among the poorest. Furthermore, the poor endure worse health within some countries when compared to others. For example, although Gross Domestic Product (GDP) is similar in Sweden and Britain, the poorest groups in Sweden still can expect to live longer than those in poorer groups in Britain (Kunst et al., 1998).

In addition, the global burden of disease is disproportionately experienced by those in lower-income countries. The HIV epidemic is disproportionately experienced by those in Southern Africa, with some reports suggesting a thousand deaths per day. Average life expectancy fell (declining to less than 40 years) in many countries such as Angola, Botswana, Rwanda and Zambia as a result of the HIV/AIDS epidemic (Macdonald, 2006). However, the latest epidemiological data indicate that globally the spread of the disease peaked in 1996 and that the epidemic has significantly stabilized since then (UNAIDS, 2009). Table 12.2 shows the variations in the incidences of HIV/AIDS cases in different parts of the world.

Table 12.2 clearly shows that Africa accounts for the majority of infections. Not only are the numbers of infected individuals unequal across the globe, the implications of such a diagnosis also vary

Table 12.2. Disparities in the global incidence of HIV/AIDS.

	Africa 2008	Latin America	North America, Western and Central Europe
People living with HIV	22.4 million	2 million	2.3 million
New infections	1.9 million	170,000	75,000
Deaths from HIV/AIDS	1.4 million	77,000	38,000

Data from UNAIDS, (2009)

massively according to location; those in lower-income countries have more negative outcomes (Macdonald, 2006). For example, anti-retro viral drugs can assist most HIV/AIDS patients to live longer and maintain quality of life. However, these drugs are not widely available to those in lower-income countries largely because of the power of the pharmaceutical industry in preventing the production of generic cheaper copies. This has resulted in the early deaths of hundreds of thousands of poor HIV/AIDS patients (Macdonald, 2008).

As well as the HIV epidemic, many other infectious and preventable diseases lead to high death rates in poorer countries; 4,500 children die every day from preventable diseases (WHO, 2007b). Malaria is a huge global killer, infecting one child in Africa every thirty seconds. Malaria is responsible for more than three hundred million acute illnesses every year and over a million deaths (Millennium Campaign News, 2006). Tuberculosis (TB) is also a massive problem. Although it does not affect as many people as malaria does, it has a far higher mortality rate with estimates of approximately one and a half million people dying from it on an annual basis. Left untreated, half of those infected with TB will die (Macdonald, 2007). Poverty is a clear risk factor in the develop-ment of TB, with the bacterium activated in those with compromised immunity associated with their societal position. Treating TB is also an issue in poorer countries where there is often a lack of drugs, a lack of well-trained medical staff and a lack of education about the importance of adherence to treatment regimes. Thus, infectious diseases remain a large global problem. Kaufmann (2009) argues that figures are simply abstract because it is impossible for most people to grasp the fact that fifteen million people die as a result of infectious diseases every year. To add to this, it is harder still to comprehend the massive loss of life-years due to sickness, disability and early death.

Financing and health care

As well as bearing a disproportionate amount of the global burden of disease, poorer countries have far less money available to spend on health care, less developed health care infrastructure, staff shortages and in many cases a lack of basic supplies such as drugs. Spending on health care is incredibly unevenly distributed, with the poorest countries spending the equivalent of $11 per year per person, com-pared to an average US spend of $2000 (WHO, 2000). The thirty most developed nations (all members of the Organization for Economic Co-operation – OCE), are made up of 20 per cent of the world's population yet they account for 90 per cent of the world's total health expenditure (WHO, 2007b). However, increased investment is not the ideal recipe for creating better health, with the USA being a case in point. Despite the largest investments in the world (based upon GDP) there are still large health inequalities across America; many people are without health insurance and have no access to basic health care. In lower-income countries what is needed are low-cost health care innovations, such as the provision of **primary health care**, access to education and improvements in sanitation and water. It is these simple solutions that arguably have been most compromised by globalization (Labonte, 2010), further increasing inequality.

People in lower-income countries tend to have far less access to modern technology and adequate health care and are often reliant upon donor aid to provide health care. Indeed, the health care systems that are found in some lower-income countries do not perform well. Thirty-five of the fifty worst health care systems are found in sub-Saharan Africa (Macdonald, 2007). Just to meet the most basic of health needs, the World Health Organization suggests that at least $66 billion should be invested in low-income countries (WHO, 2002). These sums seem incredibly large; however, to put things into global perspective, US citizens spend two billion dollars every year on whitening their teeth and spending on perfumes and cosmetics is a similar amount to the entire budget allocated for the Millennium Development Goals associated with health and health care (Kaufmann, 2009).

Learning task 12.4

Financing Health Care.

You live in a region that has approximately a quarter of a million inhabitants. The government and foreign aid are used together to finance your health care because the country is poor. Furthermore, following the recent global recession, your already limited health budget is being cut. Every year you usually receive 20 million naira to fund all services (hospital care, primary health care such as vaccination programmes and health promotion). Your district also has high incidences of HIV/AIDS. You now have to reduce your annual budget by 5 million naira. Here are some of the changes that you may consider:

● Cut hospital staff by a third – save 1.75 million
● Reduce all wages by 5% – save 1 million
● Introduce user charges for sexual health services – save 1 million
● Only prescribe essential drugs – save 2 million

1. Think about the benefits and disadvantages of these changes (list them), whilst considering the perspective of different stakeholders.
2. How might patients feel?
3. How might staff react?
4. Finally, reflect upon the difficulty of financing health care in such circumstances and keep in mind that all health care across the globe is rationed in some way in order to limit costs.

Financing health care is a complex task associated with managing difficult budgets and making ethically challenging decisions. Learning task 12.4 will help you to think about the financial decisions that are often made in relation to the provision of health care.

Health governance and policy

The forces of globalization have arguably led to an increased range of global policy actors, shaping health policy, funding and provision. Many organizations assume a role in creating and maintaining the conditions required for good health and health care on a global level (Davies 2010). These global actions affect our abilities to improve both national and local health (Labonte 2010).

Global governance has grown in recent years with several organizations becoming more important following the recognition that epidemics have no boundaries and that poverty, social inequality and disease are obviously interrelated. Consequently a number of large international organizations have made attempts to combat these issues (Kaufmann 2009). There are a number of organizations involved in ensuring that global health is achieved and delivered, with many agencies working together in partnership and via alliances to deliver health-related programmes (Walt and Buse 2006). There are governmental and non-governmental organizations such as the World Health Organization, charities such as Oxfam, private foundations and large corporations such as pharmaceutical companies. For example, Oxfam, Médecins Sans Frontières and the Gates Foundation all work globally to tackle health problems. This range of global actors drives a variety of health agendas and consequently influences priorities within individual countries, affecting the resources that are available to both workers and patients alike (Davies 2010). Therefore, recent global health priorities have been defined through several processes and by several actors (Ollilia 2005). Table 12.3 illustrates the key actors in global policy-making, the work that they engage in and some of the criticisms that they have faced.

The actors described in table 12.3 are by no means the only ones working towards changing global health. The not-for-profit sector has played a role in debates about essential drugs and breast milk substitutes. Public Health Non-Governmental organizations have also been important in shaping pharmaceutical policies (Ollila 2005). The Gates Foundation by 2002 had granted $2.8 billion of health funding, starting the Global Alliance for Vaccines and Immunization (GAVI) an independently governed initiative (Yamey 2002). Similarly, Aid agencies also continue to work in global public health. Oxfam's latest briefing paper, 21st Century Aid (2010), defends criticisms that all aid is bad and should be phased out, citing evidence to show progress related to the provision of aid. For example, in 2006 in Zambia as a result of support from international aid, health care was made free for all those living in rural areas.

Table 12.3. The key actors in global policy-making.

Organization	Remit	Health Work	Criticisms
The World Health Organization	Established in 1948 as the UN's specialist agency for health, with the mandate of attaining the highest possible level of health for all people.	• Vertical programmes such as mass immunization. • Eradication programmes such as small-pox, malaria and cholera. • Focus upon primary health care. • GOBI programme; growth monitoring to tackle malnutrition, oral rehydration to combat diarrhoeal diseases, breastfeeding and immunization (Brown et al 2006). • 2010 *World Health Report* focuses upon improving health care access across the world.	• Changing policies over the years • Lack of funding to support some programmes (such as primary health care – see Koivusalo and Ollila 1997). • Diverse leadership and many changes • Heavily influenced by neo-liberal ideology (Carpenter 2000) • No long-term development of health care systems.
The World Bank	Provides low-interest loans to low-income countries imposing policy conditions for repayment. It aims to reduce poverty by investing in people.	• Public sector reform on the basis of loans. • Imposition of user charges on health services.	• Detrimental impact of policies on health because of reducing investment in public services as part of loan conditions (Stiglitz 2006). • Some projects have caused environmental damage (Abbasi 1999). • Increases poorer countries' reliance upon external sources of incomes. • Worsened inequalities.
The World Trade Organization	Established in 1995, its role is to regulate trade.	• Promotes free trade. • No direct health remit but trade related polices have many health implications.	• Many negative consequences resulting from privatization of public services. • The erosion of workers rights, increased inequalities and making health care unaffordable for many (Yuill et al., 2010).

Table 12.3. (continued).

Organization	Remit	Health Work	Criticisms
International Monetary Fund	The IMF has had a role in shaping the global economy since the 1940s. Its remit is to encourage economic growth and stability. It works with lower-income countries to stabilize their economies and reduce poverty.	• Public sector reform via structural adjustment policies requiring countries to reduce investment in health care.	• Negative health consequences resulting from policy measures imposed.

The emergence of new powerful actors in the public health field has led to some debate about the continued need for organizations such as the WHO. However, Yamey (2002) argues that there is now more of a need than ever for an overarching health agency such as the WHO. Grouped together, global actors have delivered a number of programmes in an attempt to fight communicable diseases, with some notable successes such as the impressive global eradication of the smallpox virus by the WHO (Macdonald, 2008). The World Bank, despite many criticisms remains massively important in global health policy-making and therefore global health governance (Kumaranayake & Walker, 2002).Yet the overall impact of such organizations in shaping better health outcomes has been questioned (Fidler, 2007). As well as questioning the ideological underpinnings of organizations such as the World Bank (Macdonald, 2007), some critics have suggested that the list of global health priorities simply reflects the issues that are threatening to the interests of the industrialized Western world (Ollila, 2005). For example, Ebola, SARs, Avian flu and swine flu have all received attention because they are perceived as massive threats to the health of higher-income countries but these diseases did not cause the damage and death predicted. Moreover, global policy-making has been clearly aligned with industrial and trade policies (Ollila, 2005), arguably to the detriment of global health.

Despite these criticisms, the work of global health actors has led to large scale vaccination schemes, education and health promotion to try to combat the HIV/AIDS epidemic as well as strategies to deal with tuberculosis and malaria, with much attention given to sub-Saharan Africa, the worst affected area in relation to these problems (Kaufmann, 2009). The Millennium Development Goals defined by the UN member states are another clear example of the positive role of global governance. In 2000, a set of targets were adopted in an attempt to deal with poverty and inequality, to improve health, to develop a cleaner and more sustainable environment and promote a fairer world.

Table 12.4. Overview of the Millennium Development Goals.

Goal	Description
MDG 1	Eradicate extreme poverty and hunger. The proportion of the world's poor that live on less than $1 per day will be halved. The number of people who suffer from hunger will also be halved.
MDG 2	Universal primary education for both boys and girls.
MDG 3	Promote gender equality and strengthen the rights of women, especially educationally.
MDG 4	Reduce child mortality by two-thirds and increase the immunization of young children against measles.
MDG 5	Reduce maternal mortality by three quarters by improving medical care for women during both pregnancy and childbirth.
MDG 6	To halt and possibly begin to reverse the spread of AIDS, malaria and tuberculosis as well as other major diseases.
MDG 7	Ensure environmental sustainability. Halve the number of people unable to access or afford safe drinking water and basic sanitation a well as improving the living conditions of slum dwellers.
MDG 8	Develop global partnerships to improve debt relief initiatives and access to technology. Enable access to essential drugs at affordable prices for developing countries fighting infectious diseases.

Source: United Nations Development Programme (2010)

These goals are an attempt to promote global collective responsibility for health threats, defined in the broadest possible sense as they include poverty, preventable communicable disease and environmental degradation (Davies 2010). The goals are described in table 12.4.

These goals have been discussed within the context of human rights and linked to the human rights framework as this is seen as an important tool for achieving these targets in an equitable, just and sustainable way. However, despite increasing policy attention given to human rights within development policy and programming, many argue that in practice these concepts remain separate (UNDP, 2010). These eight goals should be met as targets by 2015, yet although progress indicators demonstrate moves in the right direction it is still unlikely that they will be fully achieved. For example, at the global level, the maternal mortality ratio fell by 34% from 1990 to 2008, with the largest changes seen in Asia and North Africa but this is still insufficient to meet the MDG target (Wilmoth et al., 2010). Oxfam (2010) argues that donors are giving far less than is needed to meet the goals. The goals themselves also remain open to interpretation for example, defining extreme poverty, measuring 'promotion' and making reductions to an unspecified level are all vaguely conceptualized. The goals have also been threatened by delays in implementation and the resistance of higher-income countries.

Furthermore, there are many locally contingent factors that compound the goals being achieved; wars, corruption and transnational corporations serving their own interests are all impeding progress (Macdonald 2007). However, on a more positive note, it has been suggested that the goals represent an attempt to prioritize health and, more specifically, the health of the poor (Lee 2009). Macdonald (2007, 2) concludes that these goals are simply 'a minimum basis for creating a global context for equity in health and other human rights'. This is a critical perspective with others arguing that great progress has been made against these goals in many countries, for example, in the reduction of HIV/ AIDS incidences and maternal mortalities.

This is not the first attempt on a global scale to achieve large health improvements. The World Health Organization outlined a target of health for all by 2000, at the Alma Ata Conference in 1978. This ambitious target, to be met by the implementation of primary health care across the globe was not remotely realized. However, the WHO's 2008 *World Health Report* again emphasizes the importance of the role of primary health care in achieving more equal health outcomes across the globe. The WHO's 2008 Report, 'Closing the Gap: Health Equity through Action on the Social Determinants of Health' (CSDH, 2008) also outlines the need to tackle social inequality, identifying that the causes of inequality and poor health are found in social and economic factors. The report also makes three recommendations:

1. Improve daily living conditions
2. Tackle the unequal distribution of power, money and resources
3. Measure and understand the problem and assess the impact of any action taken.

The report is clear in identifying areas where health threats are socially created and therefore shows that these can be tackled too on a social level. However, the question remains as to how effective such goals are and the influence of the organizations that set them has also been discussed within the broader literature. Davies (2010) argues that much more work is needed to determine how the growing number of political actors is influencing health and whether this is positive or negative.

Why is all of this important?

Health is completely related to and bound up within global relationships in a number of complex ways. Health is the outcome of a number of global processes and in many senses the processes of globalization affect our health. The increasing interconnectedness of the world affects our health in a number of ways, for example, in relation to the spread of diseases (both communicable and non-communicable), the availability of health-care staff, funding and medications, as well as the global relationships underpinning policy-making. There are also environmental considerations that need attention at the global level as our changing environment is likely to lead to additional health considerations. Therefore, as this chapter has shown, there are many global public health challenges and concerns remaining in the twenty-first century. Globalization has changed our lives and so too is changing our health and this is why it is necessary to understand the role that global processes play in influencing our health. Global policy will continue to be developed in attempts to deal with the challenges that remain in global health, attempting to tackle threats to health and to maintain good health once it is achieved. Policy-making at the global level is complex and there are many interests vested in the process, with the outcomes of such policy-making not always being beneficial to health. Despite the complexities of global policy-making '. . . the causes, cures and means of improving health the world over are bound up with the actions and decisions not of single nation states but the co-ordinated activities of people and organizations across the globe' (Yuill et al., 2010: 84). Ultimately, health for many has to be understood and discussed within a global context.

Case study

Women's powerlessness and health outcomes.

The disempowered position of women across the globe, in particular in the poorest countries, is detrimental to their health in many ways. Women in poorer countries often depend upon men for survival, are not well educated and are responsible for domestic chores. All of these factors combine to worsen their health outcomes in general. Girls can be married young from the age of fifteen and will experience many pregnancies, as they are often powerless to negotiate safe sex. Macdonald (2007) argues that early marriages limit educational opportunities, increase health risks due to pregnancies at a young age and put women at an increased risk of HIV exposure as they are often married to an older man, with a long sexual history.

A 2007 report, entitled *Because I am a Girl* summarizes evidence to show that female foetuses are more likely to be aborted, and female babies abandoned. In Asia it is estimated that 60 million women are missing as a result of such practices. Female babies are also less likely to be fed as much, experiencing malnutrition and are more likely to be illiterate by their teenage years, damaging their life chances later on. Such women are seen as the property of their fathers until they are married and become the property of their husbands, finding that they do not get to choose when to have sex or indeed under what conditions. Younger women are also more likely to be sexually assaulted and face violence.

There is a wealth of evidence to show that the powerlessness of women affects their physical and mental health, their access to health care treatment, and their right to control their own body and fertility.

Summary

- Globalization as a social process is influencing health in a number of ways, with ongoing debates about whether this is positive or negative.

- The global governance of health has expanded in recent years, with a large number of global actors working on health issues and problems. There have been some successes and targets are often set; however, the neo-liberalist framework underpinning the work of some of these organizations does not result in positive health outcomes for the poorest people in most instances.

- There are major health problems across the globe but these are spread unequally as inequality means that the global burden of disease is borne by the world's poorest inhabitants.

Questions

1. If you were a global policy-maker, what would your priorities for action be and why? Would you focus upon tackling specific diseases or would it be better to try and improve standards of living and to tackle general inequality?

2. Is globalization good? Can global capitalism and the processes of globalization associated with it be used to tackle the problems of inequality across the world?

3. In terms of reducing the health inequality of women across the world, what do you think is necessary and how might this be achieved?

Further reading

Cockerham, C. & Cockerham, W. (2010) Health and Globalization. Cambridge and Malden, Polity.
This book takes the reader through all of the key aspects of the relationship between globalization and health. Beginning with a comparison of health benefits and risks, it then covers disease, health care and the role of global actors in the governance of health care. This essentially tours the major issues associated with globalization and health.

Global Health Watch (2010) V.3 The Alternative World Health Report. London, Zed Books.
This third edition of Global Health Watch is a comprehensive and critical coverage of a range of important global health topics including access to medicines, mental health, water and sanitation, nutrition, and war and conflict. The book also covers the politics of global health and the policies and actions of key actors such as the WHO and the Global Fund to Fight AIDS, Tuberculosis and Malaria.

Macdonald, T.H. (2007) The Global Human Right to Health. Dream or Possibility? Oxford, Radcliffe.
This book provides a critical discussion around the progress (or not) towards developing the right to health for the population of the globe.

The chapters again cover a range of areas including the role of the UN, global finance, transnational corporations and literacy and education. The final chapter attempts to address the key question of whether the global right to health really is a possibility.

13 Synthesizing Perspectives: Case Studies for Action

Key learning outcomes

By the end of this chapter you should be able to:

- understand how a broad range of influences combine to determine health
- understand how different strategies can be used to tackle health problems
- synthesize and critique different approaches to conceptualizing health

Overview

This chapter draws upon material from the rest of the book to demonstrate how understanding determinants of health can aid the development of public health strategy and action. It is therefore an important chapter for those working in the public health field. Using the Dahlgren and Whitehead (1991) rainbow model, detailed case studies of contemporary health issues are used to illustrate all of their associated determinants, their levels are mapped against the model and strategies for action in relation to each case study are highlighted. There are three case studies, one on malaria, one on cervical cancer and one on neighbourhoods as settings. Each case study is used to synthesize material from earlier chapters and to discuss different strategies for promoting health, for example considering policy as an approach. The final section of this chapter discusses and evaluates the Dahlgren and Whitehead model in depth to explore it as a mechanism for understanding the social determinants of health. It explores the strengths of the rainbow model and discusses how it might be built upon to further develop understandings of health and health experience.

Case study

Malaria
- Globally malaria causes an estimated two million deaths and 300 million diagnoses annually (Walley, Webber & Collins, 2010).
- As of 2001 malaria was the second highest ranking cause of disease in the sub-Saharan African region (Mathers et al., 2005).
- There are four types of malaria that can infect humans and the potentially most deadly of these is Plasmodium Falciparum. The female mosquito hosts the malaria parasite and a bite from an infected mosquito can cause the transmission of the parasite from the saliva glands of the mosquito to the human bloodstream and then the liver, where multiplication of the parasites takes place. These are released into the bloodstream and produce toxins that cause the physical symptoms of infection – high temperature, headaches and pain (Walley, Webber & Collins, 2010). Table 13.1 gives an overview of the determinants of malaria.

Table 13.1. The determinants of malaria.

Determinants	Mechanism	References
● Socio economic status	Low rates of ITN usage in some surveys is due to a lack of nets for everyone in the household.	WHO (2010a)
	Poverty is directly linked to infant and maternal malnutrition, which that has an impact on malarial recovery rates.	Walley & Gerein (2010)
● Individual behaviour	Use of ITNs are one of the most effective ways to prevent malaria.	Beigbeder (2004) Macdonald (2007)
● Pregnancy	Pregnant women are more vulnerable to malaria.	Malaria Consortium, (2008)
● Age	People aged 5–19 years old are least likely to use an ITN compared with those in younger and older age groups.	WHO (2010a)

Strategies to tackle malaria

Effective control of malaria depends on both curative and preventive measures (Walley, Webber & Collins, 2010: 12).

Biomedical strategies

Primary prevention   Primary prevention of malaria centres on breaking the cycle of infection from mosquito bites. The World Health

Figure 13.1. Factors influencing malaria using Dahlgren and Whitehead's model as a framework for understanding determinants.

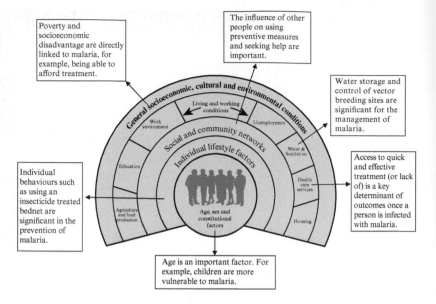

Poverty and socioeconomic disadvantage are directly linked to malaria, for example, being able to afford treatment.

The influence of other people on using preventive measures and seeking help are important.

Water storage and control of vector breeding sites are significant for the management of malaria.

Individual behaviours such as using an insecticide treated bednet are significant in the prevention of malaria.

Access to quick and effective treatment (or lack of) is a key determinant of outcomes once a person is infected with malaria.

Age is an important factor. For example, children are more vulnerable to malaria.

Organization (2010a) states that vector control (or mosquito control) is generally the most effective means of malaria prevention. Methods of vector control include 'indoor residual (household) spraying with insecticide and the promotion and use of insecticide treated bednets for protection from mosquitoes' (Walley, Webber & Collins 2010: 15) and environmental strategies such as drainage or filling-in of potential breeding sites for mosquitoes. Vector control is a key strategy for reducing infection rates by reducing possibilities of infection through mosquito bites (the mosquito is the 'vector').

Promotion of insecticide treated bednets would be categorized as a 'lifestyle intervention' and malaria is largely preventable through their use (Macdonald, 2007). Different strategies may be employed to promote the use of bednets such as promotion through rural clinics, TV and media and introducing government subsidies to reduce the cost of them to promote uptake and use. For example, social marketing has been shown to be an effective strategy for promoting bednet use in rural Tanzania (Armstrong Schellenberg et al., 2001). The methods used included community sensitization meetings, locally accepted branding of the bednets, localized distribution alongside a comprehensive information, education and communication strategy.

Primary prevention also includes such 'personal protection' strategies as using insecticide treated bednets, insect repellents and covering up exposed flesh with clothing (Walley, Webber & Collins, 2010). Taking anti-malaria medication is also a personal protection strategy but the malarial parasite is increasingly resistant to medication such that, in some parts of the world, it is totally ineffective (WHO, 2010a). There is a great deal of research being conducted on developing a

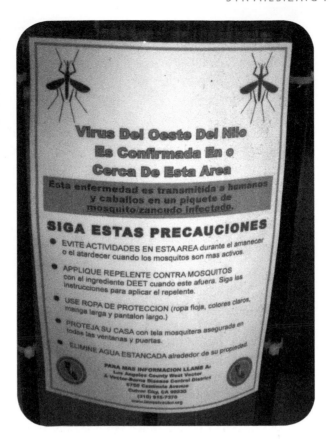

Mosquitoes are the principal vectors of a variety of diseases, such as malaria.

vaccine for malaria prevention. There is potential for effective vaccination in the next ten years or so – trials are currently underway (Macdonald, 2007; Walley, Webber & Collins, 2010).

Secondary prevention   Early detection of infection from malaria is key to reducing morbidity and mortality rates. This requires clinic facilities and access to primary health care services. 'Early detection and treatment of malaria is one of the important interventions for malaria' (Walley, Webber & Collins, 2010: 278).

Tertiary prevention   Tertiary prevention for malarial infection requires prompt drug treatment and an infected person may need hospital admission and rehabilitation. Malaria can usually be cured by a course of anti-malarial drugs (Macdonald, 2007). Global health and socio-economic inequalities are evident here. Macdonald argues that if large areas of the developed world were affected by malaria in the same way that the developing world is, then more efforts would have been made by the pharmaceutical industry to develop drugs to prevent it, given the potential profit that could be made.

Individual lifestyle/behavioural change   Changes in behaviour at an individual level require compliance and adherence to preventative behaviours as well as to drug treatment regimes for prevention and treatment. Using ITNs in hot and humid climates is not comfortable and this is often cited as a reason for non-use (see Macdonald, 2007) However, encouraging this practice among an at-risk population is vital to malaria control. Factors affecting individual behaviour are complex (as discussed in detail in chapter 6). Lay beliefs are important – what local people believe about the causes of malaria will affect what they do as well as whether, and how, they seek treatment once infected.

Education for behaviour change is also key to tackling malaria. Knowledge about the malaria infection cycle, how it is transmitted and how risk factors can be reduced, is very important.

Changing the social and economic environment   Environmental measures are extremely important in malaria prevention and control. Macdonald (2007: 158) states that 'if every person, even in the poorest communities, could spend the night in a bed covered by a net, the incidence of malaria would fall dramatically'. The key point here is that of poverty and socio-economic disadvantage. Not being able to afford bednets for all household members is often a reason for non-use (Armstrong Schellenberg et al., 2001). In addition, children suffering malnutrition are more susceptible to infection and more vulnerable during infection and recovery.

The physical environment is also important for tackling malaria. The malaria-carrying mosquito does not travel far from its breeding ground so if human dwellings are at least 50 metres from them this reduces the likelihood of being bitten (Macdonald, 2007). This appears to be a very simple measure to take. Removing standing water from inside and close to houses would also have a similar effect (by removing opportunitistic breeding places).

Lastly, as Wilkinson (2005) argues, significant environmental changes can lower incidences of malaria such as irrigation schemes, disruption to habitat, changes in land-use and population resettlement.

Policy   The prevention of malaria requires global, national and local political will. 'There is strong evidence that insecticide impregnated bednets are highly effective in preventing malaria and related morbidity. The important decision is not whether to use ITN, but how to deliver them to the whole population at risk of malaria' (Walley, Webber & Collins 2010: 59). This requires policy-level interventions and the political will to engage in distribution of bednets to whole populations. Global climate change is causing changes in malaria infection patterns as temperature rise so that certain areas are no longer protected by lower temperatures (Walley, Webber & Collins, 2010). There is a great deal of action taking place on a global level to try and tackle malaria. Reduction in malaria infection links directly to the Millennium Development Goals.

There are a number of global strategies in place, including the Roll Back Malaria campaign, the US presidential malaria initiative and the programmes supported by the Bill and Melinda Gates Foundation. Roll Back Malaria has four key areas of action – prompt access to treatment, increasing use of ITNs, prevention and control of malaria in pregnant women and emergency response (Beigbeder, 2004). The World Health Organization (2010a) reported that progress on the global burden of malaria has been seen in all WHO Regions since 2005. This is a positive trend given the impact that malaria has on global mortality and morbidity rates.

Case study

Cervical cancer
- Approximately half a million women develop cervical cancer every year, and almost half of those diagnosed die as a result (WHO, 2010b).
- Cervical cancer accounts for 1 in 10 cancers diagnosed in women worldwide (Cancer Research UK, 2010) and causes the greatest problems in low-income countries in which health care resources are limited (Bosch et al. (1995).
- Furthermore, in the UK, approximately 55 women are diagnosed with cervical cancer every week (Cancer Research UK, 2010).
- Finally, in the UK, around two-thirds of women survive the disease for five years or more, with survival rates being much higher in women diagnosed at a younger age. Women diagnosed under 40 years of age have survival rates of more than 85% (Cancer Research UK, 2010). Despite these survival rates, women diagnosed with this type of cancer die younger than in most other cases of cancer (Curtin et al., 2009). Table 13.2 gives an overview of the determinants of cervical cancer.

Strategies to tackle cervical cancer

Biomedical strategies

Primary prevention   The development of an HPV vaccination and its successful administration has the potential to reduce cases of cervical cancer on a large scale and so is argued to be largely cost-effective (WHO, 2010b). The UK HPV vaccination was introduced in schools as part of a national immunization programme in 2008, for girls aged between twelve and thirteen. Its effects are yet to be evaluated in the long term. However, preventing young women from acquiring HPV

Table 13.2. The determinants of cervical cancer.

Determinants	Mechanism	References
Sexual behaviour	A woman's total lifetime number of sexual partners and her number of regular relationships are predictive of risk. Women who have recently acquired a new partner are at much higher risk.	Deacon et al. (2000)
	Age at first intercourse: the younger a women begins then the higher the risk	Mant et al. (1988)
	Infection with sexually transmitted diseases, particularly herpes simplex virus 2, increases the risk. HPV has been detected in cervical tumours across the world. Some studies suggest that it is present in virtually all tumours.	Cancer Research UK (2010)
	Long-term use of the oral contraceptive pill increases the risk of cervical cancer	Wallboomers & Meijer (1997); Bosch et al. (1995)
Smoking	There is strong evidence to show increasing risks associated with longer periods of smoking and the more cigarettes smoked per day.	Cancer Research UK (2010)
Socio-economic status	Women living in the most deprived areas have higher rates of cervical cancer. So those in lower social classes are at higher risk.	Deacon et al. (2000)
Genetics	Women with a sister or mother who have had cervical cancer are at an increased risk of developing it themselves.	Harris et al. (1998), Currin et al. (2009)
Immunosuppression	Some meta-analyses have shown that women with HIV/AIDS have a six-fold increased risk and those who have undergone organ transplantation have more than double the risk.	Brown et al. (1997) Cancer Research UK (2010)

will ultimately reduce the incidence of cervical cancer, given that HPV is the largest known cause of the disease.

Secondary prevention   Despite the HPV vaccination now being available in a number of countries, this does not remove the need for screening because the vaccines only prevent about 70 per cent of cervical cancer cases (WHO, 2010b). Since 1988 when screening was first introduced in the UK, cervical cancer cases have significantly fallen, with screening being the most likely explanation (Raffle et al., 2003). Peto et al. (2004) argue that since the introduction of screening in England and Wales, the rate of cervical cancer has halved. Although this does not provide a reliable estimate of the effect of screening, Peto et al. (2004) argue that screening prevents approximately 4500 deaths per

Figure 13.2 Factors influencing cervical cancer using Dahlgren and Whitehead's model as a framework for understanding determinants.

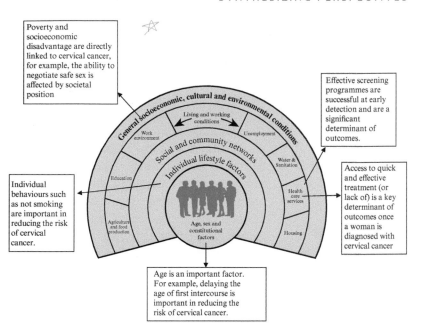

Poverty and socioeconomic disadvantage are directly linked to cervical cancer, for example, the ability to negotiate safe sex is affected by societal position

Effective screening programmes are successful at early detection and are a significant determinant of outcomes.

Individual behaviours such as not smoking are important in reducing the risk of cervical cancer.

Access to quick and effective treatment (or lack of) is a key determinant of outcomes once a woman is diagnosed with cervical cancer

Age is an important factor. For example, delaying the age of first intercourse is important in reducing the risk of cervical cancer.

year and the rate is still improving. However, successful screening is compounded by women not accessing screening services. Attendance at screening is affected by knowledge of the screening process, risk factors associated with cervical cancer and health perceptions with variable rates of screening existing across the world (Leung & Leung, 2010). In many parts of the world where screening rates for cervical cancer are low, there have been calls for the development of health promotion to increase women's awareness of their risk and to prompt attendance at screening (Twinn et al., 2007).

Tertiary approaches   There are several treatment options available for women who are diagnosed with cervical cancer, dependent upon the stage at which the cancer is diagnosed. These include surgery such as removal of parts of the cervix, total hysterectomy and more radical hysterectomy. Laser surgery may also be appropriate in some instances. Radiation therapy and chemotherapy are also treatment options that attempt to kill cancer cells or to prevent them from growing (National Cancer Institute, 2011). The suitability of each treatment and its effectiveness varies across patients.

Individual lifestyle changes in behaviour   Differences in sexual behaviour have been used to explain vast inequalities in incidences of cervical cancer across countries (Herrero, 1996) and within populations (Cooper et al., 2007). It has been argued that on an individual level women can change their behaviour to reduce their risk of cervical cancer. For example, women who don't smoke, delay the age of first sexual intercourse, who have fewer sexual partners and who protect themselves through condom usage reduce their risk. Health promotion can also be an effective tool here in terms of providing educational interventions that encourage women to adopt such lifestyle changes. Health promotion campaigns can also be used to encourage women to take up both screening and vaccination opportunities (see chapter 7 for a comprehensive discussion of health promotion). A review conducted by Shepherd et al. (2009) demonstrates that educational interventions aimed specifically at socially and economically disadvantaged women can encourage short-term sexual risk reduction behaviour (condom use), especially when complemented with sexual negotiation skill development. However, sociologists criticize this focus upon individual lifestyle change and health-seeking behaviour as placing too much emphasis upon individual choices and responsibility as well as being victim blaming. The broader structural factors that influence the daily decisions people make regarding their health and sexual behaviour ultimately need recognition.

Changing the social and economic environment Sociologists have long discussed how social factors can and do influence health behaviours and how the structure of society is detrimental to some people's health (see chapter 4 for a more detailed discussion). There is a large amount of evidence demonstrating that our health is ultimately determined by our position within the social structure; society determines our health in many ways. This is indeed true of the relationship between social class position and cervical cancer risk. There is much evidence to support the links between lower social class position and higher risk of cervical cancer. However, explaining this is complex because risk factors cluster together and make it difficult to determine the individual contribution of each variable at population level (Currin et al., 2009). For example, Mant et al. (1988) argue that social class differences in cervical cancer incidence can not simply be ascribed to more promiscuous sexual behaviour in women of lower social class status. Those from lower socio-economic groups are also less likely to take up screening opportunities. This is again linked to the broader structural factors that influence their daily lives, sometimes de-prioritizing health concerns and healthy behaviours. Psychological theories tell us that behaviour change (i.e. encouraging people to take up screening opportunities or moderating their sexual behaviour) is incredibly complex (chapter 6 discusses this in much more depth) and that health risk behaviours are also complex, with people often engaging in both health-enhancing and health-damaging behaviours simultaneously. Some health-enhancing behaviours, however, can be encouraged, for example, to successfully increase screening rates and vaccination uptake, interventions should seek to normalize behaviour such as taking part in health-promoting activities (Twinn et al., 2007).

Policy   In the UK, there is a clear policy in relation to the prevention, detection and treatment of cervical cancer, for example, the national screening programme introduced in 1988 and the introduction of the HPV schools vaccination programme in 2008. However, policy in this area is not without controversy. The vaccination is already available and in use across many different countries but the implementation of any national vaccination programme creates many difficult decisions for policy-makers. The WHO (2010) outlined several considerations for policy-makers in relation to the vaccination, including questions such as, who should receive the vaccination and at what age? The question of how such vaccination programmes are to be funded is also a concern for policy-makers. The vaccination is also most effective when administered in girls at the age of nine to thirteen years, before

Learning task 13.1

Using Dahlgren and Whitehead as an analytical tool.
Choose a health issue from the list below
- HIV/AIDS
- lung cancer
- pandemic influenza
- obesity
- depression

Now use the Dahlgren and Whitehead rainbow model to draw out some of the influences upon your chosen health issue by reflecting upon how each of the layers relates to your topic. Refer back to the detailed case studies in this chapter to see how they use the model and produce a similar diagram as a framework for understanding.

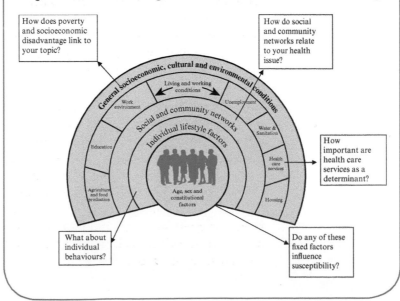

Case study

Neighbourhoods

- A 'settings approach' to health promotion came from Ottawa Charter for health promotion stating that 'Health is created and lived by people within the settings of their everyday life; where they learn, work, play and love' (WHO, 1986: 6). Instead of a topic-based approach to addressing health it was proposed that health promotion activities take place in settings and their associated systems to improve overall health. Basically investments in health are made in social systems for which health is not their primary remit (Dooris, 2004).

Neighbourhoods are a key setting for health promotion, and the health of a neighbourhood is subject to a range of complex determinants.

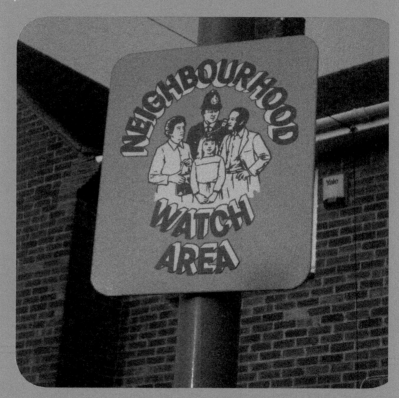

- Neighbourhoods provide a major setting in which people live and work and can be thought of as a location in which a raft of health promotion strategies can be applied. Naidoo and Wills (2009) suggest that neighbourhoods are a key setting for health promotion because physical and social environments interact with other service provision such as health care, welfare services, important hubs like pubs, shops, post offices, community centre and churches.

- The determinants of neighbourhood health are complex and intertwined by work already discussed in chapters 9, 10, 11 and 12. It is not possible to consider all determinants of neighbourhood health or indeed the multitude of actions to address these determinants. However, in the case study a flavour of initiatives are suggested that foster healthy neighbourhoods. Table 13.3 provides an overview of the determinants of unhealthy neighbourhoods.

Table 13.3. The determinants of unhealthy neighbourhoods.

Determinants	Mechanism	References
Social environment	Poor social support leads to social isolation and feelings of low self-esteem and not belonging.	Uchino (2006)
Social support from networks	Some support networks are damaging for health-related behaviour.	Mant et al. (1988)
Lack of trust between **community** networks (poor social capital)	In communities that trust each, other relations between people are likely to be more co-operative and less stressful.	Halpern (2005)
Fear of crime and safety issues	Lead to poor physical and mental health status.	Jackson & Stafford (2009)
Physical environment		
Housing and overcrowding	Leads to poor physical and mental health.	Campbell (2006)
Poor design of neighbourhoods and houses	Can lead to disputes and conflicts between neighbourhoods. Noise leads to poor sleeping patterns.	Donaldson and Scally (2009)
Transport Over-reliance on cars	Congestion and road rage.	
Pollution from transport and workplaces	Direct exposure to carcinogens and carbon monoxide.	Koplan and Fleming (2000)
Lack of green spaces for play and recreation	Not well understood but links to quality of life and relaxation.	Jackson (2003) Mitchell & Popham (2008)
Socio-economic environment	The above determinants are underpinned by a complex relationship between social class and income in which people with poorer status generally live in more deprived social and physical environments.	Stansfeld (2005)
Unemployment	Poorer material circumstances leads to less choice and fewer basic elements such as heating, shelter and food.	Lin et al. (1995)
Poorer education achievement	Higher education achievement can lead to higher incomes that in turn link to better health outcomes	Cutler and Lleras-Muney (2006)

they become sexually active. However, vaccinating young girls in the UK has led to a variety of reactions, with some parents reporting concerns about encouraging risky sexual behaviour (Waller et al., 2006). Furthermore, in many parts of the world policy has not been created to support large scale vaccination and screening programmes, leaving

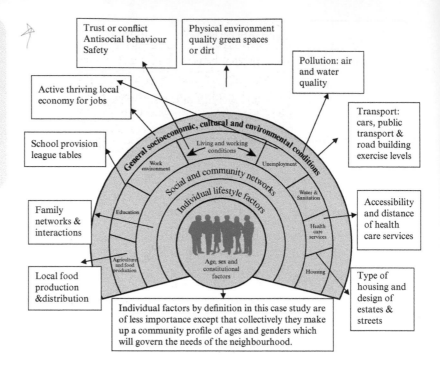

Figure 13.3. Factors influencing neighbourhood health using Dahlgren and Whitehead's model as a framework for understanding.

many women more vulnerable to negative outcomes associated with cervical cancer.

Strategies to improve neighbourhood health

Biomedical strategies   We can see using a settings approach that the major determinants of neighbourhood health cannot be adequately addressed by drawing on biomedical strategies such as screening or vaccination. That is not to downplay the role that screening or vaccination can play in health protection and prevention for specific diseases but are unlikely to address the health concerns of the neighbourhood.

Individual lifestyle / behavioural change strategies   The strategy of individual behaviour change is also less applicable to addressing neighbourhood determinants of health. Concepts such as social support and social capital imply a connectedness between people that can influence individual choice and action. However, it is possible to consider how educational approaches can be used to foster participation in neighbourhood life. Indeed, citizenship within the UK national curriculum for school-aged children has, at its heart, participation in neighbourhoods, communities and civic activities (Qualifications and Curriculum Development Agency, no date).

Changing the social and economic environment   If health is to be addressed at the level of the neighbourhood then strategies that are implemented

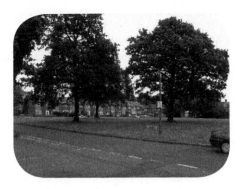

Town planning can have an impact on health in neighbourhoods through the provision of green spaces.

at that level are likely to impact on health more effectively. It is important to acknowledge that policy-related approaches outlined in the next section will provide a favourable milieu in which social, physical and economic changes can take place.

(a)   Physical environment
Transport initiatives where 'walk to work and school' schemes are nurtured or where more co-operation exists between competitive bus service provision may improve health. Fostering stronger provision of cycle-friendly environments such as adequate cycle lanes and subsidized hire of cycles may enable individuals to lead active, greener lifestyles. Architects and town planners have a role to play in making neighbourhoods desirable places to live and work with green open spaces, play areas, safe well lit areas and designing how streets and hubs are connected for greatest social and civic engagement (Thorp, 2010).
Gardening schemes linked to food co-operatives where local food is produced and then in turn sold or used in community cafes to generate income are sustainable initiatives that also serve to build links between different areas and groups in neighbourhoods.

(b)   Social environment
Fear of crime and anti-social behaviour such as noise, graffiti and threatening behaviour can reduce mental health status. These can be addressed by changes in the social environment such as providing case intervention to work with families and multi-agency working via Community Safety Partnerships (Chartered Institute of Environmental Health, 2006).
Other measures to increase social support and social capital have already been outlined at the end of chapter 9 but include mentoring programmes, family support and extensive development and investment in volunteering programmes and the voluntary sector.

Policy   Activities reducing income and status inequalities are fundamental in promoting healthy neighbourhoods. Suggested activities to address inequalities more generally are commitment to full employment and skills development for the unemployed, redistributive taxation policies and promoting subsidized childcare for working families. Strategies that encourage neighbourhood renewal, regeneration and investment into deprived neighbourhoods will also serve to engender a sense of pride and belonging.

In addition specific neighbourhood policies related to local authority planning could be utilized to design healthy spaces. For example local authorities are now beginning to limit the number of fast-food outlets in a local area in order to reduce availability of 'junk food' on the high street.

Neighbourhoods offer opportunities to utilize a settings approach for health improvement. The determinants are multi-faceted and interconnected so they require comprehensive strategies at different levels of action (from individuals, networks, neighbourhoods, regionally and nationally). Different approaches are therefore needed; from educational strategies, to building capacity in neighbourhoods, community development, generating social capital and implementing healthy public policy to shape the physical, social and economic environment within neighbourhoods.

Learning task 13.2

Strategies for tackling health problems.
Again choose a health issue from the list below
- HIV/AIDS
- Lung cancer
- Pandemic influenza
- Obesity
- Depression

1. Now list the strategies that can be used to tackle the problem. Use the same headings that the detailed case studies discuss in this chapter. Start with biomedical strategies and consider approaches that use primary prevention, secondary prevention and then tertiary prevention.
2. Consider how making changes within individual lifestyles might have an impact, and then think about the changes that could be made socially and economically in order to effectively address your health issue.
3. Finally, list the policy changes that you think are needed.

Revisiting the chapters throughout this book will help you to complete this task; for example, chapter 4 highlights social influences upon health, chapter 6 discusses individual characteristics and chapter 11 outlines policy approaches which all need considering in relation to tackling your chosen health issue.

The determinants of health 'rainbow'

This section of the chapter offers a critical consideration of Dahlgren and Whitehead's (1991) influential model depicting the determinants of health. It starts by describing the model, then discusses its key strengths, then moves onto considering the model in a more critical light with a view to how it might be improved upon to better aid understanding of the key influences on health and health experience. Before you move on, take some time to do learning task 13.3.

Learning task 13.3

Evaluating Dahlgren and Whitehead's model of determinants of health.
Look at the Dahlgren and Whitehead social determinants of health model and think about it critically.

Draw a two-column table and on one side list what is good about the model (strengths) and on the other side list any problems with the model. You might want to think about what works well as well as ways in which it could be improved.

Dahlgren and Whitehead's model highlights several of the main factors determining population health. Crucially it 'acknowledges the complex nature of health determinants' (Marks 2005: 13). The core of the model is several fixed determinants of health such as age, sex, genetics and hereditary factors. Starting from the centre and then moving outwards the surrounding layers are determinants of health that are open to modification through social policy such as behavioural factors like levels of physical activity, levels of alcohol consumption and tobacco smoking. There is a large evidence base to demonstrate that individuals faced with disadvantaged circumstances tend to exhibit higher prevalence of health-damaging behaviours such as smoking and having a poor diet. In addition they also face greater financial barriers to choosing a healthier lifestyle (WHO, 2005c).

The next layer details the importance of community and broader social influences. Social interactions and peer groups can influence individual health outcomes both positively and negatively. WHO (2005c) discusses how indicators of community organization register fewer networks and support systems available for those in lower social class groups. This disadvantage is further compounded by high levels of deprivation resulting in fewer facilities within communities and generally poorer security.

The next layer points to the importance of living and working conditions and food supply (among others) that are needed for the maintenance of health. The conditions associated with social deprivation again heighten risks for those at the lower end of the social spectrum and include poorer housing conditions, exposure to more dangerous or stressful working environments and poorer access to services (WHO, 2005c).

Finally, the economic, cultural and environmental aspects of society are identified as overall mediators of population health. These factors, which can include the overall economic state of a country, cultural attitudes and general labour market conditions (WHO, 2005c), ultimately influence all of the other layers of the model. The key point of this model is its simple emphasis upon interactions in that 'individual lifestyles are embedded in social norms and networks, and in living and working conditions, which in turn are related to the wider socio-economic and cultural environment' (Dahlgren and Whitehead, 2006b: 21). These health determinants can also be influenced either positively or detrimentally by decisions made at the individual, commercial or political level.

Key strengths of the rainbow model

Dahlgren and Whitehead's (1991) determinants of health model is an extremely useful framework for considering some of the complexities of health and the factors that impact on, and affect, health. It has been used extensively within the health literature during the last two decades and is drawn upon in a variety of different contexts.

The model has many strengths, which are well documented. These include its relative simplicity (although, conversely, this could be viewed as a limitation as it lacks explanatory value – see Bradshaw, 2008), its application to different contexts and the fact that it makes intuitive sense. It clearly demonstrates some of the complexities associated with the social determinants of health, illustrating the interconnectedness of various sociological, environmental and health-related factors that combine to influence health (WHO, 2005c). It also demonstrates that individual choices are a very small component in determining health. Indeed, Whitehead (1995) describes the layers of influence and health determinants in terms of the context of action required by policy-makers to tackle health inequalities, which further cements this point.

The model has been very effective in terms of examining how different determinants contribute to inequalities in health. Additionally it, among others, has been described as a 'useful conceptual device to identify the causal pathways that have differential impacts on health' (Exworthy, 2008: 319). It certainly helps us to appreciate the complexity of the determinants of health and how these are much wider than individual behavioural factors. The complexity of the levels of influence that permeate the model reinforce the need for a number of public health strategies, for example, at the level of the individual and more structurally at a societal level. It has also very usefully provided a framework to examine health inequalities in different regions and countries such as Europe (Dahlgren & Whitehead 2006a, 2006b, 2007), South Africa (Bradshaw, 2008) and Brazil (Cruz, 2008).

→ The model clearly recognizes and outlines the importance of the social and structural in relation to health. Graham (2004) argues that the Dahlgren and Whitehead (1991) model makes the point that health inequalities are socially produced, which is very important. The model also shows that exposure to health damaging risk factors plays a significant role in the health of the poor (Jarvis & Wardle 1999). Popay et al. (2003) also argue that the model is a convenient framework within which to discuss existing approaches to the study of social inequalities in relation to health. The model is also theoretically grounded, as it draws upon social ecological theory, which bridges several different research fields and demonstrates the importance of environmental settings having multi-faceted social, cultural and physical aspects that all influence health (Stokols, 1998).

The model, however, has been criticized and has its limitations. No one theoretical framework can provide a full picture of the determinants of health. However, there is a general tendency within the literature to reproduce the model without critique. The next section of the chapter will take a more critical look at Dahlgren and Whitehead's (1991) popular framework. It will explore its limitations and how it might be built upon to provide an even more comprehensive framework for understanding determinants of health.

How the rainbow model might be improved

Refer back to the things you considered in learning task 13.3. As part of this task you were asked to think about how the rainbow model might be improved upon. This section will consider this in more depth. The model has proved invaluable in a wide variety of situations for assessing and conceptualizing factors influencing health; however, no single framework can capture everything. The model, although widely used, has been subject to some criticism.

——> The framework tends to be more descriptive rather than analytical or critical, demonstrating the relationships between different influences on health but not really going into any depth about what the nature of these are and how they interact or co-exist to influence health outcomes. Therefore, although the model shows many of the determinants of health, it cannot demonstrate the complexities of causes. Dahlgren and Whitehead (2006b) themselves argue that the analysis of causal factors needs further development.

——> There is a lack of detail in relation to describing the extent to which the identified determinants influence health overall. So, for example, are social and community networks a more significant determinant than health care services? Dahlgren and Whitehead (2006b: 22) recognize this when stating 'in practice, making the distinction between these categories of determinants may be difficult at times'.

The model, as it stands, neglects global, political and historical determinants of health. There is no explicit identification of these as determinants of health despite a large evidence base, which, for example, demonstrates that many aspects of global society act as a health determinant.

The model does not outline the feasibility of changing specific factors, what action is needed in relation to each layer or how one layer influences another. Hence, it is not useful as a basis for action (Wainwright, 1996). Similarly, Graham (2004) argues that the model does not help policy-makers because it does not outline strategies for improving public health; hence it fails to provide any clear direction.

As a model to depict the determinants of health, rather than health inequalities, the distinction between the social factors influencing health and the social processes determining inequality can easily become confused. This may therefore lead to assumptions by policy-makers that health inequalities can be reduced by simply focusing upon the social determinants of health. The model fails to highlight that policy-makers must pay attention to the differing consequences of their policies across social groups because access to the determinants of good health are not equal (Graham, 2004).

The relationship between the different layers of the model and the way in which the different factors interact with each other could also be explored in greater detail. As Bradshaw (2008) argues, the pathways (or relationships) between each determinant and health inequalities are not necessarily linear or uncomplicated. Therefore solid, in-depth understanding is needed in order to tease out the mechanisms involved so that changes can be made and health inequalities can be tackled in effective and meaningful ways. Ecological theory asks us to consider the relationship and interactions between individuals, behaviours and the environment. The relationship between general socio-economic, cultural and environmental conditions and the individual (particularly in terms of lifestyle factors) is much more closely connected than the rather distal placement of the outer semi-circle of the model implies.

Determinants of health resulting from the lifespan are also not considered in the model with any great effect. Green and Tones (2010) give the example of the 'powerful early influence of primary socialization' (p. 89). Similarly life course influences and events are also not taken into account in this model although Dahlgren and Whitehead (2006b) do consider these in some detail in a later piece of work.

Another factor that is not given adequate attention within the model as it stands is the 'determinant' of power. Krieger (2008) argues that power is a key determinant of health and that structures of agency and resistance also need to be taken into account as well as analyses of power at different levels. Social and geographical mobility are also

Learning task 13.4

Building on the rainbow model of health.
Take some time to think about how you would conceptualize and represent the wider determinants of health, based both on your own ideas (developed in learning task 13.3) and the discussion in this section.

Next try to draw a model or framework that captures the essential factors as you see them. For example, you could use the rainbow idea and develop this further or you could start with a web diagram as a basis for representing them.

determinants not accounted for within the model, but are extremely influential on health (take processes of urbanization, social erosion and urban immigration for example).

From a health promotion perspective, whose ideological basis necessitates a move away from focusing at an individual level, the focus of the centre of Dahlgren and Whitehead's model at an individual level is called into question. Health promotion would seek to places social inequalities at the 'centre' of any framework designed to represent determinants of health. In that sense this model would be turned 'inside out'. Last but not least, the model does not directly provide us with any answers about how we might tackle inequalities in health although it does give an indication as to where action might be targeted (at, and within, the different levels) and highlights the importance of policy for improving health.

Despite these limitations the model remains an extremely useful framework. The central argument here is to do with how the model might be improved upon rather than rejecting the model as a framework; indeed, the reliance of structure of Part III of this book on the model demonstrates how useful it is and how it might be utilized to develop understanding. Dahlgren and Whitehead (2007) revised the framework in a paper published in 2007 and suggested that the framework should be viewed as an 'interdependent system for improving health and reducing health hazards' (p. 13). They go on to to suggest that the four layers of determinants can translate into four levels of policy intervention and that equity aspects can also be specifically focused in terms of the four layers (or levels).

Barton and Grant (2006b: 252) have developed the rainbow model further from its original form (see figure 3.4) based on the argument that 'the environment we live in is a major determinant of health and well-being'. The rainbow idea remains central to the framework and individuals remain at the core of it. It retains the original features of Dahlgren and Whitehead's model demonstrating the determinants of

Figure 13.4. Barton and Grant's (2006) 'health map' – an extension of Dahlgren and Whitehead's model.

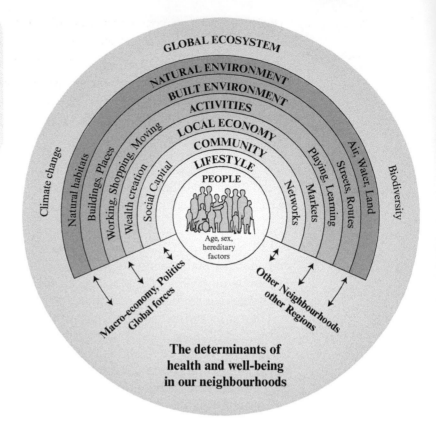

The determinants of health and well-being in our neighbourhoods

health. The key difference is that Barton and Grant's (2006) model puts the people at the centre within the wider context of the 'global ecosystem' to include factors such as climate change and sustainability. In addition, Barton and Grant's (2006) model reflects the importance of 'human habitat' – development and settlement processes, the built environment and how these impact on the natural environment and the wider global ecosystem. This framework was developed to specifically consider the role of local government and why the social determinants of health are so important. Designing the framework in this way challenges the role of health services in influencing and maintaining health demonstrating that the factors impacting on health are many, varied and complex.

In conclusion this chapter has brought together the different aspects discussed throughout this book in relation to three case studies. This has enabled us to develop deeper understanding of the multitude of issues raised and the complexity of the debates around the nature of health and our experience of it. The chapter has also provided an in-depth discussion about the rainbow model of health, noting its merits and considering how it might be built upon in order to develop our understanding. Health is complex, health is social and maintaining and promoting positive health is an ongoing challenge for us all.

Summary

- Health is extremely complex and a multitude of factors influence and impact on health, which means there are a lot of ways in which ill-health might be prevented and positive health might be promoted.

- Developing an understanding of the wider determinants of health will help us to design strategies for action drawing on different sectors of the 'public health' workforce.

- Dahlgren and Whitehead's rainbow model is a very useful framework for conceptualizing determinants of health, which can be built upon to broaden our understanding of factors influencing health.

Glossary

Glossary terms are highlighted in bold in the text at first occurrence. The definitions explain how the terms are to be understood in the context of health studies.

aetiology
This is about giving a cause to a specific outcome (determining a cause and effect relationship). For example, the aetiology of lung cancer may involve smoking as causation.

association
This is the relationship between being exposed to a risk factor and then the ensuing disease. It is a term used to express a causal relationship, for example that leads from exposure to disease. One such association is that of exposure to radiation and then a resulting cancer diagnosis.

attitude
An attitude is the feelings that someone has about an action or an object. 'There are three aspects to a person's attitude to an issue – cognitive (knowledge and information), affective (their emotions, likes and dislikes) and behavioural (their skills and competencies)' (Naidoo & Wills, 2008: 372).

autonomy
'The doctrine that the individual human will is or ought to be governed only by its own principles and laws' (Free Dictionary, nd). This is about individuals having the ability and capacity to be able to be in charge of their own actions. This relates to health because people are often constructed as autonomous in relation to health-related behaviours such as not smoking and drinking less but in reality they are also influenced by other factors (see chapters 4, 6, 9, 10, 11, 12 and 13 for discussion of the different determinants of health).

bias
This is a term often used in relation to research studies and is 'the result of any process that causes observations to differ from their true values in a systematic way' (Naidoo & Wills, 2008: 372). Bias can enter into the research process at any stage; for example, from sampling

through to analysis and the reporting of results (see chapter 3 for more detailed discussion of the research process).

biological
Biological can be defined as being related to biology. Biology has an influence upon health particularly in relation to genetics. There are a number of genetic conditions that have been identified as leading to poorer health outcomes, for example, cystic fibrosis is a genetically inherited condition that affects the internal organs of sufferers, whose lungs become clogged with thick mucus, making it hard for them to breathe and eat. Indeed, biological factors have also been linked to the development of some mental disorders, including schizophrenia.

biomedicine
This is 'the application of the principles of the natural sciences, especially biology and physiology' (Free Dictionary, nd) to the human body. Biomedicine focuses upon the causes of ill-health and disease within the physical body and the development of appropriate clinical treatments. This school of thought is associated with the medical profession and contrasts with the social model of health (see chapters 1 and 4).

British Household Survey
This survey started in 1991 and is a multi-purpose study based upon households in which every inhabitant is interviewed. These households are a representative sample of individuals who are followed for a number of years. Data from this service are available online, via the UK data archive.

census
A census is simply a count of the population. In the UK there is a census conducted every ten years that also gathers information about the population and has to be completed by every household by law. Two hundred countries across the world carry out similar censuses, often gathering information about various aspects of social life. UK census data is made available online.

characteristic
A characteristic is simply a feature or a quality that belongs to a person and therefore can be used to identify that person. As individuals, we all have health characteristics and it is possible to define the characteristics that are associated with good health.

citizenship
A citizen is an individual who is a member within a community and, as a result of that membership, can gain both rights and duties. Notions of health citizenship are often concerned with people having

self-direction and as a result are able to achieve quality of life. There is also a relationship between health and citizenship in the sense that those excluded from citizenship are likely to suffer from poorer health (Brewis & Fitzgerald, 2010).

cohort
This is a group that can be followed and tracked through time. Bowling (2009: 463) describes those in a cohort study as a population with 'a common experience or characteristic that defines the sampling'. Cohort studies are used as a research method to explore the relationship between specific risk factors and the development of diseases; for example, the consumption of food high in saturated fat and the development of specific types of cancer. Chapter 3 discusses research in depth.

collectivism
This is defined specifically as 'the principles or system of ownership and control of the means of production and distribution by the people collectively, usually under the supervision of a government' (Free Dictionary, nd). It is about the responsibility of individuals as a community (collective) to meet the needs of others. For example, the British NHS is a collective health service because it is funded by members of society via the taxes that they pay (see chapter 11 for more about the NHS and the welfare state).

communicable
This term refers to diseases that are infectious and therefore transmittable across populations. An example of a well-known communicable disease is the 'flu, which is caused by a virus. There are many other respiratory infections that are communicable such as TB and pneumonia and a broad range of other infectious diseases such as HIV, cholera and measles.

community
This is a contested concept and so is difficult to define. It usually refers to a group of people who live in the same neighbourhood (a geographic community) or a group of people who share the same interests (for example a religious community). Chapter 9 discusses the importance of community in relation to health.

concept
A concept can be described as a 'general notion' (*Oxford English Dictionary*, 1989) or as an 'idea'. In the context of this book a 'concept of health' is a notion or idea about health.

consumerism
Consumerism refers to the process by which goods and services become desired and are purchased because they are ideologically

valued and perceived as beneficial. Giddens (2009: 1114) defines a consumer society as 'a type of society that promotes the consumption of mass-produced products'. Notions of health consumerism often describe patients as being more involved in their health care, having more awareness of health and illness and buying health-related goods and services.

construct

A construct is something that is made to explain and interpret the social world. There are a number of constructs used to interpret and understand health; for example the notion of quality of life is a health-related construct. The WHO (1995) illustrates that health-related quality of life is a broad and multi-dimensional construct that includes numerous aspects, such as psychological well-being and social health.

critique

A critique is simply the critical discussion of a topic generally within an academic context. 'The term critique, meaning the critical art, or critical evaluation or analysis . . . involves evaluating strengths and weaknesses of discussions/arguments across a range of authors' (Craswell, 2005: 31–2). There are many critiques of models and theories attempting to explain and understand health.

culture

This is a widely used term and simply refers to the 'values and ways of life that characterize a given group' (Giddens, 2009). Helman (2000: 2) defines culture as '. . . an inherited "lens", through which the individual perceives and understands the world . . .'. Understanding culture is important in relation to health because we all live in a specific cultural context that can positively or negatively influence our health.

DALY

'Disability-adjusted life years' (DALY) is a measure for the overall disease burden. Originally developed by the World Health Organization, it is becoming increasingly common in the field of public health and health impact assessment (HIA). It is designed to quantify the impact of premature death and disability on a population by combining them into a single, comparable measure. In so doing, mortality and morbidity are combined into a single, common metric' (Free Dictionary, nd).

deconstructed

The process of deconstruction is one in which the language used in writing is analysed and critically examined. Put simply, it means to break down components (Free Dictionary, nd). This approach is associated with the work of Jacques Derrida, a French philosopher. As an approach it encourages readers to ask critical questions about the material that they are reading, such as what are the boundaries and limitations? This approach suggests that the material that we read is part of our culture and the world that we inhabit and, as a result, must be deconstructed to be fully understood.

definition

A definition is the explanation of a term in order to illustrate its meaning. It is not always easy to define terms, as there may be different views about the exact meaning of something. For example, chapter 1 of this book discusses the complexity associated with defining health and shows that there are many ways in which health can be defined and understood.

determinant

There are many factors influencing an individual's health, and these are often inter-related and more commonly described as determinants. The World Health Organization (2010) argues that whether people are healthy or not is determined by their circumstances and environment. Thus, factors such as where we live, our environment, our social class position and gender all have an impact upon health, ultimately determining how healthy we are. The determinants of health include the social and economic environment, the physical environment and a person's individual characteristics and behaviours (WHO, 2010).

discipline

Macdonald and Bunton (2002: 17) state that 'a discipline involves an ordered area or field of study'; several disciplines discussed in this book are important in relation to health studies, for example, sociology, anthropology and psychology. Each discipline has its own perspective, theories and different ways of understanding and finding out about things including health.

discourse

This is a term that refers to a collection of ideas about knowledge, which is often taken for granted. Discourses are a 'body of ideas, concepts and beliefs' (Bilton et al., 1996: 657) that are used as a framework from which we draw our understandings of the social world. Discourses change over time and can be powerful; for example, medical and religious knowledge are part of important knowledge systems in the world, and both inform understandings and interpretations of health.

egalitarian

Egalitarianism is a school of thought that favours equality (although defining this is not simple either) specifically 'Affirming, promoting, or characterized by belief in equal political, economic, social, and civil rights for all people' (Free Dictionary, nd). Equality is important in relation to health outcomes as discussed in several chapters of this book (see chapters 4, 11 and 12).

empirical

Empiricism is an important part of social research because it is about proving knowledge through data. Empiricism is a philosophical approach suggesting that 'the only form of valid knowledge is that which is gathered by the use of the senses' (Bowling, 2009: 464). So, an empirical research approach will offer explanations based upon observed data. There is a plethora of empirical research that contributes to our understandings of health.

empowerment

This is again a concept that is difficult to define as it is used in many ways, by a variety of commentators. 'Since people of all political persuasions have a need for a word that makes their constituents feel that they are or are about to become more in control of their destinies, *empower* has been adopted by conservatives as well as social reformers. It has even migrated out of the political arena into other fields' (Free Dictionary, nd). In health promotion (see chapter 7) it is taken to mean the process by which people are able to identify their needs and then take action in order to meet them.

environment

The environment is the area, conditions, and circumstances that surround individual people. 'The environment influences our health in many ways – through exposures to physical, chemical and biological risk factors, and through related changes in our behaviour in response to those factors. Thirteen million deaths annually are due to preventable environmental causes. Preventing environmental risk could save as many as four million lives a year, in children alone, mostly in developing countries' (WHO, 2009).

epidemic

This is 'an outbreak of a contagious disease that spreads rapidly and widely' (Free Dictionary, nd). Historically there have been several well-documented epidemics such as the plague, various flu epidemics, Ebola, and SARs, to give a few examples.

epistemology

Saks and Allsop (2007: 410) describe epistemology as 'the nature of knowledge or how we come to know certain things about the world'. Epistemology is important in research because it informs choice of research methods; researchers draw upon different epistemologies as the social world can be understood in a variety of ways, and this leads to the production of different forms of knowledge. So there are different epistemological views of how to research health and what knowledge is important in adding to understandings about health.

equity
This is about fairness and justice. It means 'The state, quality, or ideal of being just, impartial, and fair' (Free Dictionary, nd). To achieve equity does not necessarily mean that individuals have to be treated in the same way; indeed it may mean tailoring specific services to those who are most in need (see chapter 11 for further discussion of policy approaches that have operated in such a way).

ethnography
This is a research approach firmly embedded in the qualitative tradition. It has been developed by anthropologists to study culture and specific cultural groups. Moule and Goodwin (2009: 388), describe ethnography as the observation of 'behaviour, customs, rituals, interactions and practices'. Ethnographic health-related research has demonstrated interesting belief systems about health and illness and added to understandings about the provision of health care.

evidence-based practice
'Evidence-based practice' (EBP) is an approach that tries to specify the way in which professionals or other decision-makers should make decisions by identifying such evidence that there may be for a practice and rating it according to how scientifically sound it may be. Its goal is to eliminate unsound or excessively risky practices in favour of those that have better outcomes' (Free Dictionary, nd). There is further discussion of evidence and evidence-based practice in chapter 3.

experiment
Bowling (2009: 464) describes experiments as 'a scientific method used to establish cause and effect relationships between the independent and dependent variable . . . the true experimental method involves the random allocation of participants to experimental and control groups. Ideally participants are assessed before and after the manipulation of the independent variable in order to measure its effects upon the dependent variable.' Put simply this is a scientific method for testing a hypothesis.

factors
A factor is simply an influence, and there are many influences upon our health as this book demonstrates. Factors that can influence our health both positively and negatively include social factors and structural factors (see chapter 4), psychological factors (see chapter 6), environmental factors (see chapter 10), political and economic factors (see chapter 11) and cultural factors (see chapter 5).

gender

Gender is different from biological sex as it does not describe the physical attributes associated with men and women, rather it refers to 'social expectations about behaviour regarded as appropriate for members of the opposite sex' (Giddens, 2009: 1119). Gender is important in relation to differential health behaviours, understandings of health and health outcomes.

global governance

This is the process by which rules and frameworks are developed in order to tackle global problems. Global governance is implemented by a number of different and diverse organizations including governments. Global health governance has been defined as 'the collective forms of governance, from the sub-national to the global level, which addresses health issues with global dimensions' (Lee & Goodman, 2002: 115).

globalization

Giddens (2009: 126) defines globalization as 'the fact that we all increasingly live in one world, so that individuals, groups and nations become ever more dependent'. It is about the changing nature of relationships across different countries and the world. Globalization is related to health threats (see chapter 2), health inequalities and global health governance (see chapter 12).

health beliefs

These are the opinions and viewpoints of people in relation to actions and behaviours that may or may not affect health. For example, people may believe that smoking is bad for health whereas others believe that eating bread is fattening. These are related to lay beliefs (see chapters 1 and 5) and are not necessarily based upon research and evidence.

health indicator

This is a characteristic that is used to describe a particular aspect of the population's health, for example, life expectancy, disease prevalence rates and disability adjusted life years (DALYs).

health inequality

This is where the health status and health experience of different groups and sub-populations is unequal i.e. not the same. 'Health inequalities can be defined as differences in health status or in the distribution of health determinants between different population groups' (WHO, 2011).

health inequity

This is similar to health inequality, although a moral judgement is made about whether the differences are deemed to be unfair. For example many people would argue that the inequality where higher social classes have better health than lower social classes is not fair, therefore making it a health inequity.

healthy public policy

'Healthy public policy is characterized by an explicit concern for *health* and equity in all areas of policy, and by accountability for health impact. The main aim of healthy public policy is to create a *supportive environment* to enable people to lead healthy lives. Such a policy makes healthy choices possible or easier for citizens. It makes social and physical environments health enhancing' (Nutbeam, 1998: 13).

holistic

This term comes from the word 'whole'. As applied to health it means thinking about health in terms of the whole person and also encompasses a range of dimensions in health including physical, mental, social and emotional health.

HPV

This is the human papillomavirus that is an infectious virus causing skin problems and warts. This virus can lead to cancer of the cervix when it is transmitted sexually. In 2008, the UK government introduced a vaccination for young girls to help prevent them from contracting the virus and developing cancer of the cervix (see the detailed case study in chapter 13).

humanism

Humanists believe in human values and concerns, suggesting that the world can be understood through reason, shared experience and values without the need for religious interpretations and beliefs. Humanism has been used to explore experiences of health and to make arguments for health care reform. 'The medical humanism movement seeks to understand the patient as a person, focusing on individual values, goals, and preferences with respect to clinical decisions' (Hartzband & Groopman, 2009: 554).

hypothesis

A hypothesis is a tool used as part of the research process. It is the expression of a solution to a research question, which is then tested. It is a statement about what should happen 'expressed in the form of a prediction about the relationship between the dependent and independent variables' (Bowling, 2009: 465). An example of a health-related hypothesis that has been tested via the research process is the foetal origins hypothesis. This hypothesis suggests that the risk of adult morbidity and mortality is heightened by retardation in development, specifically within the womb. However, Christensen et al. (1995) found that this hypothesis is false through their research with identical twins.

identity

An individual identity refers to the specific characteristics of a person. Our individual identities are characterized by our gender, ethnicity, nationality, age and social class. Similarly, a group identity refers to the distinctive characteristics of a group. Identity can be affected by health in a number of ways.

ideology

An ideology is a particular school of thought or a shared set of beliefs or ideas. Ideologies exist in every society in the world. 'The concept of ideology has a close connection with that of power, since ideological systems serve to legitimize the differential power held by groups' (Giddens, 2009: 1121). Power and ideology are important in examining health because of the existence of widespread health inequalities.

incidence

This simply refers to the number of newly diagnosed cases during a specific time-frame. In health incidence rates of diseases are often reported to monitor changing patterns of disease and to monitor new threats (see chapter 2 for more about contemporary threats to health).

interdisciplinary

This refers to the way in which different disciplines are related and can be used together to analyse a specific issue. 'Interdisciplinarity involves researchers, students, and teachers in the goals of connecting and integrating several academic schools of thought, professions, or technologies – along with their specific perspectives – in the pursuit of a common task' (Free Dictionary, nd). Health studies adopts this approach by drawing upon numerous disciplines (see part II of the book) to analyse health.

interpretivism

This is a perspective associated with qualitative research; it is a 'theoretical perspective used to describe the lived experiences of individuals from their own viewpoints and to understand how people make sense of ("interpret") their experiences' (Kalof, Dan & Dietz 2008: 200). There has been much health-related research about people's experiences and understandings, for example, studies on lay interpretations of health and illness.

justice

This is about the application of fairness and the upholding of certain standards, for example in relation to the law. Justice comes in a variety of forms 'resource allocation (distributive justice), meeting natural rights (rights-based justice) and the law (legal justice)' (Naidoo & Wills, 2008: 377).

lay health beliefs

These are the non-professional beliefs, interpretations and under-standings about illness causation. They may contradict biomedical understandings and explanations but nevertheless co-exist alongside them (see chapters 1 and 5).

lifespan

Lifespan is 'the maximum length of life that is biologically possible for a member of any given species' (Giddens, 2009: 1124). The lifespan is important in relation to health because individuals experience a range of health issues at various points during their lifespan.

lifestyle

This describes a certain way of living based upon specific patterns of behaviour. So to adopt a healthy lifestyle an individual usually exercises, eats healthily, does not smoke and would only consume alcohol in moderate quantities. Lifestyles are assumed to be a matter of choice but may be influenced by other health determinants as this book outlines.

literature

This is the printed material forming a body of knowledge, discussion, debate and critique within all academic fields. Literature is found in aca-demic textbooks and journals, within different disciplines. For example, the *Journal of Health Education Research* publishes articles about health education and health promotion from across the world. This literature is often based upon empirical research and has been through a peer review process, in which other experts in the field review it; hence, it is consid-ered to be of high quality and to be offering new insights into the field.

macro-level

This level of analysis focuses upon higher levels of societal organiza-tion such as policy-makers (see chapter 11) and the economic context of a society. In relation to health, health care policy analysis is explor-ing what is happening at the macro-level.

mainstream

This can be defined as the dominant contemporary thought of most people within a given society at any time. For example, there are main-stream ideas about the causes of obesity reported in the media, often blaming individuals for eating too much and not exercising enough without any recognition of the broader structural and economic factors influencing individual behaviours. There are also mainstream aca-demic views within specific fields.

medicalization

This is 'the process of increased medical intervention and control in areas that hitherto would have been outside of the medical domain'

(Bilton et al., 1996: 664). Medicalization therefore refers to the increased involvement of the medical profession within aspects of social life previously not of interest or concern within the medical sphere.

meso-level
The meso-level falls between the micro and the macro-level; it is the middle layer. It refers to social actors such as local and regional governments, non-governmental organizations such as charities and private sector organizations. In terms of health, those working at the meso-level include health care and community organizations.

methodology
Methodology 'relates to the broader principles and philosophies governing research' (Saks & Allsop 2007: 412). Methodologies are therefore different approaches to research developed within a particular paradigm. Hence, quantitative and qualitative methodologies are different, leading to a variety of ways in which health data can be gathered.

methods
In research, methods describes the process of collecting and analysing data using tools such as interviews, focus groups, observations and the thematic analysis of the data.

micro-level
The micro-level refers to the very lowest level of society, which means individual components i.e. people. Interactionist theorists (see chapter 4) are concerned with examining patient interactions at the micro-level.

MMR
This is a single vaccination against three infectious diseases, measles, mumps and rubella. It protects against these three diseases, which have low incidence rates now in the UK.

model
A model is a representation of a system or a structure often used in academic terms to try to explain and understand the social world. For example, there are a number of models underpinning the discipline of health promotion (see chapter 7), and several models have been developed that try to explain health-related behaviour change (see chapter 6).

morbidity
This terms refers to 'the proportion of ill people in a population' (Kaufman 2009: 296). Generally, the term refers to the existence of a disease or health condition. Morbidity rates are officially recorded

by many governments and demonstrate the prevalence of certain conditions. Morbidity rates can also be used as a tool to compare the prevalence of diseases among different groups within populations and so contribute to the evidence base about the existence of health inequalities.

mortality

This terms refers to 'the proportion of people in a population who die' (Kaufman, 2009: 296). Mortality rates are calculated for different populations such as children, and mothers giving birth as well as broader populations such as entire countries. Mortality rates across the world are used to compare leading causes of death in different countries.

multi-disciplinary

This describes the study of a subject that applies the methods and approaches of several disciplines. It is a term also applied when professionals from different backgrounds come to work together to resolve a particular problem. Chapter 13 demonstrates the value of a multi-disciplinary approach in relation to malaria, cervical cancer and neighbourhoods as a setting.

nature

This is a term used to describe the characteristics of specific phenomena as well as those of individuals. For example, the nature of good mental health can be described through listing specific characteristics recognizable in those who experience positive mental health such as the ability to deal with stress. Similarly, within the discipline of psychology, personality theory suggests that individuals have different natures and that this can help to explain why people behave in a variety of ways.

non-communicable

This term refers to diseases that are not infectious and therefore cannot be transmitted across populations. An example of a well-known non-communicable disease is heart disease. There are many other examples of non-communicable diseases that are a problem for population health, including cancer, asthma and diabetes.

neo-liberialism

This is a form of philosophy associated with right-wing schools of thought. Giddens (2009: 1126) defines it as 'the economic belief that free market forces, achieved by minimizing government restrictions on business, provide the only route to economic growth'. Neo-liberal approaches to health care assume that health services can be run in accordance with business principles, and as such support the private provision of care. Critics argue that this enhances health inequalities.

new social movements

This term is used to characterize groups of people such as feminists, student movements and environmental campaigners who come together politically to express their shared interests in relation to certain issues. They are defined as new in the sense that they differ from earlier movements in the 1960s. In relation to health, social movements are an important political force made up of different organizations, supporters and networks. Health Social movements 'make many challenges to political power, professional authority and personal and collective identity' (Brown & Zavestoki, 2005: 1).

objective

An objective can be a goal or a target set for individuals to achieve, for example people often set several health-related objectives, aiming to eat more fruit and vegetables, to lose weight, to exercise more and to drink less alcohol. Objectives can also be set on a much larger scale than the individual level, for example policy targets are objectives that countries aim to meet. The Millennium Development Goals are global objectives that are to be met by 2015 (see chapter 12 for more detailed discussion).

objectivity

This is a term commonly associated with research and is 'an approach to knowledge acquisition that claims to be unbiased, impersonal and free from prejudice' Bilton et al., 1996: 665). This approach is associated with the positivist school of thought.

ontology

Ontology is the study of being or existence. It is the study of reality and is simply described as 'a theory of what exists' (Kalof, Dan & Dietz 2008: 202). Ontology is about the nature of knowable things.

operationalization

This term refers to the 'development of proxy measures that enable phenomena to be observed empirically (i.e. measured)' (Bowling, 2009: 466). For example, if a researcher was measuring positive mental health then they would have to operationalize the concept of positive mental health in order to measure it effectively. Hence, proxy measures need to identified or indeed developed. These may include positive emotions, engagement and purpose, which are all indicators of mental health (Seligman, 2008).

pandemic

A pandemic is an epidemic of disease that is spread through populations of people across countries and indeed the world. Historically there are many examples of pandemics, such as smallpox.

paradigm

A paradigm refers to a body of knowledge or understanding about an issue. In relation to health, an example is the scientific paradigm, which greatly influences medical understandings of health.

pathology

Pathology is simply the study and diagnosis of disease. Pathologists diagnose disease through laboratory methods. These diagnoses lead to the selection of appropriate treatment for patients. Pathogenic thus relates to the presence of disease caused by a pathogen (a virus or bacteria).

perspectives

A perspective is a viewpoint or an opinion. For example, there are cultural perspectives about health (see chapter 5), international perspectives about health (see chapter 12) and contested perspectives and understandings in relation to health (see chapter 1).

philosophy

Philosophy is the seeking of wisdom and knowledge as well as the explanation of reality. The question of what is health as explored in chapter 1 is a central philosophical debate of major importance in the contemporary literature. There are also many philosophies associated with seeking and achieving good health; for example, Buddhism focuses upon meditating as a process to develop and achieve good mental health and well-being.

policy sectors

Policy sectors are simply organizational structures dealing with particular areas of the social world that require social policy. Policy sectors include education, transport and health. These sectors all have institutions to help to develop and implement policy and they are made up of institutions that also have their own rules, customs and internal hierarchies. Health is influenced and affected by a number of policy sectors; for example, transport policy can affect our health and so can welfare policy.

political economy

Political economy perspectives are explanations that 'embrace concepts of social class, the value and division of labour, and moral sentiments' (Bilton et al., 1996: 666). Political economy is often a term associated with Marxist theorists (see chapter 4) who try to explain the social world by analysing the economic system upon which the world is based. Others too are concerned with the importance of the complex dynamics driving the world economy. Political economy of health perspectives so too analyse economics and politics as forces determining and shaping health and health care.

positivism

This is an approach to research based upon quantitative methods. 'A positivist assumes that reality is concrete and **objectivity** is achievable; the researcher can collect and interpret social facts objectively; and can produce laws and models of behaviour from social facts to predict future outcomes' (Saks & Allsop 2007: 414). Positivist approaches to health research have been used to map out disease characteristics, the prognosis of diseases and the range of factors that can influence health outcomes.

post structuralism

This is a theoretical approach in which the idea of a universal truth is not accepted. Post structuralist theorists therefore argue that 'plural interpretations of reality are inevitable' (Giddens 2009: 1128). Such theorists also argue that discourse has the power to shape reality. The work of Michel Foucault has been particularly popular within the sociological literature and is relevant to health because it includes an analysis of madness.

prevalence

This simply means 'the total number of cases of a disease in a given population at a specific time' (Free Dictionary, nd). So the prevalence of chronic disease is growing across high-income countries as a result of lifestyle changes (see chapter 2).

primary health care

This is health care located within communities, so that it is accessible and broad and includes the services of doctors and nurses as well as those of non-medical professionals.

private sector

'The private sector is that part of the economy run by private individuals or groups, usually as a means of enterprise for profit, and is not controlled by the state' (Free Dictionary, nd). The private sector includes businesses such as the pharmaceutical industry, which are important in relation to health (see chapter 12).

privatization

This refers to the process by which the ownership of business and enterprise is moved from the public sector to the private sector. 'In a broader sense, privatization refers to the transfer of any government function to the private sector – including governmental functions like revenue collection and law enforcement' (Free Dictionary, nd). The UK NHS has privatized some of its services over a lengthy period of time, for example, cleaning of hospitals is now conducted by staff from private firms.

psychological

The word psychological generally refers to the mind and mental health. Thus psychological knowledge is applied to the diagnosis and treatment of mental illness. Psychological health can also be defined and measured, for example Michie and Williams (2002) identified several key factors at work that can lead to psychological ill-health, such as long hours, pressure and lack of control at work.

public sector

'The Public Sector, sometimes referred to as the state sector, is a part of the state that deals with either the production, delivery and allocation of goods and services by and for the government or its citizens' (Free Dictionary, nd). The UK NHS is a public sector organization that for many commentators is increasingly becoming privatized.

qualitative research

There are a number of different approaches to qualitative research but in general qualitative research uses techniques to collect, analyse and interpret data based upon words and text. Mason (1996: 4) identifies a loose working definition of qualitative research as 'grounded in a philosophical position which is broadly interpretivist . . . based on methods of data generation which are flexible and sensitive to the social context in which data are produced . . . based on methods of analysis and explanation building which involve understandings of complexity, detail and context'. Qualitative health research includes the use of interviews, observations and documentary analysis methods.

quality of life

The term quality of life is used to evaluate the general well-being of individuals and is a ways of describing an individual's emotional, social and physical well-being as well as their ability to function within different contexts. The World Health Organization Quality of Life (WHOQOL) project led to the development of an international cross-culturally comparable quality of life assessment instrument (WHO, 2009). Quality of life can be measured specifically in relation to illness experiences. Specific conditions such as asthma and cancer affect an individual's quality of life in different ways.

quantitative research

This is an approach to research involving designs and data collection techniques to create numerical data, which can then be analysed via the application of statistical methods. Kalof, Dan, and Dietz (2008: 204) define quantitative research as 'methods used to understand variation in things, test causal relationships, and identify the prevalence or distribution of phenomena; also the use of statistical tools to interpret data'. Quantitative approaches to health research can include a broad range of tools including randomized control trials and social surveys.

randomized control trial

This is an experimental study in which people are selected either to receive an intervention or not. 'A randomized controlled trial (RCT) is a type of scientific experiment most commonly used in testing the efficacy or effectiveness of health care services (such as medicine or nursing) or health technologies (such as pharmaceuticals, medical devices or surgery). The key distinguishing feature of the usual RCT is that study subjects, after assessment of eligibility and recruitment, but before the intervention to be studied begins, are randomly allocated to receive one or other of the alternative treatments under study' (Free Dictionary).

rationing

This is about ensuring that excess demands are managed. It is also called prioritization, which is ultimately about putting things in order. Examples of rationing in health care include waiting lists, not pre-scribing expensive medications (or making them available to a limited population) and rationing treatments.

reductionist

This term refers to the tendency to try to explain a complex set of facts in a simplistic manner, hence reducing the explanation to something far too simple to account for the level of complexity. Biomedical approaches to the treatment of illness have often been described as reductionist as they aim to treat the problem in isolation rather than viewing the disease as affecting the whole of an individual.

relativism

This is a theoretical position suggesting that 'conceptions of truth and moral values are not absolute but are relative to the persons or groups holding them' (Free Dictionary, nd). So health beliefs can be relative in relation to their cultural context (see chapter 5)

research

Research is a complex process and so defining it is not an easy task. Bowling (2009: 1) describes research as 'the systematic and rigorous process of enquiry which aims to describe phenomena and to develop and test explanatory concepts and theories. Ultimately it aims to contribute to a scientific body of knowledge.' Research is a tool used in many different disciplines and in relation to health studies it is often concerned with improving health.

resilience

Resilience is the strength and capacity of people to cope with problems and so is an important aspect of our mental health. Neeman (2009) argues that although resilience is an elusive concept it is useful as it provides answers to why some people crumble in the face of tough times, while others do not.

risk factors

These are the factors that make an individual or population susceptible to disease and illness. These can be related to the environment (see chapter 10), lifestyle (see chapter 2) or social position (see chapters 4 and 12).

salutogenesis

Aaron Antonovsky first emphasized salutogenic approaches to health. Salutogenesis is 'understanding the origins (genesis) of health (salus) not illness'. He produced a theory to explain why some people can stay well even though they are exposed to factors of stress. The key element in the salutogenic theory is the 'sense of coherence' (SOC). This capacity for maintaining your sense of coherence can be achieved when you can assess and understand the situation you are in, when you think that your life has meaning and that you have the resources available to meet the demands of life (Lindstrom & Eriksson, 2005).

sampling

'A sample is a selection of elements (members or units) from a population' (Blaikie 2000: 198). Sampling is therefore the process of selecting participants for inclusion within the research process, using a specific technique. There are a number of approaches to sampling that can be used within health research, discussed in depth within chapter 2.

screening

This is the process when tests are used to detect illnesses. There can be blood tests to detect malaria or x-rays and scans to detect certain types of cancer. Screening is used to detect cervical cancer (discussed in chapter 13).

self-esteem

Essentially, self-esteem is about how we value ourselves and is linked with ideas about self-worth (and our self-concept – ideas about ourselves). It is to do with how much value people place on themselves (Baumeister et al., 2003). Self-esteem is strongly related to health and well-being, particularly mental health.

semantics

Semantics is the study of meaning and usually refers to the way in which words are used through language to express meaning. Understanding semantics (meanings) is important when studying health because language exists in social contexts and so different meanings and interpretations inform us about perceptions and experiences of health.

sex

Is a term used to describe the physical anatomical differences between men and women. Our physical differences relate to health in a number of ways. For example, women's anatomical differences mean that they can give birth to children, which has a number of health-related impacts.

social

The social world is an organized community in which we all live, within structures such as communities and families. There is a large amount of evidence to show that how we socially live and interact is important in relation to our health because many determinants of health are social (see chapter 4 and chapter 9).

social capital

This is a concept defined in a number of ways but essentially refers to the types of networks and trust that exist within a community and levels of community cohesion. These networks and levels of trust have been shown to be important as a health determinant (see chapter 9, which discusses this concept in depth).

social class

This is the ranking of groups according to their occupation; those with manual jobs are lower down the scale than those with professional occupations. Such a system of classification only occurred recently through the advent of capitalism. Social class is also related to status and power as well as the amount of money that people earn.

social constructionism

This is a school of thought believing that social reality is created through the interactions of people. Giddens (2009: 1132) highlights how social constructionists '. . . see social reality as the creation of the interaction of individuals and groups'. Health and illness from this perspective are seen as socially constructed with individuals' perceptions about their experiences forming a crucial aspect of the construction process.

social inequalities

These are the inequalities in income, resources, power and status that are important in relation to health. Such inequalities are maintained by those in powerful positions via institutions and social processes (Naidoo & Wills, 2008). They are discussed extensively throughout this book.

social marketing

This is a specific approach that attempts to produce behaviour change at an individual level. It involves the application of marketing with other techniques to achieve goals that are seen as socially good. It was popular in UK health policy under the last Labour government (see chapter 11 for more discussion).

stigma

Stigma refers to a negative labelling process on a societal level whereby individuals with certain characteristics are demeaned. Individuals become stigmatized via 'a process or experience in which some form of social behaviour or attribute is subject to social disapproval and becomes discredited, resulting in a spoiled identity in the eyes of others and possible exclusion from normal social interaction' (Bilton et al., 1996: 670). Certain health problems and medical conditions such as cancer and HIV arguably stigmatize sufferers.

subjective

A subjective perspective is one arising from a personal interpretation rather than any evidentiary basis. As patients, we all experience illness and health care subjectively. Subjective reporting of health and illness experiences are represented within lay perspectives (see chapter 1) and within discussions of illness narratives (see chapter 5).

subjectivity

This is another term commonly associated with research and the interpretivist paradigm underpinning qualitative research. It is an approach to gaining knowledge and data that enables the researcher to analyse the subjective meanings and interpretations of those being researched, to explore the social and culturally embedded nature of individual experiences and to examine the relationship between those being researched and those carrying out the research (Rubin & Rubin, 2005).

theory

A theory is an idea which explains a phenomenon within the social world. Researchers test theories especially when adopting quantitative approaches. Thus, theories are 'an idea about how some parts of the social world work, often taking the form of causal statements. A theory must be testable and falsifiable to be considered scientific' (Kalof, Dan & Dietz 2008: 208). Theorizing about health and health-related issues is important for understanding health and for also developing guides for action.

triangulation

Triangulation is the process of combining a number of different research methods in order to address research questions. Kalof, Dan and Dietz (2008: 208) describe it as 'a multi-faceted approach to studying a topic. Triangulation can involve the use of multiple data sources, multiple theories and/or multiple methods to provide a more well-rounded understanding of a topic.'

typology

A typology is a system of classification in which 'types' or 'attributes' are put into categories based upon their similarities and differences.

For example, there are typologies of health care system financing across the world. Some are publicly funded and some are privately funded, hence these different approaches to funding can be used to classify countries' finance approaches within an overall funding typology. The British NHS would fit into the public funded section of the typology.

universalism
This means that something is applicable in all cases. One of the founding principles of the British NHS is that it is universal, meaning that as a health care system it does not exclude anyone from using its service irrespective of their social position and ability to pay.

values
Traditionally defined as something of value, but defining value is more complex than this. Naidoo and Wills (2008: 382) demonstrate this in saying 'value may be subjective (something is valued simply because it is wanted), instrumental (something is valued because it has a useful function) or intrinsic (something is valued because it has fundamental and irreducible importance)'. Values are referred to in various chapters of this book because they underpin our notions of the importance of health and health care approaches.

variable
A variable is 'a measured/observed item or characteristic' (Kalof, Dan & Dietz, 2008: 209); for example, a person's gender or their ethnicity. Variables are important within research as they are 'an indicator assumed to represent the underlying construct or concept' (Bowling 2009: 470).

well-being
The concept of well-being in relation to health is recognizing that there is more to health than simply the absence of disease. Well-being is an important component of mental health as it is a positive dimension. According to the WHO (2009) 'Mental health is defined as a state of well-being in which every individual realizes his or her own potential, can cope with the normal stresses of life, can work productively and fruitfully, and is able to make a contribution to her or his community.'

References

Abbasi, K. (1999) The World Bank and world health: Changing sides. *British Medical Journal* 318, 865–9.

Abraham, C. & Sheeran, P. (2005) The health belief model. In Conner, M. & Norman, P., eds, *Predicting Health Behaviours*. 2nd edn. Buckingham, Open University Press. pp. 28–80.

Abraham, C., Conner, M., Jones, F. & O'Connor, D. (2008) *Health Psychology*. London, Hodder Education.

Accoron, A. & Watson, R. (2006) Burning is too good for them: Sex, retribution and 'others'. *Lesbian & Gay Psychology Review* 7 (3), 257–63.

Acheson, D. (1998) *Independent Inquiry into Inequalities in Health Report*. London, Stationery Office.

Ackroyd, S. & Hughes, J. (1992) *Data Collection in Context*. Longman, London & New York.

Acton, G.J. & Malathum, P. (2008) Basic need status and health-promoting self-care behavior in adults. *Western Journal of Nursing Research* 22, 796–811.

Aggleton, P. (1990) *Health*. London, Routledge.

Aginam, O. (2005) *Global Health Governance*. Toronto, University of Toronto Press.

Aidoo, M. & Harpham, T. (2001) The explanatory models of mental health among low-income women and health care practitioners in Lusaka, Zambia. *Health Policy and Planning* 16 (2), 206–13.

Airhihenbuwa, C.O. & Obregon, R. (2000) A critical assessment of theories/models used in health communication for HIV/AIDS. *Journal of Health Communication* 5 (Supplement), 5–15.

Albery, I.P. & Munafò, M. (2008) *Key Concepts in Health Psychology*. London, Sage Publications.

Albrecht, G.L. & Devlieger, P.J. (1999) The disability paradox: High quality of life against all odds. *Social Science and Medicine* 48, 977–88.

Angell, M. (1997) The ethics of clinical research in the third world. *New England Journal of Medicine* 337 (12), 847–9.

Antonovksy, A. (1996) The salutogenic model as a theory to guide health promotion. *Health Promotion International* 11 (1), 11–18.

Aphramor, L. & Gingras, J. (2008) Sustaining imbalance – evidence of neglect in the pursuit of nutritional health. In Riley, S., Burns, M., Frith, S., Wiggins, S. & Markula, P., eds, *Critical Bodies*. New York, Palgrave Macmillan. pp. 155–74.

Appleby, J. & Phillips, M. (2009) The NHS: Satisfied now? In Park, A., Curtice, J., Thomson, K., Phillips, M. & Clery, E., eds, *British Social Attitudes. The 25th Report*. National Centre for Social Research, London, Sage. pp. 25–51.

Armstrong Schellenberg, J.R.M., Abdulla, S., Nathan, R. et al. (2001) Effect of large-scale social marketing of insecticide-treated nets on child survival in rural Tanzania. *Lancet* 357, 1241–7.

Aronsson, G., Gustafsson, K. & Dallner, M. (2002) Work environment and health in different types of temporary jobs. *European Journal of Work and Organisational Psychology* 11 (2), 151–75.

Artazcoz, L., Benach, J., Borrell, C. & Cortès, I. (2004) Unemployment and mental health: Understanding the interactions among gender, family roles, and social class. *Journal of American Public Health* 9 (1), 81–8.

Backett. K. (1982) Taboos and excesses: Lay health moralities in middle class families. *Sociology of Health and Illness* 14 (2), 255–73.

Backett. K. & Davidson, C. (1992) Rational or reasonable? Perceptions of health at different stages of life. *Health Education Journal* 51, 55–9.

Barnoya, J. & Glantz, S.A. (2005) Cardiovascular effects of secondhand smoke. Special report. *Circulation* 111, 2684–98.

Barton, H. & Grant, M. (2006a) A health map for the local human habitat. *Journal of the Royal Society for the Promotion of Health* 126 (6), 252–61.

Barton, H. & Grant, M. (2006b) *The Determinants of Health and Well-Being In our Neighbourhoods*. The Health Impacts of the Built Environment, Institute of Public Health in Ireland.

Bauman, Z. & May, T. (2001) *Thinking Sociologically*. 2nd edn. Malden, Blackwell.

Baumeister, R.F., Campbell, J.D., Krueger, J.I. & Vohns, K.D. (2003) Does high self-esteem cause better performance, interpersonal success, happiness or healthier lifestyles? *Psychological Science in the Public Interest* 4 (1), 1–4.

BBC News (2005) Pubs in new 24-hour opening era. BBC News, 24 November 2005 [Internet] Available at: http://news.bbc.co.uk/1/hi/uk/4464284.stm [Accessed 20 October 2010].

BBC News (2010) Spending Review at a Glance. BBC News, 20 October 2010 [Internet] Available at: http://www.bbc.co.uk/news/uk-politics-11591881 [Accessed 21 October 2010].

Beattie, A. (1991) Knowledge and control in health promotion: A test case for social policy and social theory. In Gabe, J., Calnan, M. & Bury, M., eds, *The Sociology of the Health Service*. London, Routledge. Cited in Naidoo, J. & Wills, J. (2000) *Health Promotion: Foundations for Practice*. 2nd edn. Edinburgh, Bailliere Tindall.

Bebbington, P. (1996) The origins of sex differences in depressive disorder: Bridging the gap. *International Review of Psychiatry* 8, 295–332.

Beck, U. (1992) *The Risk Society: Towards a New Modernity*. Sage, London.

Beigbeder, Y. (2004) *International Public Health: Patient Rights vs. the Protection of Patients*. Aldershot, Ashgate.

Bellingham-Young, D.A. & Adamson-Macedo, E.N. (2003) Foetal origins theory: Links with adult depression and general self-efficacy. *Neuroendocrinology Letters* 6 (24), 412–17.

Bennett, P. & Murphy, S. (1997) *Psychology and Health Promotion*. Buckingham, Open University Press.

Benson, J. & Thistlethwaite, J. (2008) *Mental Health across Cultures: A Practical Guide for Health Professionals*. Oxford, Radcliffe.

Berger, P. & Luckman, T. (1967) *The Social Construction of Reality*. London, Penguin.

Berkman, L.F., Leo-Summers, L. & Horwitz, R.I. (1992) Emotional support and survival after myorcardial infarction: A prospective, population-based study of the elderly. *Annals of International Medicine* 117, 1003–9.

Berkman, L.F. & Syme, S.L. (1979) Social networks, host resistance, and mortality: A nine-year follow-up study of Alameda county residents. *American Journal of Epidemiology* 109, 186–204.

Berkman, L.F., Glass, T., Brissette, I. & Seeman, T.E. (2000) For social integration to health: Durkeim in the new millennium. *Social Science and Medicine* 51 (3), 843–57.

Berry, D. (2007) *Health Communication: Theory and Practice*. Maidenhead, Open University Press.

Bettcher, D. & Lee, K. (2002) Globalisation and public health. *Journal of Epidemiology and Public Health* 56, 8–17.

Beveridge, W.H.B. (1942) *Social Insurance and Allied Services. The Beveridge Report*. London, HMSO.

Bhopal, R. (2008) *Concepts of Epidemiology: Integrating the Ideas, Theories, Principles and Methods of Epidemiology*. 2nd edn. Oxford, Oxford University Press.

Biddle, L., Brode, A., Brookes, S.T. & Gunnel, D. (2008) Suicide rates in young men in England and Wales in the 21st century: Time trend study. *British Medical Journal* 336, 539–42.

Bilton, T., Bonnett, K., Jones, P., Skinner, D., Stanworth, M. & Webster, A. (1996) *Introduction to Sociology*. 3rd edn. Basingstoke, Macmillan Press.

Blaikie, N. (2000) *Designing Social Research*. Cambridge. Polity.

Blakemore, K. & Griggs, E. (2007) *Social Policy: An Introduction*. Maidenhead, Open University Press.

Blaxter, M. (1990) *Health and Lifestyles*. London, Routledge.

Blaxter, M. (2004) *Health*. Cambridge, Polity.

Blaxter, M. (2007) How is health experienced? In Douglas, J., Earle, S., Handsley, S., Lloyd, C.E. & Spurr, S., eds, *A Reader in Promoting Public Health*. London, Sage Publications. pp. 26–32.

Blaxter, M. & Paterson, L. (1982) *Mothers and Daughters: A Three Generation Study of Health Attitudes and Behaviours*. London, Heinemann.

Bleich, A., Gelkopf, M. & Soloman, Z. (2003) Exposure to terrorism, stress-related mental health symptoms, and coping behaviors among a nationally representative sample in Israel. *Journal of American Medical Association* 290 (5), 612–20.

Bloom, D.E. & Canning, D. (2001) The health and wealth of nations. *Science 2000* 287, 1207–8.

Blouin, C. (2007) Can the World Trade Organisation help achieve the health millennium development goals? In Cooper, A.F., Kirton, J.J. & Schrecker, T., eds, *Governing Global Health: Challenge, Response, Innovation*. Aldershot, Ashgate. pp. 87–100.

Blumhagen, D. (1980) Hyper-tension: A folk illness with a medical name. *Culture, Medicine and Psychiatry* 4, 197–227.

Borg, V., Kristensen, T.S. & Burr, H. (2000) Work environment and changes in self-related health: A five year follow-up study. *Stress Medicine* 16, 37–47.

Bosch, F.X., Manos, M.M., Munoz, N. et al. (1995) Prevalence of human papillomavirus in cervical cancer: A worldwide perspective. *Journal of the National Cancer Institute* 87 (11), 796–802.

Boseley, S. (2009) *Swine flu pandemic 'less lethal than expected'*. [Internet] Available at: http://www.guardian.co.uk/world/2009/dec/10/swine-flu-pandemic-less-lethal [Accessed 11 December 2010].

Bowling, A. (2009a) *Research Methods in Health: Investigating Health and Health Services*. Maidenhead, McGraw-Hill, Open University Press.

Bowling, A. (2009b) *Measuring Disease: A Review of Disease Specific Quality of Life Measurement Scales*. Buckingham, Open University Press.

Boyden, S. (2004) *The Biology of Civilisation: Understanding Human Culture as a Force in Nature*. Sydney, UNSW Press.

Bradby, H. (2009) *Medical Sociology: An Introduction*. London, Sage.

Bradley, F., Smith, M., Long, J. & O'Dowd, T. (2002) Reported frequency of cross sectional survey of women attending general practice. *British Medical Journal* 324 (7332), 271–5.

Bradshaw, D. (2008) Determinants of health and their trends in South Africa. In Barron, P. & Roma-Reardon, J., eds, *South African Health Review 2008*. Durban, Health Systems Trust. pp. 51–69.

Brannen, J. & Storey, P. (1996) *Child Health in Social Context: Parental Employment and the Start of Secondary School*. HEA, London.

Breakwell, G.M. (2000) Risk communication: Factors affecting impact. *British Medical Bulletin* 56, 110–20.

Brewis, R. & Fitzgerald, J. (2010) *Citizenship in Health. Self-Direction: Theory to Practice In Control Discussion Paper*. West Midlands, In Control Partnerships.

Broom, A. & Willis, E. (2007) Competing paradigms and health research. In Saks, M. & Allsop, J., eds, *Researching Health: Qualitative, Quantitative and Mixed Methods*. London, Sage Publications. pp. 16–31.

Brown, J., Harding, S. & Bethune, A. (1997) Incidence of health of the nation cancers by social class. *Population Trends*. London, Office for National Statistics.

Brown, P. & Zavestoski, S. (2005) Social movements in health: An introduction. In Brown, P. & Zavestoski, S., eds, *Social Movements in Health*. Malden, Blackwell. pp. 1–16.

Brown, T.M., Cueto, M. & Fee, E. (2006) The World Health Organization and the transition from international to global public health. *American Journal of Public Health* 96 (1), 62–72.

Brummett, B. H., Barefoot, J. C., Siegler, I. C. et al. (2001) Characteristics of socially isolated patients with coronary artery disease who are at elevated risk for mortality. *Psychosomatic Medicine* 63, 267–72.

Brundtland, G.H. (2001) Foreword: *The World Health Report 2001 – Mental Health: New Understanding, New Hope. The World Health Report*. Geneva, WHO.

Brundtland, G.H. (2003) Global Health and International Security. *Global Governance* 9, 417–23.

Bryman, A. (2001) *Social Research Methods*. Oxford, Oxford University Press.

Bryman, A. (2004) *Social Research Methods*. 2nd edn. Oxford, Oxford University Press.

Brynin, M. & Scott, J. (1996) *Young People, Health and the Family*. HEA, London.

Buckingham, A. (2009) Doing better, feeling scared: Health statistics and the culture of fear. In Wainwright, D., ed., *A Sociology of Health*. Sage Publications, London. pp. 19–37.

Bukatko, D. & Daehler, M.W. (2001) *Child Development: A Thematic Approach*. 2nd edn. New Jersey, Houlton.

Bungay, H. (2005) Cancer and health policy: The postcode lottery of care. *Social Policy and Administration* 39 (1), 35–48.

Bunton, R. & Macdonald, G. (2002) *Health Promotion: Disciplines, Diversity and Developments*. 2nd edn. London, Routledge.

Bunton, R., Baldwin, S., Flynn, D. & Whitelaw, S. (2000) The 'stages of change' model in health promotion: Science and ideology. *Critical Public Health* 10 (1), 55–70.

Burge, P.S. (2004) Sick building syndrome. *Occupational and Environmental Medicine* 61, 185–90.

Burgess, R.G. (1988) Conversations with a purpose: The ethnographic interview in educational research. In Burgess, R.G., ed., *Studies in Qualitative Methodology: A Research Annual*. Volume 1, London, JAI Press. pp.137–55.

Burgess, A. (2009) Health scares and risk awareness. In Wainwright. D., ed., *A Sociology of Health*. London, Sage Publications. pp. 56–75.

Burns, M. & Gavey, N. (2004) 'Healthy weight' at what cost? 'Bulimia' and a discourse of weight control. *Journal of Health Psychology* 9 (4), 549–65.

Burrows, L. & Wright, J. (2004) The Good Life: New Zealand Children's Perspectives on Health and Self. *Sport, Education and Society* 9 (2), 193–205.

Bury, M.R. (1982) Chronic illness as biographical disruption. *Sociology of Health and Illness* 4 (2), 167–82.

Bury, M.R. (1991) The sociology of chronic illness: A review research and prospects. *Sociology of Health and Illness* 13 (4), 451–68.

Bury, M. (2005) *Health and Illness.* Cambridge, Polity.

Busfield, J. (2000) *Health and Health Care in Modern Britain.* Oxford, Open University Press.

Busfield, J. (2010) A pill for every ill: Explaining the expansion in medicine use. *Social Science & Medicine* 70 (6), 934–41.

Cacioppo, J. & Patrick, W. (2008) *Loneliness: Human Nature and the Need for Social Connection.* New York City, W.W. Norton and Co.

Calnan, M. (1987) *Health and Illness: The Lay Perspective.* London, Tavistock Publications.

Campbell, F. (2006) *Housing and Neighbourhoods.* [Internet] Available at: http://www.idea.gov.uk/idk/core/page.do?pageId=22937822#contents-6 [Accessed 5 January 2011].

Campbell, J.C. (2002) Health consequences of intimate partner violence. *Lancet* 359, 1331–6.

Campbell, C., Williams, B. & Gilgen, D. (2002) Is social capital a useful conceptual tool for exploring community level influences on HIV infection? An exploratory case study from South Africa. *AIDS Care* 14 (1), 41–54.

Canadian Public Health Association (1996) *Action Statement for Health Promotion in Canada.* [Internet] Available at: http://www.cpha.ca/en/programs/policy/action.aspx [Accessed 18 September 2010].

Cancer Research UK (2010) *CancerStats Key Fact: Cervical Cancer.* [Internet] Available at: http://info.cancerresearchuk.org/cancerstats/types/cervix/ > [Accessed 11 January 2011].

Caplan, R. & Holland, R. (1990) Rethinking health education theory. *Health Education Journal* 49 (1), 10–12.

Carpenter, M. (2000) Health for some: Global health and social development since Alma Ata. *Community Development Journal* 35 (4), 336–51.

Carrera, P.M. & Bridges, J.F.P. (2006) Globalization and healthcare: Understanding health and medical tourism. *Expert Review of Pharmacoeconomics and Outcomes Research* 6 (4), 447–54.

Carricaburu, D. & Pierret, J. (1995) From biographical disruption to biographical reinforcement: The case of HIV-positive men. *Sociology of Health and Illness* 17 (1), 65–88.

Case, A., Fertig, A. & Paxson, C. (2005) The lasting impact of childhood health and circumstance. *Journal of Health Economics* 24, 365–89.

Chapman, N., Emerson, S., Gough, J. Mepani, B. & Road, N. (2000) *Views of Health 2000.* Save the Children, London Development Team.

Chartered Institute of Environmental Health (2006) *Taking Action: Tackling Anti-Social Behaviour: A Toolkit for Environmental Health Practitioners.* London, Chartered Institute of Environmental Health.

Child of our time (2010) *Big Personality Test – Episode One*. London, BBC2, June.

Chronin de Chavez, A., Backett-Milburn, K., Parry, O. & Platt, S. (2005) Understanding and researching well-being: Its usage in different disciplines and potential for health research and health promotion. *Health Education Journal* 64 (1), 70–87.

Christensen, K., Vaupel, J.W., Holm, V.N & Yashin, A.I. (1995) Mortality among twins after age 6: Fetal origins hypothesis versus twin method. *British Medical Journal* 310, 432.

Clark, A. (2003) 'It's like an explosion in your life . . .': Lay perspectives on stress and myocardial infarction. *Journal of Clinical Nursing* 12, 544–53.

Clarke, R., Waddell, T.K., Gallagher, J.T. et al. (2008) A postcode lottery still exists for cancer patients with 'exceptional circumstances'. *Clinical Oncology* 20 (10), 771–2.

Cobb, S. (1976) Social support as a moderator of life stress. *Pyschosomatic Medicine* 38, 300–13.

Cole, T.J., Bellizzi, M.C., Flegal, K.M. & Dietz, W.H. (2000) Establishing a standard definition for child overweight and obesity worldwide: International survey. *British Medical Journal* 320, 1240–3.

Commission for the Social Determinants of Health (CSDH) (2008) *Closing the Gap in a Generation: Health Equity through Action on the Social Determinants of Health. Final Report of the Commission on Social Determinants of Health.* Geneva, WHO.

Connell, J. (2006) Medical tourism: Sea, sun, sand and . . . surgery. *Tourism Management* 27 (6), 1093–100.

Conner, M. & Norman, P., eds (2005) *Predicting Health Behaviour*. 2nd edn. Maidenhead, Open University Press.

Cooper, D., Hoffman, M., Carrara, H. et al. (2007) Determinants of sexual activity and its relation to cervical cancer risk among South African Women. *BMC Public Health* 7, 341.

Corin, E. (1995) The cultural frame: Context and meaning in the construction of health. In Amick, B.C., Levine, S., Tarlov, A.R. & Chapman Walsh, D., eds, *Society and Health*. New York, Oxford University Press. pp. 272–304.

Courtenay, W.H. (2000) Behavioural factors associated with disease, injury and death among men: Evidence and implications for prevention. *Journal of Men's Studies* 9, 81–142.

Courtney, K.E. & Polich, J. (2009) Binge drinking in young adults: Data, definitions and determinants. *Psychological Bulletin* 135 (1), 142–56.

Cox, C.R., Cooper, D.P., Vess, M., Arndt, J., Goldenberg, J.L. & Routledge, C. (2009) Bronze is beautiful but pale can be pretty: The effects of appearance standards and mortality salience on sun-tanning outcomes. *Health Psychology* 28 (6), 746–52.

Craswell, G. (2005) *Writing for Academic Success. A Postgraduate Guide.* London, Sage.

Cribb, A. & Duncan, P. (2002) Introducing ethics in health promotion. In Bunton, R. & McDonald, G., eds, *Health Promotion: Disciples and Diversity*. 2nd edn. London, Routledge. pp. 271–83.

Crinson, I. (2009) *Health Policy: A Critical Perspective*. London, Sage.

Cross, R., Milnes, K., Rickett, B. & Fylan, F. (2010) *Risking a Stigmatised Identity: A Discourse Analysis of Young Women's Talk about Health and Risk*. BPS Qualitative Methods in Psychology Section Conference, Nottingham University. 23/25 July.

Crossley, M. (2003) 'Would you consider yourself a healthy person?': Using focus groups to explore health as a moral phenomenon. *Journal of Health Psychology* 8, 501–14.

Crowther, A. (2008) When good times turn bad. *Health Service Journal*, 4 December 2008, 20–2.

Cruz, F.O., ed. (2008) *The social causes of health inequalities in Brazil*. National Commission on Social Determinants of Health, Editora Fiocruz.

Currin, L.G., Jack, R.H., Linklater, K.M., Mak, V., Moller, H. & Davies, E.A. (2009) Inequalities in the incidence of cervical cancer in South East England 2001–2005: An investigation of population risk factors. *BMC Public Health* 9, 62.

Cutler, D. M. & Lleras-Muney, A. (2006) *Education and Health: Evaluating Theories and Evidence. NBER Working Paper No. 12352*. Cambridge MA, National Bureau Economic Research.

Dahlgren, G. & Whitehead, M. (1991) *Policies and Strategies for Promoting Social Equity in Health*. Stockholm, Institute of Futures Studies.

Dahlgren, G. & Whitehead, M. (2006a) *European Strategies for Tackling Social Inequities in Health: Levelling up Part 1*. World Health Organization, Copenhagen.

Dahlgren, G. & Whitehead, M. (2006b) *European Strategies for Tackling Social Inequities in Health: Levelling up Part 2*. World Health Organization, Copenhagen.

Dahlgren, G. & Whitehead, M. (2007) *Policies and Strategies for Promoting Social Equity in Health*. Background document to WHO – Strategy paper for Europe. Institute for Futures Studies.

Davies, S.E. (2010) *Global Politics of Health*. Cambridge and Malden, Polity.

Deacon, J.M., Evans, C.D., Yule, R. et al. (2000) Sexual behaviour and smoking as determinants of cervical HPV infection and of CIN3 among those infected: A case-control study nested within the Manchester cohort. *British Journal of Cancer* 88 (11), 1565–72.

De Boo, H.A. & Harding, J.E. (2006) The developmental origins of adult disease (Barker) hypothesis. *Australian and New Zealand Journal of Obstetrics and Gynaecology* 46, 4–14.

Dein, S. (2006) *Culture and Cancer Care: Anthropological Insights on Oncology*. Maidenhead, Open University Press.

Denzin, N. & Lincoln, Y. (1998) *Collecting and Interpreting Qualitative Data*. Sage Publications, Thousand Oaks.

Department of Health (1992) *The Health of the Nation. A Strategy for England.* London, DOH.

Department of Health (1999) *Saving Lives: Our Healthier Nation.* London Department of Health.

Department of Health (2000) *The NHS Plan.* London, Department of Health.

Department of Health (2003) *Tackling Health Inequalities: A Programme for Action.* London, Department of Health.

Department of Health (2004) *Choosing Health: Making Healthier Choices Easier.* London, HMSO.

Department of Health (2005) *Tackling Health Inequalities: Status Report on the Programme for Action.* London, Department of Health.

Department of Health (2007a) *Health Survey for England 2007.* Stationery Office, London.

Department of Health (2007b) *Health Profile for England.* London, Department of Health.

Department of Health (2010) *Healthy Lives, Healthy People: Our Strategy for Public Health in England.* London, Department of Health.

Direct Gov. (2010) *Tax Credits and Child Benefit.* [Internet] Available at: http://www.direct.gov.uk/en/index.htm [Accessed 20 October 2010].

Ditchfield, J. (1994) *Family Ties and Recidivism. Home Office Research Bulletin. No.36.* London, Home Office.

Dixey, R. & Woodall, J. (Forthcoming) The significance of 'the visit' in an English category-B prison: Views from prisoners, prisoners' families and prison staff. *Community, Work and Family.*

Donaldson, L. & Scally, L.J. (2009) *Donaldson's Essential Public Health.* 3rd edn. Oxford, Radcliffe.

Donnelly, L. (2010) Taxpayer should fund 'bribes' for obese and smokers. *Daily Telegraph,* 26 September 2010. [Internet] Available at: http://www.telegraph.co.uk/health/healthnews/8025014/Taxpayer-should-fund-bribes-for-obese-and-smokers.html [Accessed 1 October 2010].

Dooris, M. (2004) Joining up settings for health: A valuable investment for strategic partnerships? *Critical Public Health* 14, 37–49.

Downie, R.S., Tannahill, C. & Tannahill, A. (1996) *Health Promotion Model and Values.* 2nd edn. Oxford, Oxford University Press.

Downie, R. & Macnaughton, J. (2001) Images of health. In Heller, T., Muston, R., Sidell, M. & Lloyd, C., eds, *Working for Health.* London, Sage Publications. pp. 11–15.

Doyal, L. (1998) *Women and Health Services: An Agenda for Change.* Buckingham, Open University Press.

Dubourg, R., Hamed, J. & Thorns, J. (2005). *The Economic and Social Costs of Crime against Individuals and Households.* London, Home Office.

Duncan, P. (2007) *Critical Perspectives on Health.* Basingstoke, Palgrave Macmillan.

Earle, S. (2007a) Exploring Health. In Earle, S., Lloyd, C.E., Sidell, M. & Spurr, S., eds, *Theory and Research in Promoting Public Health*. London, Sage. pp. 37–66.

Earle, S. (2007b) Promoting public health: Exploring the issues. In Earle, S., Lloyd, C.E., Sidell, M. & Spurr, S., eds, *Theory and Research in Promoting Public Health*. London, Sage. pp. 1–36.

Easton, M. (2010) *Happiness Index 'Could Lead to Policy Changes.'* [Internet] Available as http://www.bbc.co.uk/news/uk-politics-11842673 [Accessed 1 December 2010].

Eckersley, R. (2005) Is modern western culture a health hazard? *International Journal of Epidemiology* 35 (2), 252–8.

Emslie, C. & Hunt, K. (2008) The weaker sex? Exploring lay understandings of gender differences in life expectancy: A qualitative study. *Social Science and Medicine* 67, 808–16.

Entwistle, V.A., Renfrew, M.J., Yearley, S., Forrester, J. & Lamont, T. (1998) Lay perspectives: Advantages for health research. *British Medical Journal* 316, 463–6.

Epstein, Y. (2008) Sick building syndrome. *Harefuah*, July 147 (7), 607–8.

Esping-Anderson, G. (1990) *The Three Worlds of Welfare Capitalism*. Cambridge, Polity.

Evans, J., Hyndman, S., Stewart-Brown, S., Smith, D. & Petersen, S. (2000) An epidemiological study of the relative importance of damp housing in relation to adult health. *Journal of Epidemiology and Community Health* 54, 677–86.

Evans-Pritchard, E.E. (1937) *Witchcraft, Oracles and Magic among the Azande*. Oxford, Clarendon Press.

Ewles, L. & Simnett, I. (2003) *Promoting Health: A Practical Guide*. 5th edn. London, Bailliere Tindall.

Exworthy, M. (2008). Policy to tackle the social determinants of health: Using conceptual models to understand the policy process. *Health Policy and Planning* 23, 318–27.

Feacham, R.G.A. (2001) Globalisation is good for your health, mostly. *British Medical Journal* 323, 504–6.

Fenton, S. & Sadiq-Sangster, A. (1996) Culture, relativism and the expression of mental distress: South Asian women in Britain. *Sociology of Health & Illness* 18 (1), 66–85.

Fidler, D.P. (2007) Architecture amidst anarchy: Global health's quest for governance. *Global Health Governance* 1 (1), 1–17.

Finkelstein, J. (1990) Women, pregnancy and childbirth. In Schutt, J.A., ed., *Baby machine: Reproductive Technology and the Commercialisation of Motherhood*. London, Green Print. pp. 12–32

Fitzpatrick, R., Newman, S., Archer, R. & Shipley, M. (1991) Social support, disability and depression: a longitudinal study. *Social Science and Medicine* 33, 605–11.

Fleming, D.M. (1999) Weekly returns service of the Royal College of General Practitioners. *Communicable Disease Public Health* 2, 96–100.

Flick, U. (2003) Editorial: Health concepts in different contexts. *Journal of Health Psychology* 8 (5), 483–4.

Food and Agriculture Organization of the United Nations (2003) *Trade Reforms and Food Security: Conceptualizing the Linkages.* Rome, ,FAO.

Foster, P. (1995) *Women and the Health Care Industry; An Unhealthy Relationship?* Buckingham, Open University Press.

Foucault, M. (1976) *The Birth of the Clinic: An Archaeology of Medical Perception.* London, Tavistock.

Foucault, M. (1979) *The History of Sexuality. Volume 1.* London, Allen Lane.

French, C. & Webster, J. (2002) The cycle of conflict. In Adams, L., Amos, M. & Munro, J., eds, *Promoting Health: Politics and Practice.* London, Sage Publications. pp. 5–12.

Friedli, L. (2009) *Mental Health, Resilience and Inequalities.* Geneva, WHO.

Fuchs, V. (1974) *Who Shall Live? Health, Economics and Social Choice.* New York, Basic Books.

Fukuyama, F. (1999) *The Great Disruption: Human Nature and the Reconstitution of Social Order.* Free Press, New York.

Furbey, R., Dinham, A., Farnell, R., Finneron, D. & Wilkinson, D. (2006) *Faith as Social Capital: Connecting or Dividing?* Bristol, Policy Press.

Furedi, F. (2008) Medicalisation in a therapy culture. In Wainwright, D., ed., *A Sociology of Health.* London, Sage. pp. 97–114.

Galdas, P.M., Cheater, F. & Marshall, P. (2005) Men and health help-seeking behaviour: Literature review. *Journal of Advanced Nursing* 49 (6), 616–23.

Geiger, J.H. (2001) Terrorism, biological weapons and bonanzas: Assessing the real threat to public health. *American Journal of Public Health* 91(5), 708–9.

Geller, A.C., Colditz, G., Oliveria, S. et al. (2002) Use of sunscreen, sunbathing rates and tanning bed use among more than 10,000 US children and adolescents. *Pediatrics* 109 (6), 1009–14.

Germond, P. & Cochrane, J.R. (2010) Healthworlds: Conceptualizing landscapes of health and healing. *Sociology* 44 (2), 307–24.

Giddens, A. (1999) Risk and responsibility. *Modern Law Review* 62 (1), 1–10.

Giddens, A. (2009) *Sociology.* 6th edn. Cambridge, Polity.

Gillick, M.R. (1985) Common-sense models of health and disease. *New England Journal Medicine* 313, 700–3.

Gjonca, A., Tomassinic, C., Toson, B. & Smallwood, S. (2005) Sex differences in mortality, a comparison of the UK and other developed countries. *Health Statistics Quarterly* 26, London, Office for National Statistics.

Glanz, K., Basil, M., Maibach, E., Goldberg, J. & Snyder, D. (1998) Why Americans eat what they do: Taste, nutrition, cost, convenience and weight control as influences on food consumption. *J Am Diet Association* 98 (10), 1118–26.

Glennerster, H. (2003) *Understanding the Finance of Welfare. What Welfare Costs and How to Pay for it.* Bristol, Policy Press.

Gluckman, P.D., Hanson, M.A., Cooper, C. & Thornburg, K.L. (2008) Effect of in utero and early life conditions on adult health and disease. *New England Journal of Medicine* 359, 61–73.

Goffman, E. (1963) *Stigma.* London, Penguin.

Gottlieb, S. (2002) 1.6 million elementary school children have ADHD says report. *British Medical Journal* 324, 1296.

Government Office for Science (2007) FORESIGHT: *Tackling Obesities: Future Choices – Obesogenic Environments – Evidence Review.* October 2007 London, Department of Innovation, Universities and Skills.

Graham, H. (1987) Women's smoking and family health. *Social Science and Medicine* 1, 47–56.

Graham, H. (2000) *Understanding Health Inequalities.* 2nd edn. Buckingham, Open University Press.

Graham, H. (2004) Social determinants and their unequal distribution: Clarifying policy understanding. *Milbank Quarterly* 82, 101–24.

Graham, H. (2010) Poverty and health: Global and national patterns. In Douglas, J., Earle, S., Handsley, S., Jones, L., Lloyd, C.E. & Spurr, S., eds, *A Reader in Promoting Public Health.* London, Sage. pp. 39–51.

Graham, H. & Kelly, M.P. (2004) *Health Inequalities: Concepts, Frameworks and Policy.* London, Health Development Agency.

Graham, H. & Power, C. (2004) *Childhood Disadvantage and Adult Health: A Life Course Framework.* London, Health Development Agency.

Gray, J.A.M. (1997) *Evidence-Based Health Care: How to Make Health Policy and Management Decisions.* New York and London, Churchill Livingstone.

Green, L.W., Simons-Morton, D.G. & Potvin, L. (1997) Education and life-style determinants of health and disease. In Detels, R., Holland, W.W., McEwen, J. & Omenn, G.S., eds, *Oxford Textbook of Public Health.* Vol. 1, 3rd edn. Oxford, Oxford University Press. pp. 125–39.

Green, J. & Tones, K. (1999) For debate: Towards a secure evidence base for health promotion. *Journal of Public Health* 21 (2), 133–9.

Green, J. & Tones, K. (2010) *Health Promotion: Planning and Strategies.* 2nd edn. London, Sage.

Gregg, J. & O'Hara, L. (2007) Values and principles evident in current health promotion practice. *Health Promotion Journal of Australia* 18 (1), 7–11.

Grulich, A.E., Van Leeuwen, M.T., Falster, M.O. & Vajdic, C.M. (2007) Incidence of cancers in people with HIV/AIDS compared with immunodeficiency syndrome patients: A meta analysis. *Lancet* 370 (9581), 59–67.

Grundy, E. & Bowling, A. (1991) The sociology of ageing. In Jacoby, R. & Oppenheimer, C., eds, *Psychiatry in the elderly*. Oxford, Oxford University Press. pp. 24–36.

Guterres, A. (2009) *World Refugee Day: 42 Million Uprooted People Waiting to Go Home*. UN Refugee Agency, 19 June 2010. [Internet] Available at: http://www.unhcr.org/4a3b98706.html [Accessed 12 August 2010].

Halpern, D. (2005) *Social Capital*. Cambridge. Polity.

Hammond, C. (2004) The impacts of learning on well-being, mental health and effective coping. In Schuller, T., Preston, J., Hammond, C., Brassett-Grundy, A. & Bynner, J., eds, *The Benefits of Learning: The Impact of Education on Health, Family Life and Social Capital*. London, Routledge. pp. 37–56.

Hanlon, P., Carlisle, S., Lyon, A., Hannah, M. & Reilly, D. (2010) *Disease: The Modern Epidemics. Obesity and Modern Life*. [Internet] Available at: http://www.afternow.co.uk/papers [Accessed 28 June 2010].

Hanlon, P., Carlisle, S., Lyon, A., Hannah, M. & Reilly, D. (no date) *New Wave: The Next Revolution in Society. 1.1 Four Waves of Public Health*. Glasgow, University of Glasgow.

Hardey, M. (1998) *The Social Context of Health*. Buckingham, Open University Press.

Harper, R. & Kelly, M. (2003) *Measuring Social Capital in the United Kingdom*. London, Office for National Statistics.

Harris, J., Crawshaw, J.G. & Millership, S. (2003) Incidence and prevalence of head lice in a district health authority area. *Commun Dis Public Health* 6, 246–9.

Harris, V., Sandridge, A.L., Black, R.J., Brewster, D.H. & Gould, A. (1998) *Cancer Registration Statistics: Scotland 1986–1995*. Edinburgh, ISD Scotland Publications.

Harrison, S. & Macdonald, R. (2008) *The Politics of Healthcare in Britain*. London, Sage Publications.

Hartzband, P. & Groopman, J. (2009) Keeping the patient in the equation – humanism and health care reform. *New England Journal of Medicine* 361, 554–5.

Hawkes, C. & Ruel, M. (2006) The links between agriculture and health: an intersectoral opportunity to improve the health and livelihoods of the poor. *Bulletin of the World Health Organization* 84 (12), December, 984–92.

Health Development Agency (2003) *Health Equity Audit Made Simple*. London, Health Development Agency.

Health Development Agency (2004a) *Social Capital*. London, Health Development Agency.

Health Development Agency (2004b) *Promoting Healthier Communities and Narrowing Health Inequalities: A Self Assessment Tool for Local Authorities*. London, HDA, NHS.

Health Protection Agency (2010) *What the HPA does*. [Internet] Available at: http://www.hpa.org.uk [Accessed 18 September 2010].

Healy, D. (2006) The latest mania: Selling bipolar disorder. *Public Library of Science- Medicine* 3 (4), 441–4.

Helman, C.G. (1991) Limits of biomedical explanation. *Lancet* 337, 1080–3.

Helman, C.G. (2000) *Culture, Health and Illness.* 4th edn. London, Hodder Arnold.

Helman, C.G. (2007) *Culture, Health and Illness.* 5th edn. London, Hodder Arnold.

Henderson, P. & Oldfield, S. (1993) The first victim of mad cow disease? *Daily Mail,* 12 March, 1/5.

Hendryx, M.S., Ahern, M.M., Lovrich, N.P. & McCurdy, A.H. (2002), Access to health care and community social capital, *Health Services Research* 37 (1), 85–101.

Hennick, M., Hutter, I. & Bailey, A. (2011) *Qualitative Research Methods.* London, Sage.

Hernandez, L.M. & Blazer, D.G., eds (2006) *Genes, Behavior and the Social Environment: Moving Beyond the Nature/Nurture Debate.* National Academies Press, USA. [Internet] Available at: http://books.nap.edu/catalog.php?record_id=11693#toc [Accessed 25 August 2010].

Herrero, R. (1996) Epidemiology of cervical cancer. *Journal of National Cancer Institute* 21, 1–6.

Hicks, J. & Allen, G. (1999) *A Century of Change: Trends in UK statistics since 1900.* RESEARCH PAPER 99/11. London, House of Commons.

Hill, M. (1997) *The Policy Process in the Modern Society.* 3rd edn. London, Prentice Hall.

Hill, K., Thomas, K., Abouzahr, C. et al. (2007) Estimates of maternal mortality worldwide between 1900 and 2005: An assessment of available data. *Lancet* 370, 1311–19.

Hinrichsen, D. & Robey, B. (2000) *Population and the Environment: The Global Challenge.* Baltimore, Johns Hopkins University.

Hogwood, B.W. & Gunn, L.A. (1984) *Policy Analysis for the Real World.* Oxford, Oxford University Press.

House, J.S. (1981) *Work, Stress and Social Support.* Reading MA, Addison Wesley.

Hovell M.F., Wahlgren, D.R. & Russos, S. (1997) Preventive medicine and cultural contingencies: The great natural experiment. In Lamal P.A., ed., *Cultural Contingencies: Behavior Analytic Perspectives on Cultural Practices.* Westport, Connecticut, Praeger Publications. pp. 1–29.

Hu, F.B., Manson, J.E. & Willett, W.C. (2001) Types of dietary fat and risk of coronary heart disease: A critical review. *Journal of American College of Nutrition* 20 (1), 5–19.

Hubley, J. & Copeman, J. (2008) *Practical Health Promotion.* Cambridge, Polity.

Hudson, J., Kuhner, S. & Lowe, S. (2008) *The Short Guide to Social Policy.* Bristol, Policy Press.

Hughner, R.S. & Kleine, S.S. (2004) Views of health in the lay sector: A compilation and review of how individuals think about health.

Health: An Interdisciplinary Journal for the Social Study of Health, Illness and Medicine 8 (4), 395–422.

Husbands, J. (2007) Promoting healthy lifestyles. In Wills, J., ed., Vital Notes for Nurses: Promoting Health. Oxford, Blackwell. pp. 129–53.

IDeA (2010) Big Society Policy [Internet] available at http://www.idea.gov.uk/idk/core/page.do?pageId=23536490> [Accessed 13 December 10].

Illich, I. (1976) Limits to Medicine. Harmondsworth, Pelican.

Jaakkola, J.J. & Gissler, M. (2004) Maternal smoking in pregnancy, fetal development and childhood asthma. American Journal of Public Health 94 (1), 136–40.

Jackson, L.E. (2003) The relationship of urban design to human health and condition. Landscape and Urban Planning 64 (15), 191–200.

Jackson, L. (2007) Health and health promotion. In Wills, J., ed., Vital Notes for Nurses: Promoting Health. Oxford, Blackwell. pp. 11–27.

Jackson, J. & Stafford, M. (2009) Public health and fear of crime: A prospective cohort study. British Journal of Criminology 49, 832–47.

Jarvis, M.J. & Wardle, J. (1999) Social patterning of health behaviours: The case of cigarette smoking. In Marmot, M. & Wilkinson, R.G., eds, Social Determinants of Health. Oxford, Oxford University Press. pp. 255–340.

Jarvis, M.J., Wardle, J., Waller, J. & Owen, L. (2003) Prevalence of hardcore smoking in England and associated attitudes and beliefs: Cross sectional study. British Medical Journal 326 (7398), 1061–6.

Jenkins, R. (1996) Social Identity. 2nd edn. London, Routledge.

Jenkins, W.I. (1978) Policy Analysis: A Political and Organisational Perspective. Oxford, Martin Robertson.

Johnson, B. (2003) Psychological addiction, physical addiction, addictive character, and addictive personality disorder: A nosology of addictive disorders. Canadian Journal of Psychoanalysis 11, 135–60.

Johnson, G. & Helman, C. (2004) Remedy or cure? Lay beliefs about over-the-counter medicines for coughs and colds. British Journal of General Practice 54 (499), 98–102.

Johnson, C. (2007) Creating Health for Everyone: Principles, Practice and Philosophy. Morrisville. NC, USA, Lulu Press.

Jones, C. (2002) Foetal programming and coronary heart diseases in later life. British Journal of Nursing 11 (12), 822–6.

Jones, L. & Earle, S. (2010) Introduction in Douglas, J., Earle, S., Handsley, S., Jones, L., Lloyds, C.E., & Spurr, S. (eds) A Reader in Promoting Public Health. London, Sage, pp. 5–9.

Jones, O. (2011) CHAVs: The Demonization of the Working-Class. London, Verso Books.

Kaiser Family Foundation (2009) Health Coverage and the Uninsured: Trends in Health Coverage. [Internet] Available at: www.kff.org/uninsured/tredns.cfm [Accessed 19 September 2009].

Kalof, L., Dan, A. & Dietz, T. (2008) *Essentials of Social Research.* Maidenhead, McGraw-Hill, Open University Press.

Kangas, I. (2002) 'Lay' and 'expert': Illness knowledge constructions in the sociology of health and illness. *Health: An Interdisciplinary Journal for the Social Study of Health, Illness and Medicine* 6 (3), 301–4.

Kaufmann, S. (2009) *The New Plagues. Pandemics and Poverty in a Globalised World.* London, Haus.

Kawachi, I., Kennedy, B.P., Lochener, K. & Prothrow-Stith, D. (1997), Social Capital, Income Inequality and Mortality, *American Journal of Public Health* 87, 1491–8.

Kelly, M.P. & Charlton, B. (1995) The modern and post modern in health promotion. In Bunton, R., Nettleton, S. and Burrows, R., eds, *The Sociology of Health Promotion: Critical Analyses of Consumption, Lifestyle and Risk.* London, Routledge. pp. 78–90.

Kennedy, B.P., Kawachi, I. & Brainerd, E. (1998) The role of social capital in the Russian mortality crisis. *World Development* 26 (11), 2029–43.

Kessler, R.C., Turner, J.B. & House, J.S. (2009) Intervening processes in the relationship between unemployment and health. *Psychological Medicine* 17, 849–961.

Khan, M.J., Partridge, E.E., Wang, S.S. & Schiffman, M. (2005) Socioeconomic status and the risk of cervical intraepithelial neoplasia grade 3 among oncogenic human papillomavirus DNA-positive women with equivocal or mildly abnormal cytology. *Cancer* 104, 61–71.

Kickbusch, I. (2003) The contribution of the World Health Organization to a new public health and health promotion. *American Journal of Public Health* 93 (3), 383–8.

Kindhauser, M.K. (2003) *Communicable Diseases 2002: Global Defence Against the Infectious Disease Threat,* WHO/CDS/2003.15, Geneva, WHO.

King, M. & Street, C. (2005) Mad cows and mad scientists: What happened to public health in the battle for hearts and minds of the Great British beef consumer? In King, M. & Watson, K., eds, *Representing Health.* Basingstoke, Palgrave Macmillan, pp. 115–32.

Kingfisher, C. & Millard, A. (1998) 'Milk makes me sick but my body needs it': Conflict and contradiction in the establishment of authoritative knowledge. *Med Anthropology Quarterly* 12, 447–66.

Kirmayer, L. (2004) The cultural diversity of healing: Meaning, metaphor and mechanism. *British Medical Bulletin* 69, 33–48.

Kitzmann, K.M., Dalton, W.D., Stanley, C.M. et al. (2010) Lifestyle interventions for youth who are overweight: A meta-analytic review. *Health Psychology* 29 (1), 91–101.

Klein, R. (2006) *The New Politics of the NHS.* 5th edn. Oxford, Radcliffe.

Klein, R. (2010) *The New Politics of the NHS. From Creation to Reinvention.* 6th edn. Oxford, Radcliffe.

Kleinman, A. (1977) Depression, somatisation and the 'New Cross Cultural Psychiatry'. *Social Science and Medicine* 11, 3–10.

Kleinman, A. (1989) *The Illness Narratives: Suffering, Healing and the Human Condition*. New York, Basic Books.

Knutsson, A. (2003) Health disorders of shift workers. *Occupational Medicine* 53, 103–108.

Kohler-Flynn, H. (2003) Self-esteem theory and measurement: A critical review. *Thirdspace*, 3 (1), no page numbers.

Koivusalo, M. & Ollila, E. (1997) *Making a Healthy World: Agencies, Actors and Policies in International*. Health London, Zed Books.

Koos, E. (1954) *The Health of Regionville: What People Thought and Did about it*. New York, Columbia University Press.

Koplan, J.P. & Fleming, D.W. (2000) Current and future public health challenges. *JAMA* 284 (13), 1696–8.

Korkman, M., Kettunen, S. & Autti-Rämö, I. (2003) Neurocognitive Impairment in early adolescence following prenatal alcohol exposure of varying duration. *Child Neuropyschology* 9 (2), 117–28.

Kreiger, N. (2008) Proximal, distal and the politics of causation: What's level got to do with it? *American Journal of Public Health* 98 (2), 221–30.

Krumeich, A. (1994) *The Blessings of Motherhood. Health, Pregnancy and Child Care in Dominica*. Amsterdam, Het Spinhuis.

Kumanyika, S.K. (2008) Environmental influences on childhood obesity: Ethnic and cultural influences in context. *Physiology & Behavior* 94 (1), 61–70.

Kumaranayake, L. & Walker, D. (2002) Cost effectiveness analysis and priority setting: Global approach without local meaning? In Kelley, L., Buse, K. & Fustukian, S., eds, *Health Policy in a Globalising World*. Cambridge, Cambridge University Press. pp.140–58.

Kunst, A.E., Groenhof, F., Mackenbach, J.P. & EU Working Group on Socioeconomic Inequalities in Health (1998) Mortality by occupational class among men 30–64 years in 11 European countries. *Social Science and Medicine* 46 (11), 1459–76.

Labonte, R. (2010) Health promotion, globalisation and health. In Douglas, J., Earle, S., Handsley, S., Jones, L., Lloyd, C.E. & Spurr, S., eds, *A Reader in Promoting Public Health*. London, Sage. pp. 235–45.

Lansley, A. (2010) *Speech to Faculty of Public Health*. [Internet] Available at http://www.dh.gov.uk/en/MediaCentre/Speeches/DH_117280> [Accessed 10 October 10].

Laverack, G. (2004) *Health Promotion Practice: Power and Empowerment*. London, Sage.

Laverack, G. (2007) *Health Promotion Practice: Building Empowered Communities*. Maidenhead, Open University Press.

Lawton, J. (2003) Lay experiences of health and illness: Past research and future agendas. *Sociology of Health and Illness* 25, 23–40.

Lawton, J., Peel, E., Parry, O., Araoz, G. & Douglas, M. (2005) Lay perceptions of type 2 diabetes in Scotland: Bringing health services back in. *Social Science and Medicine* 60, 1423–35.

Lawton, R., Connor, M. & McEachan, R. (2009) Desire or reason:

Predicting health behaviour from affective and cognitive attitudes. *Health Psychology* 28 (1), 56–65.

Leach, B., Paluzzi, J.E. & Munderi, P. (2005) *Prescription for Healthy Development: Increasing Access to Medicines.* London, Earthscan.

Lee, J.H.J. (1996) transforming society, transforming medicine: Lay medical perceptions and self-medication among contemporary Koreans. In Subedi, J. & Gallagher, E.B., eds, *Society, Health and Disease: Transcultural Perspectives.* New Jersey, Prentice Hall. pp. 25–46.

Lee, K. & Collin, J. (2005) *Global Change and Health.* Maidenhead, Open University Press.

Lee, K. & Goodman, H. (2002) Global policy networks: The propagation of health care financing reform since the 1980s. In Lee, K., Buse, K. & Fustukian, S., eds, *Health Impacts of Globalisation: Towards Global Governance'* Basingstoke, Palgrave Macmillan.

Lee, Y. & McCormick, B. (2004) Subjective well-being of people with spinal cord injury: Does leisure contribute? *Journal of Rehabilitation* 70 (3), 5–12.

Lee, K. (1998) Shaping the future of global health co-operation: Where do we go from here? *Lancet* 351, 899–902.

Lee, K. (2009) *The World Health Organization.* Oxford, Routledge.

Lee, K. & Goodman, H. (2002) Global policy networks: The propagation of health care financing reform since the 1980s. In Kelley, L., Buse, K. & Fustukian, S., eds, *Health Care Policy in a Globalising World.* Cambridge, Cambridge University Press. pp. 97–119.

Leonardi, G., McKee, M. & Powerleau, J. (2005) Drains, dustbins and diseases. In Powerleau, J. & McKee, M., eds, *Issues in Public Health.* Maidenhead, Open University Press. pp. 208–16.

Leung, S.S.K. & Leung, I. (2010) Cervical cancer screening: Knowledge, health perception and attendance rates among Hong Kong Chinese Women. *International Journal of Women's Health* 2, 221–8.

Lin, P., Simoni, J.M. & Zemon, V. (2005) The health belief model, sexual behaviours and HIV risk among Taiwanese immigrants. *AIDS Education and Research* 17 (5), 469–83.

Lin, R.L., Shah, C.P. & Svoboda, T.J. (1995) The impact of unemployment on health: A review of the evidence. *Canadian Medical Association Journal* 153 (5), 528–40.

Lindstrom, B., and Eriksson, M. (2005) Glossary: Salutogenesis. *J Epidemiol Community Health* 59, 440–2.

Lloyd, L. (2000) Dying in old age: Promoting well-being at the end of life. *Mortality* 5, 171–88.

Lowcock, D. & Cross, R.M. (2011) Health and health promotion. In Jones, P. & Walker, G., eds, *Children's Rights in Practice.* London, Sage. pp. 140–61

Lucas, K. & Lloyd, B. (2005) *Health Promotion: Evidence and Experience.* London, Sage Publications.

Lupton, D. (1993) Risk as moral danger: The social and political functions of risk discourse in public health. *International Journal of Health Services* 23 (3), 425–35.

Lupton, D. (1994) *Medicine as Culture. Illness, Disease and the Body in Western Societies.* London, Sage.

Lupton, D. & Peterson, A. (1996) *The New Public Health.* London, Sage.

Lyon, R.M., Cobbe, S.M. & Bradley, J.M. (2004) Surviving out of hospital cardiac arrest at home: A postcode lottery? *Emergency Medicine* 21, 619–24.

Lyons, A.C. & Chamberlain, K. (2006) *Health Psychology.* Cambridge, Cambridge University Press.

Macartney, J. (2009) Two are sentenced to death over toxic milk scandal. *The Times* [Internet], 22 January. Available from: <senhttp://www.timesonline.co.uk/tol/news/world/asia/article5570314.ece> [Accessed 11 August 2010].

Macdonald, T. (2006) *Health, Trade and Human Rights.* Oxford, Radcliffe.

Macdonald, T. (2007) *The Global Human Right to Health: Dream or Possibility?* Oxford, Radcliffe.

Macdonald, T. (2008) *Health, Human Rights and the United Nations: Inconsistent Aims and Inherent Contradictions.* Oxford, Radcliffe.

MacDonald, G. & Smith, P. (2001) Collaborative working in primary care groups: A case of incommensurable paradigms. *Critical Public Health* 11 (3), 253–66.

McKenzie, K. & Harpham, T. (2006) Meaning and uses of social capital in the mental health field. In McKenzie, K. & Harpham, T., eds, *Social Capital and Mental Health.* London, Jessica Kingsley Publishers. pp. 11–23.

McKeown, T. (1979) *The Role of Medicine: Dream, Mirage or Nemesis?* Oxford, Blackwell.

McKinlay, J.B. (1979) A case for refocusing upstream: The political economy of health. Cited in Jaco E.G. ed., *Patients, Physicians and Illness.* Basingstoke, Macmillan. pp. 234–48.

McMath, B.F. & Prentice-Dunn, S. (2005) Protection motivation theory and skin cancer risk: The role of individual differences in responses to persuasive appeals. *Journal of Applied Social Psychology* 35 (3), 621–43.

McQueen, D.V. (2002) Strengthening the *evidence base* for health promotion. *Health Promotion International* 16 (3), 261–8.

Macready, N. (2007) Developing Countries Court Medical Tourists. *Lancet* 369, 1849–50.

Malaria Consortium (2008) *Malaria Consortium's Statement for International Women's Day.* 7 May 2008. [Internet] Available at: http://www.malariaconsortium.org/ffimalaqkmt/news.php?id=43> [Accessed 1 November 2010].

Maltby, S.E. (1918) Manchester and the movement for national elementary education, Manchester, Manchester University Press. Cited in Webster, C. & French, J. (2002) The cycle of conflict: The history of the public health and health promotion movements. In

Adams, L., Amos, M. & Munro, J., eds, *Promoting Health: Politics and Practice*. London, Sage. pp. 5–12.

Mameli, M. (2007) Reproductive cloning, genetic engineering and the autonomy of the child: The moral agent and the open future. *Journal of Medical Ethics* 33, 87–93.

Mann, N., Hosman, C.M., Schaolma, H.P. & DeVreis, N.K. (2004) Self-esteem in a broad spectrum approach for mental health promotion. *Health Education Research* 19 (4), 357–72.

Mant, D., Vessey, M. & Loudon, N. (1988) Social class differences in sexual behaviour and cervical cancer. *Community Medicine* 10 (1), 52–6.

Marks, D.F. (2002) Editorial essay: Freedom, responsibility and power: Contrasting approaches to health psychology. *Journal of Health Psychology* 7 (1), 5–19.

Marks, D.F., Murray, M., Evans, B. & Willig, C. (2000) *Health Psychology: Theory, Research and Practice*. London, Sage Publications.

Marks, D.F., Murray, M., Evans, B., Willig, C. Woodall, C. & Sykes, C.M. (2005) *Health Psychology: Theory, Research and Practice*. 2nd edn. London, Sage Publications.

Marmot, M.G., Smith, G.D., Stansfeld, S. et al. (1991) Health inequalities among British civil servants: The Whitehall II study. *Lancet* 337 (8754), 1387–93.

Marmot, M. (2004) *The Status Syndrome. How Social Standing Affects our Health and Longevity*. New York, Owl Books.

Marmot, M. & Wilkinson, R.G. (2001) Psychosocial and material pathways in the relation between income and health: A response to Lynch et al. *British Medical Journal* 322 (7296), 1233–6.

Marmot Review Team (2010) *Fair Society, Healthy Lives: The Marmot Review*. London, The Marmot Review.

Marsella, A. (2007) Culture and psychopathology. In Kitayama, S. & Cohen, D., eds, *Handbook of Cultural Psychology*. New York; Guilford Publications. pp. 734–59.

Martin, G.P. (2008) 'Ordinary people only': Knowledge, representativeness, and the publics of public participation in healthcare. *Sociology of Health and Illness* 30 (1), 35–54.

Mason, J. (1996) *Qualitative Researching*. Sage, London.

Mathers, C.D., Ma Fat, D., Inoue, M., Rao, C. & Lopez, A.D. (2005) Counting the dead and what they died from: An assessment of the global status of cause of death data. *Bulletin of the World Health Organization*, March.

May, P.A. & Gossage, J.P. (2001) Estimating the Prevalence of Fetal Alcohol Syndrome: A summary. *Alcohol Research & Health* 25, 346–50.

Mehrotra, S. (2000) *Integrating Economic and Social Policy: Good Practices from High Achieving Countries*. Innocenti Working Paper No 80, Florence, Italy, UNICEF.

Michie, S. & Williams, S. (2002) Reducing work related psychological ill health and sickness absence: A systematic literature review. *Occupational Environmental Medicine* 60, 3–9.

Mielewczyk, F. & Willig, C. (2007) Old clothes and an older look: The case for a radical makeover in health behaviour research. *Theory & Psychology* 17, 811–37.

Miles, A. (1991) *Women, Health and Medicine.* Buckingham, Open University Press.

Miles, M.B & Huberman, A.M. (1994) *Qualitative Data Analysis: An Expanded Source-Book.* Sage Publications, Newbury Park.

Millennium Campaign News (2006) *Goal 6: Combat HIV/AIDS, Malaria and other Diseases.* [Internet] Available at: www.millenniumcampaign.org/site/Pp asp? C=grKVL2NLEs [Accessed 1 July 2006].

Mills, C.W. (1970) *The Sociological Imagination.* Oxford, Oxford University Press.

Milne, S., Sheeran, S. & Orbell, S. (2000) Prediction and intervention in health-related behaviour: A meta-review of protection motivation theory. *Journal of Applied Social Psychology* 30, 106–43.

Mitchell, R. & Popham, F. (2008) Effect of exposure to natural environment on health inequalities: An observational population study. *Lancet* 372, 1655–60.

Moore, A. (2008) The times of their lives. *Health Service Journal,* 30 October, 20–22.

Morgan, D. (2006) School food and the public domain: The politics of the public plate. *Political Quarterly* (77) 3, 379–87.

Morse, J. (2000) Determining sample size. *Qualitative Health Research* 10, 3–5.

Moule, P. & Goodwin, M. (2009) *Nursing Research: An Introduction.* London, Sage.

Moynihan, C. (1998) Theories in health care and research: Theories of masculinity. *British Medical Journal* 317, 1072–5.

Muir Gray, J.M. (1996) *Evidence Based Healthcare.* London, Churchill Livingstone.

Murray, C.J.L., King, G., Lopez, A.D., Tomijima, N. & Krug, E.G. (2002) Armed conflict as a public health problem. *British Medical Journal* 324 (7333), 346.

Murray, M., Pullman, D. & Heath Rodgers, T. (2003) Social representations of health and illness among 'baby-boomers' in Eastern Canada. *Journal of Health Psychology* 8 (5) 485–99.

Naidoo, J. & Wills, J. (2000) *Health Promotion: Foundations for Practice.* 2nd edn. London, Bailliere Tindall.

Naidoo, J. & Wills, J. (2008) *Health Studies. An Introduction* Basingstoke, Palgrave Macmillan.

Naidoo, J. & Wills, J. (2009) *Health Promotion: Foundations for Practice.* 3rd edn. London, Bailliere Tindall.

Nasreen, H-E., Kabir, Z.N., Forsell, Y. & Edhborg, M. (2010) Low birth weight in offspring of women with depressive and anxiety symptoms during pregnancy: Results from a population based study in Bangladesh. *BMC Public Health* 10, 515.

National Cancer Institute (2011) *Treatment Option Overview*. [Internet] Available at: http://www.cancer.gov/cancertopics/pdq/treatment/cervical/Patient/page4 [Accessed 11 January 2011].

National Centre for Social Research and University College London. Department of Epidemiology and Public Health, *Health Survey for England, 1991–2008*. Colchester, Essex, UK Data Archive.

Navarro, V. (1979) *Medicine under Capitalism*. London, Croom Helm.

Navarro, V. & Shi, L. (2001) The political context of social inequalities and health. *Social Science & Medicine* 52 (3), 481–91.

Neeman, M. (2009) *Developing Resilience. A Cognitive Behavioural Approach*. USA, Routledge.

Nettleton, S. & Watson, J., eds (1998) *The Body in Everyday Life*. London, Routledge.

Newman, S. (1997) Masculinities, men's bodies and nursing. In Lawler. J., ed., *The Body in Nursing*. Melbourne, Churchill Livingstone. pp. 135–53.

NICE (2006) *Public Health Intervention Guidance no. 2. Four commonly used methods to increase physical activity: Brief interventions in primary care, exercise referral schemes, pedometers and community-based exercise programmes for walking and cycling*. London, NICE.

Nolte, E., McKee, M. & Pomerleau, J. (2005) The impact of health care on population health. In Powerleau, J. & McKee, M., eds, *Issues in Public Health*. Maidenhead, Open University Press. pp. 105–26.

Norman, P., Boer, H. & Seydel, E.R. (2005) Protection motivation theory. In Conner, M. & Norman, P., eds, *Predicting Health Behaviour*. 2nd edn. Maidenhead, Open University Press. pp. 81–126.

North, F.M., Syme, S.L., Shipley, M. & Marmot, M. (1996) Psychosocial work environment and sickness absence among British civil servants: The Whitehall II study. *American Journal of Public Health* 86 (3), 332–40.

Nutbeam, D. (1998) *Health Promotion Glossary*. Geneva, WHO.

Oakley, A. (1984) *The Captured Womb: A History of the Medical Care of Pregnant Women*. Oxford, Blackwell.

Oakley, A. (1993) *Women, Health and Medicine*. Edinburgh, Edinburgh University Press.

Office of Health Economics (2007) *Life Expectancy in England and Wales*. Available at: www.ohe.org/page/knowledge/schools/appendix/life_expectancy.cfm [Accessed 3 March 2010].

Office of National Statistics (2003) *Guide to Social Capital*. [Internet] Available at: http://www.statistics.gov.uk/CCI/nugget.asp?ID=314 [Accessed 14 December 2010].

Office for National Statistics (2010) News Release. Healthy life expectancy is shorter in manual social classes. *Health Statistics Quarterly* 45, Newport, Office for National Statistics.

Ogden, J. (1996) *Health Psychology: A Textbook*. Buckingham, Open University Press.

Oliver, M. (1990) *The Politics of Disablement*. Basingstoke, Macmillan Press Ltd.

Ollila, E. (2005) Global health priorities – priorities of the wealthy? *Globalisation and Health* 1 (6), 1–6.

Oxfam (2010) 21st *Century Aid. Recognising success and tackling failure*. Oxfam Briefing Paper, Oxfam International.

Pallant, J. (2010) *SPSS Survival Manual: A Step by Step Guide to Data Analysis Using SPSS*. Maidenhead, McGraw-Hill.

Parliamentary Office of Science and Technology (2007) *Postnote, 276. Ethnicity and Health*. London, Parlimentary Office of Science and Technology.

Parker, E.A., Baldwin, G.T., Israel, B. & Salinas, M. (2004) Application of health promotion theories and models for environmental health. *Health Education and Behaviour* 31 (4), 491–509.

Parsons, T. (1951) Illness and the role of the physician: A sociological perspective. *American Journal of Orthopsychiatry* 21 (3), 452–60.

Patton, M.Q. (2002) *Qualitative research & evaluation methods*. London, Sage.

Peterson, A. & Lupton, D. (1996) *The New Public Health: Health and Self in the Age of Risk*. St Leonards, Australia, Allen & Unwin.

Peto, J. Gilham, C., Fletcher, O. & Matthews, F.E. (2004) The cervical cancer epidemic that screening has prevented in the UK. *Lancet* 364, 249–56.

Petticrew, M. & Roberts, H. (2003) Evidence, hierarchies and typologies: Horses for courses. *J Epi and Comm Health* 57 (7), 527–9.

Phillips, C.B. (2006) Medicine goes to school: Teachers as sickness brokers for ADHD. *Public Library of Science-Medicine* 3 (4), 182.

Piccinelli, M. & Wilkinson, G. (2000) Gender differences in depression. *The British Journal of Psychiatry* 177, 486–92.

Pierson, P. (2004) *Politics in Time: History, Institutions and Social Analysis*. Princeton NJ, Princeton University Press.

Piko, B. (2000) Health-related predictors of self-perceived health in a student population: The importance of physical activity. *Journal of Community Health* 25, 125–37.

Pilgrim, D. & Rogers, A. (1994) *A Sociology of Mental health and Illness*. Buckingham, Open University Press.

Pill, R. & Stott, N.C.H. (1982) Concepts of illness causation and responsibility: Some preliminary data from a sample of working class mothers. *Social Science and Medicine* 16, 43–52.

Pinto-Foltz, M.D. & Logsdon, C.M. (2009) Reducing stigma related to mental disorders: Initiatives, interventions and recommendations for nursing. *Archives of Psychiatric Nursing* 32 (1), 32–40.

Plan (2007) *Because I am a Girl: State of the World's Girls 2007*. [Internet] Available at: www.becauseiamagirl.org [Accessed 7 July 2010].

Polit, D. & Beck, C. (2006) *Essentials of Nursing Research: Methods,*

Appraisal and Utilization. 6th edn. Lippincott Williams & Wilkins, Philadelphia.

Popay, J., Bennett, S., Thomas, C., Williams, G., Gatrell, A. & Bostock, L. (2003) Beyond 'beer, fags, egg and chips'? Exploring lay understandings of social inequalities in health. *Sociology of Health and Illness* 25 (1), 1–23.

Popay, J., Williams, G., Thomas, C. & Gatrell, T. (1998) Theorising Inequalities in health: The place of lay knowledge. *Sociology of Health & Illness* 20 (5), 619–44.

Pope, V. (2008) Met Office's bleak forecast on climate change: The head of the Met Office centre for climate change research explains why the momentum on emissions targets must not be lost. *The Guardian*, [internet] Available at: www.guardian.co.uk/environment/2008/oct/01/climatechange.carbonemissions [Accessed 13 January 2010].

Pote, H.L. & Orrell, M.W. (2002) Perceptions of Schizophrenia in Multi-Cultural Britain. *Ethnicity and Health* 7 (1), 7–20.

Pridmore, P. & Stephens, D. (2000) *Children as Partners for Health: A Critical Review of the Child-to-Child Approach.* Zed Books, London.

Prior, L. (2003) Belief, knowledge and expertise: The emergence of the lay expert in medical sociology. *Sociology of Health & Illness* 25, 41–57.

Productivity Commission (2003) *Social Capital: Reviewing the Concept and its Policy Implications.* Canberra, AusInfo.

Pronyk, P.M., Harpham, T., Busza, J. et al. (2008) Can social capital be intentionally generated? A randomized trial from rural South Africa. *Social Science & Medicine* 67 (3), 1559–70.

Prout, A. (1996) Actor-network theory, technology and medical sociology: An illustrative analysis of the metered dose inhaler.'*Sociology of Health and Illness* 18, 198–219.

Pupavac, V. (2009) Changing concepts of international health. In Wainwright, D., ed., *A Sociology of Health.* London, Sage. pp. 173–93.

Putnam, R.D. (1993) *Making Democracy Work: Civic Traditions in Modern Italy.* Princeton New Jersey, Princeton University Press.

Putnam, R.D. (1995) Tuning in, tuning out: The strange disappearance of social capital in America. *Political Science and Politics* 28 (1), 1–20.

Putnam, R. (2000) *Bowling Alone: The Collapse and Revival of American Community.* New York, Simon & Schuster.

Qualifications and Curriculum Development Agency (no date) *Citizenship* [Internet] Available at: http://curriculum.qcda.gov.uk/key-stages-1-and-2/subjects/citizenship/index.aspx [Accessed 5 January 2011].

Raffle, A.E., Alden, B., Quinn, M., Babb, P.J. & Brett, M.T. (2003) Outcomes of screening to prevent cancer: Analysis of cumulative incidence of cervical abnormality and modelling of cases and deaths prevented. *British Medical Journal* 326, 901.

Raleigh, V.S. & Polato, G.M. (2004) *Evidence of health inequalities.* London, Healthcare Commission.

Ramos, D. & Perkins, D. (2006) Goodness of fit assessment of an alcohol intervention program and underlying theories of change. *Journal of American College Health* 55 (1), 57–64.

Rao, M. (2009) Climate change is deadly: The health impacts of climate change. In Griffiths, J., Rao, M., Adshead, F. & Thorpe, A., eds, *The Health Practitioner's Guide to Climate Change – Diagnosis and Cure.* London & Sterling VA, Earthscan. pp. 33–62.

Rawson, D. (1992) The growth of health promotion theory and its rational reconstruction. In Bunton, R. & McDonald, G., eds, *Health Promotion: Disciplines and Diversity.* London, Routledge. pp. 202–24.

Rawson, D. (2002) The growth of health promotion theory and its rational reconstruction. In Bunton, R. & McDonald, G., eds, *Health Promotion: Disciplines and Diversity.* 2nd edn. London, Routledge. pp. 249–70.

Reblin, M. & Uchino, B.N. (2008) Social and emotional support and its implication for health. *Curr Opin Psychiatry* 21 (2), 201–5.

Roberts, R., Towell, T. & Golding, J.F. (2001) *Foundations of Health Psychology.* Basingstoke, Palgrave.

Robertson, S. (2006) 'Not living life in too much of an excess': Lay men understanding health and well-being. *Health: An Interdisciplinary Journal for the Study of Health, Illness and Medicine* 10 (2), 175–89.

Rogers, R.W. (1975) A protection motivation theory of fear appeals and attitude change. *Journal of Psychology* 91, 93–114.

Rogers, R.W. (1983) Cognitive and physiological processes in fear appeals and attitude change: A revised theory of protection motivation. In Cacippo, J.R. & Petty, R.E., eds, *Social Psychology: A Source Book.* New York, Guilford Press. pp. 153–76.

Rose, R. (1973). Comparing public policy: An overview. *European Journal of Political Research* 1, 67–94.

Ross, C. & Wu, C. (1995) The links between education and health. *American Sociological Review,* October 60, 719–45.

Rubin, H. & Rubin, I. (2005) *Qualitative Interviewing: The Art of Hearing Data.* 2nd edn. London, Sage.

Sachs, J.D. (2001) *Macroeconomics and Health: Investing in Health for Economic Development. Report on the Commission on Macroeconomics and Health.* Geneva, WHO.

Saks, M. & Allsop, J. (2007) *Researching Health: Qualitative, Quantitative and Mixed Methods.* London, Sage.

Salin, D. (2003) Ways of explaining workplace bullying: A review of enabling, motivating and precipitating structures and processes in the work environment. *Human Relations* 56 (10), 1213–32.

Sanders, D. (2005) *Primary Healthcare and Health System Development: Strategies for Revitalisation.* Paper presented to the People's Health Assembly, July, Ecuador.

Sarafino, E. (2005) *Health Psychology: Biopsychosocial Interactions.* 4th edn. Chichester, John Wiley & Sons.

Scheff, T. (1966) *Being Mentally Ill: A Sociological Theory.* Chicago, Aldine.

Schoenberg, N., Drew, E.M., Palo Stroller, E. & Kart, C.S. (2005) Situating stress: Lessons from lay discourses on diabetes. *Medical Anthropology Quarterly* 19 (2), 171–93.

Schoon, I. & Bartley, M. (2008) The role of human capability and resilience. *The Psychologist* 21 (1), 24–7.

Schneider, J.A. (2004) *The Role of Social Capital in Building Healthy Communities.* Baltimore, Annie E. Casey Foundation.

Scholte, J.A. (2000) *Globalization: A Critical Introduction.* Basingstoke, Palgrave Macmillan.

Schwandt, T.A. (2001). *Dictionary of Qualitative Inquiry.* 2nd edn. Thousand Oaks, CA: Sage.

Scott, A.J. (2000) Shift work and health. *Primary Care* 4, 1057–79.

Scottish Community Development Centre (2010) *Supporting Best Practice in Community Development.* [Internet] Available at: http://www.scdc.org.uk [Accessed on 18 September 2010].

Scrambler, G. & Higgs, P. (1999) Stratification, class and health: Class relations and health inequalities in high modernity. *Sociology* 33 (2), 275–96.

Scuklenk, U. (2003) Intellectual property rights, compulsory licensing and the trips agreement: Some ethical issues. *Monash Bioethics Review* 22 (2), 63–8.

Seale, C. (2004) *Researching Society and Culture.* 2nd edn. London, Sage.

Seedhouse, D. (1986) *Health: The Foundations for Achievement.* Chichester, Wiley.

Seedhouse, D. (2001) *Health: The Foundations for Achievement.* 2nd edn. Chichester, Wiley.

Seligman, M.E.P. (2008) *Positive Health. Applied Psychology. An International Review* 57, 3–18.

Semple, S., Maccalman, L., Atherton Naji, A. et al. (2007) Bar workers' exposure to second-hand smoke: The effect of Scottish smoke-free legislation on occupational exposure. *Annals of Occupational Hygiene,* 1–10.

Sen, A. (1999) *Development as Freedom.* Oxford University Press, Oxford.

Shah, A. (2010) *Poverty Facts and Stats. Global Issues.* [Internet] Available at: http://www.globalissues.org/article/26/poverty-facts-and-stats [Accessed 11 August 2010].

Sharma, V. (2000) Diagnostic co-morbidity, attentional measures, and neuro-chemistry in children with ADHD. In Greenhill, L. & Osman, B., eds, *Ritalin, Theory and Practice.* Larchmont MD, Liebert. pp. 605–613.

Shaw, I. (2002) How lay are lay beliefs? *Health: An Interdisciplinary Journal for the Social Study of Health, Illness and Medicine* 6 (3), 287–99.

Shepherd, S. (2008) No smoking please, we're British. *Health Service Journal*, 24 July 2008, 20–3.

Shepperd, J., Peersman, G. & Napuli, I. (2009) *Interventions for Encouraging Sexual Lifestyles and Behaviours Intended to Prevent Cervical Cancer.* Cochrane Database of Systematic Reviews 4.

Shields, M. (2002) Shift work and health. *Health Reports,* July 13 (4), 11–34.

Sidell, M. (2010) Older People's health: Applying Antonovsky's salutogenic paradigm. In Douglas, J., Earle, S., Handsley, S., Jones, L., Lloyd, C. & Spurr, S., eds, *A Reader Promoting Public Health, Challenge and Controversy.* 2nd edn. London, Sage Publications. pp. 27–32.

Simpson, J. & Weiner, E. (1989) *Oxford English Dictionary.* 2nd edn. Oxford, Oxford University Press.

Skrabenek, P. & McCormick, J. (1989) *Follies and Fallacies in Medicine.* Tarragon Press, London.

Smith, J.A., Braunack-Mayer, A., Wittert, G. & Warin, M. (2008) 'It's sort of like being a detective': Understanding how Australian men monitor their health prior to seeking help. *BMC Health Services Research* 8, 56.

Smylie, L., Medaglia, S. & Maticka-Tyndale, E. (2006) The effect of social capital and socio-demographics on adolescent risk and sexual health behaviours. *The Canadian Journal of Human Sexuality* 15 (2), 95–112.

Sontag, S. (1989) *Illness as Metapor/AIDs and its Metaphors.* New York, Anchor.

Spector, S.J. (2009) Western Sahara and the self-determination debate. *Middle East Quarterly* 16 (3), 33–43

Spencer, N. & Logan, S. (2002) Social influences on birth weight. *Archives of Disease in Childhood Fetal and Neonatal Edition* 86, F6–F7.

Stainton-Rogers, W. (1991) *Explaining Health and Illness: An Exploration of Diversity.* London, Harvester/Wheatsheaf.

Stanley, N. (2009) *Time to 'Reclaim the Night' for Sleep.* BBC News. 11 February 2009 [Internet] Available at: http://news.bbc.co.uk/1/hi/7880583.stm [Accessed 6 October 2010].

Stansfeld, S. (2005) Social support and social cohesion. 2nd edn. In Marmot, M. & Wilkinson, R.G., eds, *Social Determinants of Health.* Oxford, Oxford University Press. pp. 155–78.

Stephens, C. (2008) *Health Promotion: A Psychosocial Approach.* Maidenhead, Open University Press.

Stephenson, J.M., Strange, V., Forrest, S. et al. (2004) Pupil-led sex education in England (RIPPLE study): Cluster-randomised intervention trial. *Lancet* 364 (9431), 338–46.

Stewart, J. (2001) The impact of health status on the duration of unemployment spells and the implications for studies of the impact of unemployment on health status. *Journal of Health Economics* 20, 781–96.

Stewart, J. & Thomas, S. (2004) Health promotion in context. *Environmental Health Journal,* December, 382–4.

Stiglitz, J. (2006) *Making Globalization Work. The Next Steps to Global Justice.* London, Allen Lane.

Stokols, D. (1998) Translating social ecological theory into guidelines for community health promotion. *American Journal of Health Promotion* 10 (4), 282–98.

Stone, D. (2009) Health and the natural environment. In Griffiths, J., Raos, M., Adshead, F. & Thorpe, A., eds, *The Health Practitioner's Guide to Climate Change: Diagnosis and Cure.* Earthscan, London & Sterling VA.

Straub, R.O. (2007) *Health Psychology: A Biopsychosocial Approach.* 2nd edn. New York, Worth Publishers.

Strömland, K., Mattson, S.N., Adnams, C., Autti-Ramö, M., Riley, E. P. & Warren, K.R. (2005) Fetal alcohol spectrum disorders: An international perspective. *Alcoholism: Clinical and Experimental Research* 29 (6), 1121–6.

Summerhayes, C. (2010) *Climate Change – An Emerging Issue in Health.* World Health Organization's Global Health Histories Seminar. [Internet] Available at: http://www.who.int/global_health_histories/seminars/presentation39a.pdf> [Accessed 11 October 2010].

Szmigin, I., Griffin, C., Mistral, W., Bengry-Howell, A., Weale, L. & Hackley, C. (2008) Re-framing 'binge-drinking' as calculated hedonism: Empirical evidence from the UK. *International Journal of Drug Policy* 19, 359–66.

Tafarodi, R.W. & Swann, W.B. (2001) Two-dimensional self-esteem; theory and measurement. *Personality and Individual Differences* 31 (5), 653–73.

Tait, N. (2006) Cancer sufferer loses drug fight. *Financial Times,* 16 February. p. 5.

Tannahill, A. (1985) What is health promotion? *Health Education Journal* 44, 167–8.

Tannahill, A. (2009) Health promotion: The Tannahill model revisited. *Public Health* 123, 396–9.

Tarnapol Whitacre, P., Tsai, P. & Mulligan, J. (2009) *The Public Health Effects of Food Deserts: Workshop Summary.* Washington DC, The National Academies Press.

Taylor, G. & Hawley, H. (2010) *Key Debates in Health Care.* Maidenhead, Open University Press.

The Free Dictionary (nd) *Definition of a model.* [Internet] Available at: http://www.thefreedictionary.com/model [Accessed on 3 February 2008].

The Queen's Nursing Institute (2007) *Briefing No 8: Health and Homelessness.* November 2007. London, The Queen's Nursing Institute.

The Say No to Mill Road Tesco campaign (2010) Home page. [Internet] available at http://www.nomillroadtecso.org [Accessed 20 September 2010].

Theorell, T., Blomkvist, V., Jonsson, H., Schulman, S., Berntorp, E. & Stigendal, L. (1995) Social support and the development of immune function in human immunodeficiency virus infection. *Psychosomatic Medicine* 57, 32–6.

Thirlaway, K. & Upton, D. (2009) *The Psychology of Lifestyle: Promoting Healthy Behaviours.* London, Routledge.

Thomas, L. (2006) Social capital and mental health of women living in informal settlements in Durban and Lusaka, Zambia. In McKenzie, K. & Harpham, T., eds, *Social Capital and Mental Health.* London, Jessica Kingsley Publishers. pp. 124–37.

Thomas, B., Dorling, D. & Davey Smith, G. (2010) Inequalities in premature mortality in Britain observational study from 1921 to 2007. *British Medical Journal* 341, 36–9.

Thorogood, N. (2002) What is the relevance of sociology for health promotion? In Bunton, R. & Macdonald, G., eds, *Health Promotion: Disciplines and Diversity.* 2nd edn. London, Routledge. pp. 53–79.

Thorp, J. (2010) *Improving livability in cities.* [Internet] Available at: http://www.youtube.com/watch?v=CtfV1V_eJ60 [Accessed 8 January 2011].

Tiefer, L. (2006) Female sexual dysfunction: A case study of disease mongering and activist resistance. *Public Library of Science Medicine* 3 (4), 178.

Timimi, S. (2005) *Naughty Boys. Anti-Social Behaviour, ADHD and the Role of Culture.* Hampshire, Palgrave Macmillan.

Tones, B.K. (1986) Health education and the ideology of health promotion: A review of alternative approaches. *Health Education Research* 1, 3–12.

Tones, K. & Green, J. (2004) *Health Promotion: Planning and Strategies.* London, Sage Publications.

Tones, K. & Tilford, S. (1994) *Health Education: Effectiveness, Efficiency and Equity.* 2nd edn. London, Chapman Hall.

Tones, K. & Tilford, S. (2001) *Health Promotion: Effectiveness, Efficiency and Equity.* 3rd edn. Cheltenham, Nelson Thornes.

Townsend, P. & Davidson, N. (1982) *Inequalities in Health: The Black Report.* London, Penguin.

Trifiletti, L.N., Gielen, A.C., Sleet, D.A. & Hopkins, K. (2005) Behavioural and social sciences theories and models: Are they used in unintentional injury prevention research? *Health Education Research* 20 (3), 298–307.

Trochim, W.M.K. (2006) *Research Methods Knowledge Base.* [Internet] available at http://www.socialresearchmethods.net/kb/. [Accessed 4 November 2010].

Twinn, S.F., Holroyd, E., Fabrizo, C., Moore, A. & Dickenson, J.A. (2007) Increasing knowledge about and uptake of cervical cancer screening in Hong Kong Chinese women over 40 years. *Hong Kong Medical Journal* 13 (2), 16–20.

Uchino, B.N. (2006) Social support and health: A review of physiological processes potentially underlying links to disease outcomes. *Journal of Behavioral Medicine* 29 (4), 377–87.

UNAIDS (1997) *The Female Condom and AIDS*. UNAIDS Best Practice Collection. April 1997.

UNAIDS (2007) *AIDS Epidemic Update: December 2007*. Geneva, UNAIDS and WHO .

UNAIDS (2009) *09 Aids Epidemic Update: November 2009*. Geneva, UNAIDS and WHO.

UNDP (2003) *Human Development Report 2003*. New York, United Nations Development Programme.

UNDP (2010) *Human Development Report 2010. Act Now, Act Together, Act Differently*. New York, United Nations Development Programme.

UNICEF (2010) *Progress on Sanitation and Drinking-Water. 2010 Update*. Geneva, WHO.

UNICEF (nd) *Goal: Improve Maternal Health*. [Internet] Available at: http://www.unicef.org/mdg/maternal.html [Accessed 12 August 2010].

United Nations (nd) *UN Data: A World of Information*. [Internet] Available at: http://data.un.org/Data.aspx?d=PopDiv&f=variableID%3A77 [Accessed 3 March 2010].

United Nations (2007) *Millennium Development Goals Report*. New York, United Nations.

UK Data Archive at the University of Essex (2009) *Survey Question Bank*. [Internet] available at http://surveynet.ac.uk/sqb/ [Accessed 6 November 2010].

Van Doorslaer, E., Masseria, C. & Koolman, X. (2006) Inequalities in access to medical care by income in developed countries. *CMAJ* 174 (2), 177–83.

Van Teijlingen, E. (2000) Maternity home care assistants in the Netherlands. In Van Teijlingen, E., Lowis, G., McCaffery, P. & Porter, M., eds, *Midwifery and the Medicalisation of Childbirth*. New York, Nova Science. pp. 163–72.

Vedung, E. (1988) *Carrots, Sticks and Sermons*. New Jersey, Transaction Press.

Vicary, D. & Westerman, T.G. (2004) 'That's just the way he is': Some implications of Aboriginal mental health beliefs. *Australian e-Journal for the Advancement of Mental Health* 3 (3), [Internet] Available at: http://auseinet.flinders.edu.au/journal/vol3iss3/vicarywesterman.pdf [Accessed January 2008].

Vostanis, P. (2007) Mental health and mental disorders. In Coleman, J. & Hagell, A., eds, *Adolescence, Risk and Resilience*. Chichester, John Wiley and Sons. pp. 89–106.

Wade, T. D. & Kendler, K. S. (2000) The relationship between social support and major depression: Cross-sectional, longitudinal, and genetic perspectives. *Journal of Nervous and Mental Disease* 188, 251–8.

Wainwright, D. (1996) The political transformation of the health inequalities debate. *Critical Social Policy* 49 (16), 67–82.

Wainwright, D. (2009a) Illness behaviour and the discourse of health.

In Wainwright, D., ed., *A Sociology of Health*. London, Sage. pp. 76–96.

Wainwright, D. (2009b) The changing face of medical sociology. In Wainwright, D., ed., *A Sociology of Health*. London, Sage. pp. 1–18.

Walboomers, J.M.M. & Meijer, C. (1997) Do HPV-negative cervical carcinomas exist? *Journal of Pathology* 181, 253–4.

Waller, J., Marlow, L.A.V. & Wardle, J. (2006) Mothers' attitudes towards preventing cervical cancer through human papillomavirus vaccination: A qualitative study of cancer. *Epidemiology, Biomarkers and Prevention* 15, 1257–61.

Wallerstein, N. (1992) Powerlessness, empowerment, and health: Implications for health promotion programs. *American Journal of Health Promotion* 6 (3), 197–205.

Walley, J. & Wright, J. (2010) *Public Health: An Action Guide to Improving Health*. Oxford, Oxford University Press.

Walley, J. & Gerein, N. (2010) Maternal, neonatal, and child health. In Walley, J. & Wright, J., eds, *Public Health: An Action Guide to Improving Health*. Oxford, Oxford University Press. pp. 181–213.

Walley, J., Webber, R. & Collins, A. (2010) Controlling major communicable diseases. In Walley, J. & Wright, J., eds, *Public Health: An Action Guide to Improving Health*. Oxford, Oxford University Press. pp. 259–87.

Wallston, K.A. & Wallston, B.S. (1982) Who is responsible for your health? The construct of health locus of control. In Sanders, G. & Suls, J., eds, *Social Psychology of Health and Illness*. Hillsdale, NJ. Erlbaum. pp. 65–95.

Walt, G. & Buse, K. (2006) Global cooperation in international public health. In Merson, M.H., Black, R.E. & Mills, A.J., eds, *International Public Health: Diseases, Programs, Systems and Policies*. Boston, Jones and Bartlett Publishers. pp. 649–80.

Walters, R., Gottlieb, D.J. & O'Connor, G.T. (2000) Environmental and genetic risk factors and gene-environmental interactions in the pathogenesis of chronic obstructive lung disease. *Environmental Health Perspectives* 108, Supplement 4. August, 733–833.

Wang, S., Moss, J.R. & Hiller, J.E. (2005) Applicability and transferability of interventions in evidence-based public health. *Health Promotion International* 21 (1), 76–83.

Wanless, D. (2002) *Securing Our Future Health*. London, Treasury.

Wanless, D., Appleby, J., Harrison, A. & Patel, A. (2007) *Our Future Health Secured? A Review of NHS Funding and Performance*. London, The Kings Fund.

Waters, E. & Doyle, J. (2002) Evidence-based public health practice: Improving the quality and quantity of the evidence. *Journal of Public Health Medicine* 24 (3), 227–9.

Weaver, L.T. (2001) The child is father of the man: Paediatricians should be more interested in adult disease. *Clinical Medicine* 1, Jan/Feb, 38–43.

Webster, C. & French, J. (2002) The cycle of conflict: The history of the public health and health promotion movements. In Adams, L., Amos, M. & Munro, J., eds, *Promoting Health: Politics and Practice*. London, Sage. pp. 5–12.

Welshman, J. (2002) The cycle of deprivation and the concept of the underclass. *Benefits* 35 (10), Issue 3, 199–206.

White, J. (2009) *What is the Future for Health Promotion?* Leeds, Centre for Health Promotion Research, Leeds Metropolitan University.

White, C. & Edgar, G. (2010) Inequalities in healthy life expectancy by social class and area type: England, 2001–03. *Health Statistics Quarterly* 45, Spring 2010 London, Office for National Statistics.

Whitehead, M. (1988) *The Health Divide*. London, Pelican Books.

Whitehead, M. (1995) Tackling health inequalities: A review of policy initiatives. In Benzeval, M., Judge, K. & Whitehead, M., eds, *Tackling Inequalities in Health: An Agenda for Action*. London, Kings Fund, 1995. pp. 22–52.

Whitley, R., Kirmayer, L. & Groleau, D. (2006) Understanding immigrants' reluctance to use mental health services: A qualitative study from Montreal. *Canadian Journal of Psychiatry* 51, 205–9.

Wilkinson. P. (2005) Global environmental change and health. In Scriven, A. & Garman, S., eds, *Promoting Health: Global Perspectives*. Basingstoke, Palgrave Macmillan. pp. 129–38.

Wilkinson, R. (1996) *Unhealthy Societies: The Afflictions of Inequality*. London, Routledge.

Wilkinson, S. & Kitzinger, C. (2000) Thinking differently about thinking positive: A discursive approach to cancer patients' talk. *Social Science and Medicine* 50, 797–811.

Wilkinson, R. & Pickett, K. (2009) *The Spirit Level: Why Equal Societies Almost Always Do Better*. London, Allen & Unwin.

Wilkinson, R.G. & Pickett, K. (2010) *The Spirit Level: Why Equality is Better for Everyone*. London, Allen Lane.

Williams, J.S., Gabe, J. & Davis, P. (2009) The sociology of pharmaceuticals: Progress and prospects. In Williams, J.S., Gabe, J. & Davis, P., eds, *Pharmaceuticals and Society: Critical Discourses and Debates*. US, Wiley Blackwell. pp. 1–13.

Wilmoth, J., Mathers, C., Say, L. & Mills, S. (2010) Maternal death drop by one-third from 1990–2008: A United Nations analysis. *Bulletin World Health Organization* 88.

Winter, I. (2000) *Towards a Theorised Understanding of Family Life and Social Capital*. Melbourne, Australian Institute of Family Studies.

Wisker, G. (2001) *The Postgraduate Research Handbook. Succeed with Your MA, MPhil and PhD*. Palgrave Study Guides, Hampshire.

Woodall, J., Dixey, R., Green, J. & Newell, C. (2009) Healthier prisons: The role of a prison visitors' centre. *International Journal of Health Promotion and Education* 47 (1), 12–18.

Woodall, J., Raine, G., South, J. & Warwick-Booth, L. (2010) *Empowerment* and *Health & Well-Being Evidence Review*. Leeds Centre for Health Promotion Research, Leeds Metropolitan University.

World Bank (nd) *World Bank Indicators*. [Internet] Available at: http://data.worldbank.org/indicator [Accessed 3 March 2010].

World Bank (2002) *World Development Indicators CD-ROM*. Washington DC, World Bank.

World Bank (2003) *World Development Indicators CD-ROM*. Washington DC, World Bank.

World Bank (2008) *World Development Indicators*. August 2008 [Internet] Available at http://data.worldbank.org/indicator> [Accessed 11 August 2010].

World Food Programme (2009) *Food Crisis Fact Sheet: Weathering the Storm*. World Food Programme. 29 April 2009. [Internet] Available at: http://documents.wfp.org/stellent/groups/public/documents/newsroom/wfp197596.pdf> [Accessed 11 August 2010].

World Health Organization (nd) *Global Health Observatory Botswana*. [Internet] Available at: http://www.who.int/gho/countries/bwa/en/ [Accessed 3 March 2010].

World Health Organization (1986) *Ottawa Charter for Health Promotion: First International Conference on Health Promotion*. Geneva, WHO.

World Health Organization (1991) *Sundsvall Statement on Supportive Environments for Health: Third International Conference on Health Promotion*. Geneva, WHO.

World Health Organization (1995a) *The World Health Report 1995: Bridging the Gaps*. Geneva, WHO.

World Health Organization (1995b) The WHOQOL Group. The World Health Organization quality of life assessment position paper from WHO. *Social Science and Medicine* 41, 1403–9.

World Health Organization (2000) *The World Health Report*. Geneva, WHO.

World Health Organization (2001) *The World Health Report 2001. Mental Health: New Understanding, New Hope*. Geneva, WHO.

World Health Organization (2002) *Global Crises – Global Solutions: Managing Public Health Emergencies of International Concern through the Revised International Health Regulation*. Geneva, WHO.

World Health Organization (2004) *Summary of Probable SARs Cases with Onset of Illness from 1 November 2002 to 31 July 2003* http://www.who.int/csr/sars/country/table2004_04_21/en/index.html (accessed 12.7.2011)

World Health Organization (2005a) *Climate and Health. Fact Sheet*. July 2005 [Internet] Available at: www.who.int/globalchange/news/fsclimandhealth/en/print.html [Accessed 13 January 2010].

World Health Organization (2005b) *Ecosystems and Human Well-Being: Health Synthesis. Report of the Millennium Ecosystem Assessment*. Geneva, WHO.

World Health Organization (2005c) *Draft Discussion Paper for the Commission on Social Determinants of Health*. 5 May 2005, Geneva, WHO.

World Health Organization (2005d) *The Bangkok Charter for Health Promotion in a Globalised World*. Geneva, WHO.

World Health Organization (2006) *The Definition of Health*. Geneva, WHO.

World Health Organization (2007) *Ageing*. [Internet] Available at: http://www.who.int/topics/ageing/en/ [Accessed 8 December 2010].

World Health Organization (2007a) *The World Health Report 2007: A Safer Future: Global Public Health Security in the 21st Century*. Geneva, WHO.

World Health Organization (2007b) *World Health Statistics, 2007*. Geneva, WHO.

World Health Organization (2008) *The Global Burden of Disease: 2004 Update*. Geneva, WHO.

World Health Organization (2008a) *The Right to Health. Fact Sheet 31*. Geneva, WHO.

World Health Organization (2008b) *Protecting Health from Climate Change – World Health Day 2008*. Geneva, WHO.

World Health Organization (2009) *Global Health Risks. Mortality and Burden of Disease Attributable to Selected Major Risks*. Geneva, WHO.

World Health Organization (2009a) *Public Health and Environment. Health through a Better Environment* [internet] Available from: http://www.who.int/phe/en/ [Accessed 19 November 2010].

World Health Organization (2009b) *Mental Health: A State of Well-Being*. [Internet] Available at: http://www.who.int/features/factfiles/mental_health/en/index.html [Accessed 17 November 2010].

World Health Organization (2009) *The Determinants of Health*. [Internet] Available at: http://www.who.int/jia/evidence/doh/en/> [Accessed 10 November 2010].

World Health Organization (2010a) *World Malaria Report 2010*. Geneva, WHO.

World Health Organization (2010b) Vaccinating against cervical cancer. [Internet] Available at: http://www.who.int/bulletin/volumes/85/2/07–020207/en/index.html [Accessed 10 January 2011].

WHO (2011) Health Impact Assessment Glossary [Internet] Available at http://www.who.int/hia/about/glos/en/index1.html [Accessed 10.01.2011].

Wray, R. (2010) Russian drought could push up food prices. *Guardian*, 9 August 2010 [Internet] Available from: http://www.guardian.co.uk/business/2010/aug/09/russian-drought-wheat-prices [Accessed 11 August 2010].

Wright, O. (2003) Ritalin use and abuse fears. *The Times* (UK) 28, 3 July, p. 3.

Wright, J. & Walley, J. (2010) Future trends in global public health. In Walley, J. & Wright, J., eds, *Public Health: An Action Guide to Improving Health*. Oxford, Oxford University Press. pp. 319–56.

Yamey, G. (2002) Why does the world still need WHO? *British Medical Journal* 325, 1294–1298.

Yount, K.M. & Gittelsohn, J. (2008) Comparing reports of health seeking behaviour form the integrated illness history and a standard child morbidity survey. *Journal of Mixed Methods Research* 2 (1), 23–62.

Yuill, C., Crinson, I. & Duncan, E. (2010) *Key Concepts in Health Studies.* London, Sage.

Zborowski, M. (1952) Cultural components in responses to pain. *Journal of Social Issues* 8, 16–30.

Zola, I. K. (1972) Medicine as an institution of social control. *Sociological Review* 20, 487–503.

Index

access to services, 192, 242, 254, 275, 284, 288
acupuncture, 117, 118, 119
addiction, 103, 135, 142, 185, 186, 246
aetiology, 101, 294
ageing/ageing population, 37, 42, 43, 47, 182, 235, 236
agency, xxv, 47, 90
agriculture and food production, 214–17, 226
alcohol
  addictive personality, 186
  Beattie's model of health, 156
  binge-drinking, 27
  cultural influences on health, 124
  death rates from associated diseases, 83
  determinants of health 'rainbow', 287
  drink driving, 158
  Foetal Alcohol Syndrome, 178, 179
  gender differences, 45
  global health, 253
  health-risk behaviours, 134
  homelessness, 219
  illness associated with over-consumption, 29
  legislative changes, 157, 245
  lifestyle factors, 103, 133, 304
  shifting patterns of use, 47
  social capital, 201
  social class differences, 48
  social inequalities, 246
  social policy, 233, 234, 235
  unemployment, 222
alternative treatments, 117–18
anthropology, xxiv, 109–10, 113–15, 117, 122, 126–9, 298
  see also culture
artefact explanation, 101, 102
association, 34, 58, 64, 227, 294
attention deficit hyperactivity disorder (ADHD), 95, 98, 127
attitudes
  to cancer, 120–1
  to chlamydia, 57
  cultural influences, 111, 112–13, 116, 117–19, 123, 125, 126, 288
  definition of, 294

  to disability, 98, 99
  domestic violence, 170
  gendering of mental health, 106
  health education, 155
  health promotion, 158
  ideology, 239, 241–2
  lifestyle factors, 47
  to medicine, 129
  motivation, 187
  professional, 110
  qualitative research, 75
  to risk, 96
  safe sex, 188
  stigma, 93
  surveys, 60
  Theory of Planned Behaviour, 139, 140, 141
autonomy, 77, 167, 174, 294
Ayurvedic approaches, 120

Barton and Grant health map, 291–2
Beattie's model of health, 154, 155–8, 159
bias, 70, 73, 113, 145, 294–5
Big Society debate, 208
biographical disruption, 92, 94
biological determinism, 115
biological factors, 135, 189
  biopsychosocial model of health, 16
  definition of, 295
  health promotion, 152
  holistic model of health, 16
  medical anthropology, 110
  medical model of health, 13, 15
  pain, 82
  risk-taking behaviour, 186
  social model of health, 14
  social support, 197
  threats to health, 31
biological sex, 181–3, 191, 193, 311–12
biomedical model see medical model of health
biomedicine, 81, 113, 115, 119, 125, 127, 295
biopsychosocial model of health, 16–17
Black Report, 99, 100, 101, 240
brain drain, 254–5
British Household Survey, 59, 200, 295

cancer
  ageing population, 235
  anti-cancer drugs, 237
  breast, 159
  cervical, 168, 181, 277–84, 302, 306, 312
  changing patterns of, 38
  cultural context, 120–2
  'epidemiological transition', 35
  genetic factors, 184
  health care services, 224
  lifestyle factors, 133, 253
  lung, 45, 58, 131, 243, 252, 281, 286, 294
  media attention, 231
  patient research, 56, 83
  radiation exposure, 294
  skin, 41, 124, 147
  social class differences, 48
  social support, 198
  testicular, 138, 181–3
  working environment, 220–1
capitalism, 94, 270
Caplan and Holland's model of health, 154, 162–4, 170
census, 59, 60, 295
cervical cancer, 168, 181, 277–84, 302, 306, 312
characteristics, xxv, 3, 174, 176–93
  age, 181
  biology and biological sex, 181–3
  definition of, 295
  foetal development, 177–80
  gender, 183
  health-seeking strategies, 118
  heredity and genetic factors, 183–4
  HIV/AIDS, 191
  lifespan perspective, 189–92
  nature/nurture debate, 188–9
  personality, 184–7
  psychological, 138
  sampling, 62, 73, 74
  self-esteem, 187–8
childbirth, 97, 112–13, 181, 182, 224, 267
chronic illness, 90, 92, 93, 235, 243
citizenship, 18, 284, 295–6
class *see* social class
climate change, 33, 40–1, 49, 50, 161, 225, 259, 276, 292
clinical trials, 258
coalition government, 153, 208, 239, 247
cohort studies, 56, 81, 296
collectivism, 296
commercialization, 118
Commission on the Social Determinants of Health, 100
communicable diseases, 2, 35–7, 219, 220, 266, 267, 268, 296
community, xxvi, 3
  Alt Valley Community Trust, 203
  Barton and Grant health map, 292

community-led total sanitation, 217
  Dahlgren and Whitehead model, 173, 174, 274, 279, 281, 287
  definition of, 296
  empowerment, 159, 162
  health career, 190
  health promotion, 151, 152, 157–8, 163, 167, 171, 172
  mental health, 123
  neglect of community health, 31
  neighbourhoods, 282–6
  networks, 194, 195–8, 200, 204–7, 209, 211, 289, 313
  quantitative research, 61
  rituals, 119
  social capital, 198, 199, 200
  social well-being, 9
  Zambian Open Community Schools, 210
concept of health, xxiii, 2, 7–28, 106
  definition of, 296
  definitions of health, 7–12, 26
  lay perspectives, 18–25
  theoretical perspectives, 12–18
  threats to health, 30
conservatism, 240
constructs/construction, 3, 13, 189
  ADHD, 127
  behaviour change models, 142, 145
  definition of, 297
  gender, 96, 112, 178, 183, 191
  healthworlds, 118
  Locus of Control, 136
  medicine, 126, 129
  motivation, 187
  personality, 184, 185
  psychological constructs, 191, 193
  qualitative research, 76
  quantitative research, 58
  self-esteem, 187
  see also social constructionism
consumerism, 9, 105, 296–7
consumption
  alcohol, 124, 222, 233, 234, 245, 253, 287
  consumer society, 297
  environmental threats, 259
  food, 116, 143, 215, 217, 253, 256, 296
  lifestyle diseases, 29, 47
contraception, 36–7, 141, 188
corporations, 256, 258, 264, 268, 271
critical appraisal, 79–80
critical health psychology, 148
critique, 20, 89, 102, 104–5, 297
culture, xxiv, 2, 109–29
  behaviour change models, 145
  cultural influences on health, 124–6
  cultural representations, 120–2, 123
  definition of, 297
  determinants of health, 242
  domestic violence, 170

ethnography, 110, 300
experience of illness, 115–16
gendering of mental health, 106
health career, 190
lay understandings of health, 20–2, 25
mental illness, 122–3
pain, 82
social anthropology, 109–10
social constructionism, 17
social networks, 203
treatment, 117–20

Dahlgren and Whitehead model, xxv,
    xxvi, xxvii, 3, 14, 173–5, 272
as analytical tool, 281
cervical cancer, 279
evaluation of, 287–92, 293
global environment, 251
individual characteristics, 176, 189
malaria, 274
neighbourhood health, 284
physical environment, 212, 225
social and community characteristics,
    194, 201
social model of health, 15
social policy, 229
threats to health, 33
DALYs (disability adjusted life years), 50,
    297, 301
deconstruction, 98, 297–8
demographics, 60, 138, 140, 235
determinants of health, 12, 175, 287–92,
    293
    Barton and Grant health map, 291–2
    behaviour, 133, 134–6, 145
    community development, 157
    culture, 111, 128
    definition of, 298
    environmental, 152, 153, 158–9, 171
    global environment, xxvii, 251
    health promotion, 164, 165, 169, 171
    health services, 242–3
    inequalities, 301
    lifestyles, 304
    neighbourhood health, 282–4, 286
    policy, 161, 233–4, 236, 244, 247–9
    social, xxvi, 37, 44, 47, 103, 152, 158–9,
        211, 221, 268, 292, 313
    social capital, 209
    society, 99–104
    structural, 47, 171
    threats to health, 30–3, 50
    see also Dahlgren and Whitehead
        model
diabetes, 32, 57, 235, 243
diet, 184, 287
    children's understandings of health,
        22
    cultural identity, 135
    health inequalities, 102
    high fat, 31, 48, 134

illness metaphors, 121
lay health beliefs, 116
lifestyle choices, 103, 133
obesity, 124
policy, 234
poverty, 225
Stages of Change Model, 143
disability, 10, 30, 33, 125
    age inequalities, 45
    chronic illnesses, 243
    concepts of health, 24
    depression, 252
    disability adjusted life years, 50, 297,
        301
    Foetal Alcohol Syndrome, 179
    social class, 104
    social constructionism, 98, 99
    social model of, 92
    stigma, 93
    TB, 262
disciplines, 2, 26, 85–6, 104, 110, 132
    definition of, 298
    health promotion, 169, 171
    interdisciplinarity, 1, 85, 171, 303
    multi-disciplinarity, 1, 85, 149, 306
discourse, 31, 32
    binge-drinking, 27
    definition of, 298
    global, 253
    health beliefs, 115
    'healthy weight', 21
    HIV/AIDS, 35
    mainstream, 13, 20
    medicine, 125
    metaphorical, 120
    post structuralism, 98–9
    professional, 18
    risk, 47
    social constructionism, 17
disease
    alcohol associated, 83, 235
    association, 294
    biological differences, 181, 183
    biomedicine, 295
    changing patterns of, 38, 43, 50
    climate change impact on, 40, 41
    cohort studies, 296
    communicable, 2, 35–7, 219, 220, 266,
        267, 268, 296
    conflict and war, 44
    culture and, 112, 113, 119, 120–2
    definitions of health, 12
    fear of, 34
    foetal programming, 178, 179
    globalization, 251, 252, 253, 254,
        256–68, 270
    health as absence of, 2, 5, 8, 9, 10, 164
    health indicators, 301
    health psychology, 131, 133
    heredity and genetic factors, 183–4
    illness distinction, 115

disease (*cont.*)
  infectious, 35–8, 40, 46–7, 49–50, 220,
    235, 243, 254, 256–7, 260–2, 267,
    296, 305
  lifestyle, 47–8
  malnourishment, 214–15
  medical anthropology, 110
  medical model, 13, 15, 16
  morbidity, 305–6
  NHS model of health care, 243
  non-communicable, 2, 35–7, 47, 268,
    306
  old age, 23, 43
  pathology, 308
  personality, 185
  positivism, 309
  prevalence, 47, 287, 301, 306, 309
  prevention, 154, 159, 233
  quantitative data, 59
  reductionism, 311
  risk, 312
  sexually-transmitted, 278
  social capital, 201
  social construction of, 102
  social determinants of health, 44–5,
    103
  social support, 196–7
  sociology, 95
  threats to health, 30, 31–3
  urbanization, 219
  welfare state, 238
  see also cancer; epidemics; incidence;
    pandemics
dissertations, 6
domestic violence, 63, 170
downstream approaches, 203, 243
drugs
  access to, 261, 267
  ADHD, 127
  cancer, 231
  financing, 262, 263
  hallucinogenic, 126
  HIV/AIDS, 191, 262
  lifestyle conditions, 95
  malaria, 275, 276
  Marxist perspective, 94
  NICE role, 237
  recreational use/addiction, 47, 121,
    126, 178, 185, 186, 219, 246
  TB, 47
  testing, 61
  TRIPs, 257
  WHO Essential Drugs List, 258

ecological theory, 289, 290
education, 21, 223–4
  health promotion, 152, 153, 155,
    160–1, 169
  investment in, 260
  malaria, 276
  neighbourhood health, 283, 286

policy, 229
  welfare state, 238
  see also health promotion
egalitarianism, 203, 298–9
empirical research, 19, 69, 133, 134, 140,
  201, 299
empowerment, 10, 157, 159, 160–2,
  166–7, 171, 188, 291, 299
environment, xxvi, 3, 177, 189, 192,
  212–28, 249
  agriculture and food production,
    214–17, 226
  Barton and Grant health map, 292
  behaviour change models, 145
  cervical cancer, 279, 280
  cultural, 118, 122, 288
  Dahlgren and Whitehead model, 173,
    174, 288–92
  definition of, 299
  determinants of health, 32, 102–3, 298
  education, 223–4
  family, 186
  foetal development, 178–9
  global, 251, 258–9, 266–9
  Health Action Model, 146
  health care services, 224, 226
  health career, 190
  health promotion, 152, 153, 158–9,
    161–4, 169, 171
  housing, 218–20, 226
  interaction with genetic factors, 183,
    184, 193
  malaria, 274, 276
  medical model of health, 13
  National Children's Study, 180
  nature/nurture debate, 188
  neighbourhoods, 282, 283, 284–5, 286
  obesogenic, 124
  policy impact on, 233
  social model of health, 14, 15
  understandings of health, 22, 25, 116
  unemployment, 221–2
  water and sanitation, 217–18, 226
  work, 104, 220–1, 226, 244, 288
  World Bank projects, 265
  see also climate change
environmentalism, 241
epidemics, 27, 37, 46, 47, 51, 264
  definition of, 299
  fear of, 34
  HIV/AIDS, 261–2, 266
  migration, 254
epistemology, 56, 83, 299–300
equity, 161, 167, 168, 171, 268, 291, 300
  see also inequity
ethics, 77–8, 84, 167–8, 258
ethnography, 110, 300
ethnomedicine, 110
evaluation, 166, 172, 297
evidence, xxiii, 56, 78–81, 83–4, 300
  abortion of girls, 269

ADHD, 127
birth weight and later disease, 179
breastfeeding, 256
childbirth, 97
cultural interpretations of illness, 113
disadvantaged individuals, 287
family ties, 204
gender differences, 183
global health, 252, 253–4, 290
Health Belief Model, 139
health care services, 224, 242
health inequalities, 99–103, 105,
    246–7, 306
health problems of modernity, 125
health promotion, 166, 169, 171
health-related behaviours, 131, 133–4
housing and ill health, 219
impact of education on health, 223
individual differences, 189
lifestyle interventions, 146, 234
malaria, 276
MMR vaccine, 128
NICE, 237
personality, 185, 186, 187, 193
pharmacological treatments, 120
resilience, 123
smoking, 278
social capital, 200, 201–2, 207, 209
social democracy, 241
social differences, 114–15
social structure, 99, 280, 313
social support, 196, 209
threats to health, 40, 41, 43, 44, 47–8
unemployment and ill health, 222
vCJD, 49
evidence-based practice (EBP), xxiii,
    78–81, 83, 166, 300
expectations, 118, 129, 230, 301
cultural, 112, 115, 124, 126
men, 100, 222
modern treatment, 95, 235–6
experiments, 56, 58, 61, 76, 81, 145, 179,
    300

Fabians, 241
factor, definition of, 300
faith-based organizations, 205–6
family ties, 204–5
fatalism, 142
fear, 34, 43, 126, 142
cancer, 121
crime, 283, 285
epidemics, 46
'mad cow disease', 49
MMR vaccine, 231
moral panics, 35
terrorism, 44
femininity, 183, 222
feminism, 89, 96, 97, 126, 241, 307
fiscal policy, 246–7
focus groups, 56, 69, 70, 71, 76, 82, 305

Foetal Alcohol Syndrome (FAS), 178, 179
foetal development, 177–80
foetal origins hypothesis, 302
folk medicine, 118, 122
free trade, 256, 265
functionalism, 90–1
functionality, 114, 115

gender, 105, 115, 174, 178, 183, 189
cultural factors, 112
definition of, 301
determinants of health, 298
domestic violence, 170
feminism, 96, 241
functionalism, 90
Health Belief Model, 138
health inequalities, 45, 99, 100
health-seeking behaviour, 118
healthy eating, 57
HIV/AIDS, 191
interventions, 192
levels of measurement, 65
Marxism, 96
mental health, 106
Millennium Development Goals, 267
risk-taking behaviour, 185
sampling methods, 62, 73
social model of health, 14
understandings of health, 19, 20,
    23–4, 27
unemployment, 222
women's health, 193
genetic factors, 178, 183–4, 192
global consciousness, 253
global governance, 253, 264, 266, 270,
    301
global society, 4, 175, 251–2, 253, 290
globalization, xxvi–xxvii, 4, 175, 251,
    252–4, 263, 268–70
definition of, 301
environmental damage, 258–9
food production, 216
global policy, 264–8
trade, 255–8

hallucinogenic drugs, 126
healing, 110, 118, 122–3, 128
Health Action Model (HAM), 144–6, 184,
    187, 188
health behaviour, 130–48
cervical cancer, 279–80
cultural factors, 112, 115, 124, 127–8
gender differences, 301
health damaging behaviour, 124, 280,
    287
health enhancing behaviour, 133, 134,
    280
individual differences, 189, 192
mothers, 182
responsibility for, 242
social networks, 203

health behaviour, 130–48 (cont.)
  sociology, 99, 105
  victim blaming, 165–6
  see also psychological factors
Health Belief Model, 136, 137–9, 140
health beliefs, 18–25, 111, 115–17, 119–20,
    126–8, 276, 301, 304
health care services, 224, 226, 233,
    242–3, 275, 284
health care systems, 241–2, 249–50, 255,
    263, 265
health career, 190, 192
Health Field Concept, 214
health indicators, 40, 301
health inequality see inequality
health inequity see inequity
health promotion, xxv, 150–72
  cervical cancer, 279–80
  contribution of, 169–71
  critiques of, 104–5, 168–9
  Dahlgren and Whitehead model, 291
  definitions of health, 26
  empowerment, 299
  environmental factors, 225, 226–7
  global, 266
  health behaviour, 133, 146–8
  Health Belief Model, 138
  HIV/AIDS, 266
  individual responsibility, 18
  Lalonde Report, 213–14
  lay understandings of health, 20
  models, 154–64, 305
  origins of, 152–4
  personality, 185
  policy, 233, 243
  principles and values, 164–8
  'settings' approach, 226, 227, 228, 282
  social capital, 209
  social model of health, 14–15, 104
health scares, 34
health threats, xxiii, 29–51, 267–8, 301
  climate change, 40–1
  diseases, 35–8, 46–8
  magnitude and severity, 33
  media construction and moral panics,
    33–5
  mental health, 45
  nature and determinants of health,
    30–3
  population growth, 41–3
  poverty and inequality, 44–5
  safety, security and fear, 43–4
health tourism, 255
healthworlds, 118
healthy public policy, 153, 160–2, 169,
    171, 174, 243–4, 249, 286, 302
heredity, 178, 183–4
HIV/AIDS, 30, 33, 46, 257, 263, 281, 286,
    296
  Africa, 252, 260, 261–2
  CD$_4$ cell count, 59, 198

cervical cancer, 278
early marriages, 269
education, 223
health promotion, 266
individual characteristics, 191
life expectancy, 37
low-income countries, 45
Millennium Development Goals, 268
moral panics, 35
social capital, 201
stigma, 93, 121, 314
TB relationship, 47
women's vulnerability to, 183
Zambian Open Community Schools,
    210
holistic approaches, 17, 209
  cultural beliefs, 126
  definition of, 302
  definitions of health, 8, 12
  health behaviour, 132, 133, 145
  holistic model of health, 16
  lay understandings of health, 115
  mental health, 45
  policy, 246
  social capital, 201
  social model of health, 15
  threats to health, 43
homeopathy, 118, 119
housing, 102, 218–20, 226, 238, 283,
    284, 288
HPV, 277–8, 281, 302
human rights, 10, 43, 249, 267, 268
humanism, 10, 12, 163–4, 170, 302
hypotheses, 58, 66–7, 68, 76, 178, 300,
    302

identity, 92–3, 94, 125
  alcohol use, 124
  cultural, 135
  definition of, 303
  education, 223
  indigenous people, 118
  national, 240
  social capital, 198
ideology, 174, 239–42, 249, 265, 303
idleness, 238
ignorance, 238
illness complaints, 115
illness experiences, 93, 112, 115–16, 122,
    129, 310, 314
illness metaphors, 121
illness problems, 115
incidence
  alcoholism, 124
  cervical cancer, 278, 279, 280
  definition of, 303
  headlice, 33
  HIV/AIDS, 33, 191, 261, 268
  malaria, 276
  mental health, 123
  smoking and heart-attack, 243

individual characteristics *see* characteristics
inequality, 99–104, 105, 227
  access to services, 20
  cervical cancer, 279
  Dahlgren and Whitehead model, 288–9, 290, 291
  definition of, 301
  democratic societies, 203
  GAVI, 257–8
  gender, 96, 170, 270
  global, 251, 253, 259–62, 263, 264, 301
  government agenda, 205
  health promotion, 152–3, 165, 167, 291
  ideological positions, 240, 241, 303
  inequity, 301–2
  malaria prevention, 275
  Marxist perspective, 94
  Millennium Development Goals, 266
  morbidity rates, 306
  neo-liberalism, 306
  policy, 161, 230, 233, 244, 246–7, 285–6, 288
  research, 83
  social, 103, 126, 247, 264, 268, 289, 291, 313
  social capital, 201, 202
  social model of health, 14, 15
  threats to health, 44–5
  WHO report, 268
  World Bank, 265
inequity, 45, 50, 167, 242, 301–2
infectious diseases, 35–8, 40, 46–7, 49–50, 220, 235, 243, 254, 256–7, 260–2, 267, 296, 305
interdisciplinarity, 1, 85, 171, 303
interest groups, 231
interpretivism, 54–5, 56, 57, 82, 303, 314
interviews, 57, 69, 70, 74, 76, 78, 305
ITNs (insecticide treated nets), 273, 274, 276, 277

Jamie's School Dinners campaign, 160, 161
justice, 83, 159, 167, 170, 300, 303

labelling, 121, 122, 314
Lalonde Report, 213–14
lay health beliefs, 18–25, 115–17, 119–20, 126–8, 276, 304
liberalism, 240
life expectancy
  ageing populations, 43
  decreases in, 201
  gender differences, 23, 100
  health indicators, 301
  health promotion, 171
  improvement in, 34, 37, 38
  income relationship, 39
  inequalities, 244, 246, 259–60, 261

life-course, 116, 181, 182, 189–92, 193, 290
lifespan, 189–92, 304
lifestyle
  Barton and Grant health map, 292
  behaviour change, 146, 286
  cervical cancer, 279–80
  changing patterns, 132–3
  cholesterol levels, 184
  cultural factors, 121, 125
  Dahlgren and Whitehead model, 173, 288, 290
  definition of, 135, 304
  diseases, 35, 47–8
  education, 223
  financial barriers, 287
  gender differences, 183
  globalization of unhealthy, 253
  happiness, 187
  Health Field Concept, 214
  health promotion, 151, 153, 164, 169, 171
  ideological beliefs, 242
  low-income countries, 256
  malaria, 274, 275–6
  neighbourhood health, 284
  policy, 231, 234, 235–6
  social model of health, 14
  sociological perspective, 95, 101–2, 103, 104
  understandings of health, 19
literature, 25, 53–4, 56, 80, 304
Locus of Control, 136–7
long-term conditions, 235

macro-level, 87–8, 89, 198, 304
'mad cow disease', 49
mainstream, 13, 17, 20, 148, 149, 304
malaria, 30, 37, 265, 266, 270, 273–7
  Africa, 44, 262
  climate change impact on, 40, 41
  Millennium Development Goals, 267
  multi-disciplinary approach, 306
  pharmaceuticals, 257
  poverty, 260
  pregnant women, 183
  screening, 312
malnutrition, 179, 214–15, 219, 265, 276
  climate change impact on, 40
  deaths from, 41, 252
  'epidemiological transition', 35
  female babies, 269
  health promotion, 152
  poverty, 260, 273
marginalized populations, 33, 126
markets, 255, 292
Marxism, 46, 89, 93, 94–6, 163, 240, 308
masculinity, 106, 183, 222
material deprivation, 44, 103
  see also poverty
ME, 114

media
  climate change, 40
  crime and terrorism, 43
  cultural representations, 120, 121, 123, 128
  fossil fuels, 245
  health beliefs, 115, 116
  health career, 190
  health promotion, 151, 158, 160
  inequities in access to health services, 242
  infectious diseases, 46
  lifestyle diseases, 48
  malaria interventions, 274
  MMR, 231
  policy, 231–2, 235, 249
  research evidence, 83
  starvation, 219
  threats to health, 30, 33–5, 36, 50
  vCJD, 49
medical (biomedical) model of health, 13–14, 15, 16, 17, 20, 162
  cultural factors, 111, 113, 115–16, 119, 129
  sociological critique of, 101, 106
medicalization, 95–6, 97, 106, 107, 125–6, 127, 152, 304–5
medicine
  access to, 257, 270
  childbirth, 97
  critiques of, 89, 94–5, 129
  cultural factors, 112, 117–18, 119–20, 122, 125–6, 127–8
  expectations about modern, 235–6
  feminism, 96
  health psychology, 132
  medical anthropology, 110
  NICE, 237
  see also biomedicine
mental health, 30, 45
  alcohol use, 134
  biological factors, 295
  Buddhism, 308
  climate change impact on, 41
  cultural factors, 21, 122–3
  education, 223
  gendering of, 106, 183
  global, 252, 270
  holistic approaches, 302
  homelessness, 218, 219
  indigenous people, 118
  neighbourhood health, 283, 285
  personality, 187
  policy, 235, 243, 246
  population growth, 42
  positive, 306, 307
  powerlessness of women, 269
  psychological factors, 309–10
  self-esteem, 188, 312
  social capital, 201–2
  social model of health, 15
  social processes, 209

social support, 196, 197
stigma, 93
understandings of health, 22, 28, 30–1
unemployment, 222
well-being, 315
working environment, 220
meso-level, 201, 202, 203, 305
methodology, 34, 56, 57, 79–81, 82, 83, 305
methods, 56, 83, 84
  cohort studies, 56, 81, 296
  definition of, 305
  epistemology, 299
  evidence-based practice, 78–81, 166
  experimental, 300
  exploratory, 82
  health promotion, 170–1, 172
  health psychology, 132, 145
  mixed methods, 55, 61, 71, 76–7
  philosophical frameworks, 54
  research questions, 57, 81
  see also qualitative research; quantitative research
micro-level, 87–8, 89, 305
migration, 47, 219, 254–5, 258–9
Millennium Development Goals, 33, 223, 263, 266–8, 276, 307
mixed methods, 55, 61, 71, 76–7
MMR, 34, 128, 231, 305
models, 13–17
  critiques, 143–4
  definition of, 154, 305
  Health Action Model, 144–6, 184, 187, 188
  Health Belief Model, 136, 137–9, 140
  health promotion, 154–64
  policy making, 232
  Protection Motivation Theory, 136, 139, 140–2
  Stages of Change Model, 142–3
  Theory of Planned Behaviour, 136, 139–40, 141
  welfare, 236–8
  see also Dahlgren and Whitehead model; medical model of health; social model of health
moral panics, 34, 35, 43
morality, 17–18
morbidity, 33, 38
  class differences, 100, 102, 103, 107, 114
  climate change impact on, 40
  DALY, 297
  definition of, 305–6
  foetal origins hypothesis, 302
  malaria, 275, 276, 277
  mental health, 45
  mixed method approach, 77
  reducing, 32
mortality, 12, 33, 50
  childhood, 37, 38, 179, 244, 246, 267

class differences, 100, 102, 103, 107
climate change impact on, 40, 41
DALY, 297
definition of, 306
foetal origins hypothesis, 302
malaria, 275, 277
maternal, 96, 261, 267, 268
mixed method approach, 77
reducing, 32
self-reported health, 221
social capital, 201
social inequalities, 247
social support, 196
TB, 262
motivation, 187
multi-disciplinarity, 1, 85, 149, 306

Naidoo and Wills's typology, 154, 158–9
'nanny state', 169
National Health Service (NHS), 38, 152,
    240, 241, 242–3, 296
contraceptive implants, 36
foreign staff, 255
funding, 246, 248
health promotion, 154
inequalities, 100, 244
MMR vaccine, 231
NICE regulation, 237
policy, 230, 233, 235–6, 247, 250
universalism, 315
values, 249
nationalism, 240
nature, definition of, 306
nature/nurture debate, 188–9
needs, 26, 83, 235
age-related changes, 181, 192
collectivism, 296
community, 157, 159, 207
disability, 98
elderly people, 43
empowerment, 159, 299
energy, 220
environmentalism, 241
low-income countries, 263
social policy, 249
threats to health, 41, 43
welfare state, 237, 238
neighbourhoods, 208, 282–6, 292, 306
see also community
neo-liberalism, 240, 256, 270, 306
individual responsibility, 13, 18
NHS reforms, 247
United States, 241
WHO, 265
networks
alcohol use, 124
Barton and Grant health map, 292
Dahlgren and Whitehead model, 3,
    288, 289
neighbourhood health, 283, 284, 286
policy communities, 232

sampling, 73
social and community, 194, 195–8,
    200, 203, 204–7, 209, 289, 313
social class, 104, 287
women, 170
New Labour, 233, 244, 247
new social movements, 92, 307
NICE, 166, 237
non-communicable diseases, 2, 35–7,
    47, 268, 306
non-governmental organizations
    (NGOs), 264, 305

obesity, 18, 95, 217, 281, 286
age inequalities, 45
cultural factors, 124, 125
Health Survey for England, 83
lifestyles, 47–8
mainstream ideas about, 304
policy, 233, 235, 236, 246
refusal of treatment for, 231
as risk factor for disease, 131
social inequalities, 103
threats to health, 30, 31
obesogenic environment, 124, 217
objectives, 307
objectivity, 55, 307, 309
observation, 56, 58, 69, 71, 74, 76, 82
ontology, 54–5, 56, 82, 167, 307
operationalization, 186, 199, 307

pandemics, 33, 34, 37, 38, 46, 50, 257,
    307
paradigms, 13, 25, 54, 57, 76, 163, 164,
    305, 308
pathology, 13, 308
personality, 178, 184–7, 193, 306
cultural factors, 123
Health Action Model, 146
Health Belief Model, 138
nature/nurture debate, 188
sexual behaviour, 191
perspectives, 308
pharmaceutical industry, 34, 94–5, 264
global health, 257, 258
HIV/AIDS, 262
malaria prevention, 275
Marxist perspective, 96
political economy perspective, 46
private sector, 309
see also drugs
philosophy, 17, 54–5, 308
physical environment see environment
placebo effect, 118, 120
policy, xxvi, 174, 229–50
British Welfare State, 236–9
cervical cancer, 281–4
current issues, 235–6
Dahlgren and Whitehead model, 287,
    288, 290, 291
definition of, 230

policy (cont.)
  as determinant of health, 233–4, 247–8
  environmental factors, 225
  fiscal, 246–7
  global, 264–8, 269, 270
  health care services, 242–3
  health promotion, 158, 159, 160–2, 169
  healthy public, 153, 160–2, 169, 171, 174, 243–4, 249, 286, 302
  ideological and political values, 239–42
  individual behaviour, 132
  macro-level, 304
  'mad cow disease', 49
  malaria, 276–7
  neighbourhood health, 285–6
  objectives, 307
  social and community characteristics, 206–9
  social marketing, 313
  sociology influence on, 105
policy agenda, 231, 232
policy communities, 232
policy environment, 174, 229, 239, 244–5, 248
policy making, 230, 232–3, 239, 243, 249, 264–6, 268–9
policy sectors, 174, 206, 233–4, 245–6, 247, 249, 308
political economy, 46, 94, 308
pollution, 41, 48, 178, 220, 225, 244, 259, 283, 284
populations
  ageing, 37, 42, 43, 47, 182, 235, 236
  census, 295
  cervical cancer, 279, 280
  childhood mortality, 37
  climate change impact on, 40
  cohort studies, 296
  Dahlgren and Whitehead model, 173–4, 287, 288
  DALY, 297
  democratic societies, 203, 241
  displacement of, 44
  equity, 167
  fiscal policy, 246–7
  food contamination, 216
  health care services, 224
  health indicators, 301
  health promotion, 152, 153, 156–8, 169
  inequalities, 301
  malaria treatment, 276
  MMR vaccination, 128
  morbidity, 305–6
  mortality, 306
  obesity, 217
  pandemics, 307
  perceptions and behaviour of, 113
  population growth, 41–3, 50
  prevalence of disease, 309

qualitative research, 69, 73
quantitative research, 58, 59–62, 66
risk factors, 312
threats to health, 33, 35, 47–8
urbanization, 219–20
positivism, 54–5, 56, 57, 81, 113, 309
post structuralism, 98–9, 309
poverty, 103, 179, 203, 225, 281
  ageing population, 43
  capabilities and resilience, 186
  cervical cancer, 278
  'epidemiological transition', 35
  global governance, 264, 265
  globalization, 253
  infectious diseases, 47
  malaria, 273, 274, 276
  Millennium Development Goals, 266, 267
  mortality due to, 252, 260–1
  policy, 244, 245
  social model of health, 14
  TB, 262
  threats to health, 30, 33, 37, 44–5, 48, 50
  welfare state, 238, 239
  see also socio-economic factors
power, 126, 129, 268, 290
  anthropology, 127
  Caplan and Holland's model of health, 163
  class differences, 104, 313
  communities, 211
  critical health psychology, 148
  discourse, 99
  functionalism, 90
  gender and, 96, 170, 183, 191
  ideology and, 303
  inequalities, 313
  Marxism, 94
  medical profession, 153
  pharmaceutical industry, 257, 258, 262
  policy making, 232–3, 250
  practitioners, 164
  research, 75, 83
  sociology, 89
  workplaces, 221
powerlessness, 46, 251, 260, 269
prevalence, 47, 287, 301, 306, 309
prevention, 152, 154–5, 158, 159, 161, 170, 286
  biomedical, 170
  cervical cancer, 277–9, 281
  HIV/AIDS, 46
  malaria, 273–5, 276
  upstream approaches, 165, 168
primary health care, 263, 265, 268, 275, 309
private sector, 237, 240, 305, 309
privatization, 240, 255, 265, 309
progressive taxation, 246

Protection Motivation Theory (PMT), 136, 139, 140–2
psychological factors, xxiv–xxv, 2–3, 130–49, 189, 280, 300
addiction, 135, 186
ADHD, 127
alcohol use, 134
biopsychosocial model of health, 16–17
definition of, 309–10
determinants of health, 134–6
education, 223
family ties, 204
Foetal Alcohol Syndrome, 179
Health Belief Model, 138
holistic model of health, 16
inequalities, 102, 103–4, 202
medical model of health, 13, 119
mental health, 45
motivation, 187
sexual behaviour, 191
social model of health, 14
social support, 197, 198
sunbeds, 147
traditional treatments, 118
trauma and fear, 44
well-being, 9, 297
working environment, 221
see also health behaviour; personality
psychosocial factors, 20, 22, 44, 102, 103, 115, 124, 147, 174, 203
public health, 172, 175, 272, 293
climate change impact on, 259
Dahlgren and Whitehead model, 288, 290
DALY, 297
environmentalism, 241
global governance, 264, 266
globalization, 255–6, 269
health promotion, 20, 152–3
individual behaviour, 132
Lalonde Report, 213–14
multi-disciplinary, 85
policy, 233, 236, 245, 249
sanitation improvements, 218, 219
social model of health, 15
threats to, 29–51
public sector, 208, 239, 248, 265, 266, 309, 310

qualitative research, 67–76, 83, 149, 305, 310
interpretivism, 54, 55, 303
mixed methods, 77
research questions, 81
subjectivity, 314
quality of life, 9, 171, 235, 259, 297
citizenship, 296
community empowerment, 159
definition of, 310
disability, 98

evidence-based practice, 79
HIV/AIDS patients, 262
mental health, 45
physical environment, 283
threats to health, 33
quantitative research, 58–67, 69, 74, 75–6, 82, 149, 305, 310
choice of, 72
mixed methods, 77
positivism, 54, 55, 309
research questions, 81
social capital, 198–9
theory, 314

rainbow model see Dahlgren and Whitehead model
randomized control trials (RCTs), 61, 76, 78, 79, 81, 166, 310, 311
rationing, 236, 237, 248, 249, 311
recession, 30, 218, 248, 263
redistribution, 159, 161, 202, 241, 285–6
reductionism, 13, 15, 19, 145, 311
relativism, 311
religion, 205–6
research, xxiii–xxiv, 52–84, 311
definition of, 53
ethics of, 77–8
evidence-based practice, xxiii, 78–81, 83, 166, 300
literature reviews, 53–4
philosophical frameworks, 54–5, 82
see also methods; qualitative research; quantitative research
research questions, 53, 55–8, 59, 69, 72, 75, 80–1, 83, 314
resilience, 123, 171, 186, 223, 311
responsibility, 10
behaviour change models, 145
collective, 267, 296
gender differences, 24
health promotion, 20, 105, 152, 168
lay understandings of health, 116
lifestyle factors, 103, 125, 235, 280
medical model of health, 13, 15
neo-liberal notions of, 18, 240
sick role, 91
risk/risk factors
adolescence, 182
association, 294
binge-drinking, 27
cervical cancer, 278, 279–80
class differences, 100, 102
climate change, 41
cohort studies, 296
cultural factors, 122
Dahlgren and Whitehead model, 287–8, 289
definition of, 312
diet, 31
evidence-based practice, 300
focus on, 32

risk/risk factors (cont.)
Foetal Alcohol Syndrome, 179
gender differences, 24, 45, 183, 269
genetic factors, 184
health education, 169, 171
health promotion, 105
'health-risk behaviours', 133–4
HIV transmission, 191
homelessness, 218, 219
lay understandings of health, 115
low-income countries, 224, 260, 262
malaria, 276
medicalization, 96
moral panics, 35
obesity, 217
personality, 185–6, 187
primary prevention, 159
'risk transition', 35–7
sexual behaviour, 253, 278, 280, 283
smoking, 131, 220
sunbeds, 124, 147
threats to health, 33–4, 40, 43–9, 50
Western culture, 126
working environment, 220–1, 226

salutogenesis, 16, 30, 168, 170–1, 312
sampling, 56, 59–63, 69–74, 79, 80, 84,
    294, 296, 312
screening
cervical cancer, 168, 278–9, 280, 281–4
definition of, 312
genetic, 192
health behaviour, 133
Health Belief Model, 137
health career, 190
neighbourhood health, 284
primary prevention, 158, 170
secondary prevention, 159
seatbelts, 132, 133, 169, 171, 245
self-esteem, 9, 134, 187–8, 198, 223, 283,
    312
self-medication, 119
semantics, 154, 312
'settings' approach, 227, 228, 282
sex/sexual behaviour
addiction, 186
cervical cancer, 278, 279, 280, 283,
    302
condom use, 141
cultural norms, 112
female sexual dysfunction, 95
Health Belief Model, 137
HIV/AIDS, 46, 121, 183, 191
lifestyles, 47
motivation levels and safe sex, 188
risky/unsafe, 29, 44, 121, 134, 182,
    185–6, 201
sex education, 61, 155
sexual violence, 44
sexually-transmitted infections, 235,
    253, 260

user charges for sexual health services,
    263
women's powerlessness, 269
see also biological sex
sick role, 90, 91
sickness service, 243
smoking, 23, 121, 134, 135, 184, 203
Bangladesh, 256
cervical cancer, 278, 279
children's understandings of health,
    22
class differences, 48, 102, 103
cultural influences, 111
disadvantaged individuals, 287
education, 223
Health Belief Model, 137
health beliefs, 301
ideological beliefs, 242
legislation against, 156, 243
lung cancer, 58, 131, 252, 294
passive, 220
during pregnancy, 179, 180, 234
refusal to stop, 231
Tannahill's model, 154
social anthropology, xxiv, 109–10
see also anthropology
social capital, xxvi, 198–203, 209, 211
Barton and Grant health map, 292
Big Society debate, 208
community development, 157
definition of, 313
empowerment, 159
faith-based organizations, 205–6
families, 204
health promotion, 168
neighbourhood health, 283, 284, 285,
    286
policy development, 206–7
Zambian Open Community Schools,
    210
see also society
social class
cervical cancer, 278, 280
community networks, 287
definition of, 313
determinants of health, 298
elites, 232
Health Belief Model, 138
health-seeking behaviour, 114–15,
    118
identity, 303
inequalities, 45, 94, 99–100, 102,
    302
lifestyle factors, 103
Marxism, 94
neighbourhoods, 283
ordinal data, 64, 65
political economy, 308
psychological health, 103–4
understandings of health, 19, 20, 21,
    27

unemployment, 222
    see also socio-economic factors
social cohesion, 103, 211, 240
social constructionism, 17, 96–8, 107,
    110, 165, 313
    culture, 123
    disability, 98, 99
    illness and disease, 102, 110
    pain, 82
    social model of health, 14, 15
social divisions, 96, 99–101, 105, 202
social inequalities, 103, 126, 247, 264,
    268, 289, 291, 313
social marketing, 233, 274, 313
social model of disability, 92
social model of health, 14–16, 19, 31, 101,
    104, 110, 152, 295
social networks *see* networks
social norms, 91, 111, 121, 163, 164, 288
social security, 238
social selection, 101, 102
social support, 196–8, 202, 209, 211, 223,
    283, 284, 285
socialism, 240
society, 87–8, 99–104, 105, 107
    Big Society debate, 208
    Caplan and Holland's model, 162–4,
        170
    cultural factors, 118, 123, 125–6
    culture and, 110–11
    functionalism, 90
    Marxism, 94–6
    medicalization, 95–6, 106, 127
    moral panics, 35
    'risk society', 48
    social anthropology, 109–10
    social constructionism, 96–8
    stigma, 93
    structure and agency, 90
    symbolic interactionism, 91–2
socio-economic factors, 90, 164, 171
    Caplan and Holland's model, 163
    cervical cancer, 278, 280
    Dahlgren and Whitehead model, 288,
        290
    Foetal Alcohol Syndrome, 179
    Health Action Model, 146
    health career, 190
    health promotion, 153
    healthy public policy, 161
    lay understandings of health, 22
    lifestyle choices, 104
    malaria, 275, 276
    neighbourhood health, 283
    risks to health, 37
    well-being, 31
    see also poverty; social class
squalor, 238
Stages of Change Model (SCM), 142–3
standards of living, 254, 270
stigma, 33, 45, 91–2, 93, 94, 121, 123, 314

subjectivity, 25, 102, 214
    Caplan and Holland's model of health,
        162, 163, 170
    definition of, 314
    definitions of health, 12
    experience of health and illness, 19, 91
    health behaviour, 132
    interpretivism, 55
    self-reported health, 125
    'subjective norm', 139, 140, 144
sunbeds/sunbathing, 124, 147
surveys, 56, 58, 60, 65, 76, 78, 81, 310
symbolic interactionism, 91–2

Tannahill's model of health, 154–5
taxation, 151, 161, 202, 241, 244, 285–6
    progressive, 246
    social change approach, 159
    welfare state, 238, 239
teratogens, 178
terrorism, 43, 44, 48
theory, 67, 76, 147–8, 149
    behaviour change models, 143–4
    definition of, 314
    sociology, 88, 90–9
    see also research
Theory of Planned Behaviour, 136,
    139–40, 141
Tones and Tilford's empowerment model,
    160–2
trade, 216, 253, 255–8, 265, 266
Trans Theoretical Model, 142–3
transnational corporations (TNCs), 256,
    258, 268, 271
transport policy, 229, 245, 285, 308
treatment
    antibiotics, 152
    cervical cancer, 279
    culture and, 115, 116, 117–20, 122–3,
        127–8
    domestic violence, 170
    equality in, 240, 241
    evidence-based practice, 79
    experiments, 61
    health care services, 242–3
    health tourism, 255
    malaria, 274, 275, 276, 277
    Marxist perspective, 94–5
    medical model of health, 13
    mental illness, 45, 309–10
    NHS, 236
    NICE role, 237
    policy issues, 235
    rationing, 248, 311
    refusal of, 48, 231
    social support, 197
    TB, 47, 262
    women's powerlessness, 269
    see also drugs; prevention
triangulation, 77, 314
TRIPs, 257

tuberculosis (TB), 47, 219, 257, 262, 266, 267, 270, 296
typologies
    Busfield, 213, 214
    definition of, 314–15
    health inequalities, 102
    health promotion, 154, 158–9, 162
    research designs, 81

unemployment, 102, 221–2, 283, 285
universalism, 315
upstream approaches, 165, 169, 202, 203, 243

values
    culture, 110, 124, 297
    definition of, 315
    family, 204
    Health Action Model, 187
    health promotion, 104, 105, 152, 164–8, 171
    humanism, 302
    motivation, 188
    policy, 229, 230, 239–42, 248–9
    positivism, 55
    qualitative research, 75
    quantitative research, 60, 64
    relativism, 311
    social model of health, 15
    women, 170
variables
    definition of, 315
    experimental method, 300
    Health Action Model, 144

Health Belief Model, 137, 138, 139
quantitative research, 58, 60, 65, 66
tan seeking behaviours, 147
Theory of Planned Behaviour, 139, 140

Wanless Report, 236
water and sanitation, 217–18, 226, 260, 270
welfare state, 169, 202, 236–9, 241
well-being
    adolescence, 182
    Barton and Grant health map, 291–2
    Buddhism, 308
    cultural factors, 124, 125
    definition of, 315
    definitions of health, 8, 9
    family ties, 204–5
    global health, 251–2
    health education, 155
    lay understandings of health, 20, 22, 23
    policy, 246–7
    quality of life, 297, 310
    self-esteem, 312
    social networks, 195
    socio-economic factors, 31
    socio-political environment, 225
    stigma, 93
    sunbeds, 147
working environment, 104, 220–1, 226, 244, 288

Zambian Open Community Schools, 210